Strategies to Improve Modifiable Factors of Athletic Success

Strategies to Improve Modifiable Factors of Athletic Success

Guest Editors

Vincent Dalbo
Michael D. Roberts
David H. Fukuda

MDPI

Basel • Beijing • Wuhan • Barcelona • Belgrade • Novi Sad • Cluj • Manchester

Guest Editors
Vincent Dalbo
School of Health, Medical and Applied Sciences
Central Queensland University
Rockhampton
Australia

Michael D. Roberts
School of Kinesiology
Auburn University
Auburn
USA

David H. Fukuda
School of Kinesiology and Physical Therapy
University of Central Florida
Orlando
USA

Editorial Office
MDPI AG
Grosspeteranlage 5
4052 Basel, Switzerland

This is a reprint of the Special Issue, published open access by the journal *Sports* (ISSN 2075-4663), freely accessible at: https://www.mdpi.com/journal/sports/special_issues/5JIG5F8656.

For citation purposes, cite each article independently as indicated on the article page online and as indicated below:

Lastname, A.A.; Lastname, B.B. Article Title. *Journal Name* **Year**, *Volume Number*, Page Range.

ISBN 978-3-7258-7456-9 (Hbk)
ISBN 978-3-7258-7457-6 (PDF)
https://doi.org/10.3390/books978-3-7258-7457-6

Contents

sports

MDPI

Article

Fecal Microbiota and Associated Metabolites Are Minimally Affected by Ten Weeks of Resistance Training in Younger and Older Adults

Anthony Agyin-Birikorang [1], Sarah Lennon [2], Kristen S. Smith [3], William Van Der Pol [4], Morgan A. Smith [5], Casey L. Sexton [6], Donald A. Lamb [2], Kaelin C. Young [7], Christopher Brooks Mobley [1], Kevin W. Huggins [2], Michael D. Roberts [1] and Andrew Dandridge Frugé [8,*]

1 School of Kinesiology, Auburn University, Auburn, AL 36849, USA
2 Department of Nutritional Sciences, Auburn University, Auburn, AL 36849, USA
3 Ocean Spray Cranberries, Inc., Middleboro-Lakeville, MA 02347, USA
4 Biomedical Informatics, UAB Center for Clinical and Translational Science, The University of Alabama at Birmingham, Birmingham, AL 35294, USA
5 School of Medicine, Stanford University, Palo Alto, CA 94304, USA
6 Department of Medicine, Division of Gerontology, Geriatrics and Palliative Care, University of Alabama at Birmingham, Birmingham, AL 35294, USA
7 Department of Physiology, Pacific Northwest University of Health Sciences, Yakima, WA 98901, USA
8 College of Nursing, Auburn University, Auburn, AL 36849, USA
* Correspondence: fruge@auburn.edu

Abstract: Preclinical evidence suggests that short chain fatty acids (SCFAs) produced by gut microbiota may impact body composition and muscle growth. While aging is implicated in negative alterations to the gut microbiome, exercise may mitigate these changes. Limited human evidence indicates that resistance training (RT) does not appreciably alter the gut microbiome in older adults, and no human study has examined whether resistance training differentially alters the gut microbiome and associated SCFAs between younger and older individuals. Therefore, we examined whether 10 weeks of RT differentially altered fecal microbiota composition, fecal and circulating SCFAs, and serum markers associated with gastrointestinal integrity in two cohorts of adults. Fecal and serum samples were obtained from untrained younger (22 ± 2 years, n = 12) and older (58 ± 8 years, n = 12) participants prior to and following 10 weeks of supervised twice-weekly full-body RT. Outcome measures immediately before (PRE) and after the intervention (POST) included dual X-ray absorptiometry for body composition, ultrasound for vastus lateralis (VL) thickness, 16S rRNA gene sequencing fecal microbiome data, serum and fecal SCFAs measured by gas chromatography, and serum intestinal fatty acid-binding protein 2 (FABP2), lipopolysaccharide-binding protein (LBP), and leucine-rich alpha-2 glycoprotein (LRG-1) quantified by enzyme-linked immunosorbent assays. Main effects and interactions were measured by repeated measures analysis of variance (group × time; G × T) for all dependent variables, and Spearman correlations were used to explore relationships among changes in relevant outcomes. The intervention significantly increased VL thickness and lean body mass ($p < 0.05$) equally in both groups. Although group differences in microbiome beta diversity were identified, no effects of age, time, or their interaction were observed for the alpha diversity measures. Seven SCFAs were detected in the fecal samples, albeit no significant age, time, or interaction effects were evident. In serum, acetic acid was the only SCFA detected, with no significant age, time, or interaction effects. Serum LRG1 decreased for all participants ($p = 0.007$) with higher levels in younger adults ($p = 0.015$), but no G × T interactions were observed for this marker, serum FABP2, or LBP. No significant correlations were observed among RT-induced changes in muscle mass-related outcomes and changes in fecal microbiome diversity, total or individual SCFAs, or serum

FABP2/LBP/LRG-1. These results highlight that 10 weeks of RT largely does not affect fecal microbiota, associated SCFAs, or select markers of gastrointestinal integrity in untrained younger or older adults.

Keywords: short-chain fatty acids; fecal microbiome; resistance training; aging

1. Introduction

The human gut contains a diverse array of microorganisms, including bacteria, viruses, fungi, and archaea, which inhabit the gastrointestinal tract. The colon hosts the richest microbial community in the human body [1]. Through symbiotic relationships, the gut microbiota contributes to digestion, vitamin synthesis, immune regulation, and protection against pathogens [2]. Environmental factors, including diet, exercise, xenobiotics, stress, and trauma, have been hypothesized to modify the gut microbiome [3–5]; interventions may optimize bacteria–host symbiosis to mitigate disease progression [6].

In 2007, Bäckhed et al. [7] used germ-free mice to investigate resistance to diet-induced obesity. It was the first study to suggest the presence of a gut–muscle axis. Others have reported that six weeks of *Lactobacilli plantarum* (*L. plantarum*) supplementation significantly increased grip strength, swimming time to exhaustion, normalized muscle weight, and the percentage of Type I myofibers in mice [8]. Yan et al. [9] subsequently found that the skeletal muscle fiber type was associated with microbiota. Fernandez et al. [10] demonstrated that endurance training increased the number of taxa in 8-week-old mice, which correlated with physical performance. However, neither resistance training (RT) nor endurance training (ET) altered the phyla and family compositions [10]. Cullen et al. [11] reported that RT induced mixed changes in the gut microbiomes of sedentary young adults. These collective results suggest that intestinal microbiota may communicate with skeletal muscle to, in part, regulate the adaptive responses to exercise training.

Acetate, propionate, and butyrate are the most abundant short-chain fatty acids (SCFAs) in humans and are microbial metabolites produced through the fermentation of dietary fibers and resistant starches [12]. Acetate is a bacterial product of the genera *Bifidobacteria*, *Lactobacilli*, *Clostridium*, and *Akkermansia* [13]. Propionate is largely produced by intestinal bacteria of the genera *Bacteroides*, *Ruminococcus*, and *Roseburia* [14]. *Faecalibacterium prausnitzii*, *Eubacterium rectale*, and *Roseburia* spp. produce most colonic butyrate [15]. SCFAs provide an apparent direct link between microbiome-derived metabolites and skeletal muscle physiology [16,17]. In this regard, Lahiri et al. [18] presented evidence of SCFAs regulating skeletal muscle mass and function in germ-free (GF) mice by treating the GF mice in vivo with a cocktail of SCFAs, thus partly reversing skeletal muscle impairment. Interestingly, studies in rodents and humans indicate that ET or combined ET+RT training modulates fecal SCFA content [19–22]. However, to our knowledge, no study has examined whether RT alone alters fecal and circulating SCFAs in humans.

Although the aforementioned results are promising, there are human data indicating that resistance training may minimally affect gut microbiome outcomes. For instance, our group recently published a study in older individuals indicating that six weeks of resistance training does not affect microbiome diversity or abundances of various taxa [23], and this agrees in principle with other resistance training interventions demonstrating null effects [24,25]. However, our prior results may have been due to either the shorter-term nature of the intervention and/or only examining older individuals who demonstrate a limited capacity to experience changes in the gut microbiome [26].

We previously performed two investigations examining the effects of a peanut protein supplement on training outcomes in younger and older adults [27,28], and both studies indicated that training (but not supplementation) promoted increases in measures of skeletal muscle hypertrophy and strength. Given our interest in determining if longer-term training and/or aging affects gut microbiome adaptations, we leveraged banked fecal specimens and remaining blood sera from 12 younger and 12 older participants in these studies to examine if 10 weeks of RT altered the gut microbiome, fecal and serum SCFAs, and serum markers of gastrointestinal integrity. Our secondary aim was to determine if changes in these outcomes were associated with indices of muscle hypertrophy. We hypothesized that RT would improve alpha diversity in all participants and alter fecal and serum SCFAs in younger, but not older, participants. However, we adopted the null hypothesis that microbiome and SCFA outcomes would not be associated with training outcomes.

2. Materials and Methods

2.1. Ethical Approval and Participant Eligibility

Here, we report a secondary analysis of 12 younger adults and 12 older adults who completed 10 weeks of resistance training. Both studies were conducted under a single approved protocol by the Institutional Review Board (IRB) at Auburn University (AU) (Protocol # 19-249 MR 1907), and both studies were pre-registered clinical trials (NCT04015479 registered 11 July 2019 [28]; NCT04707963 registered 13 January 2021 [27]). All participants signed written informed consent. This sample size was selected from the original 47 younger participants and 17 older participants who finished the 10-week interventions because only these 24 total individuals had enough fecal and blood materials to perform the analyses described in the following paragraphs. See Figure 1.

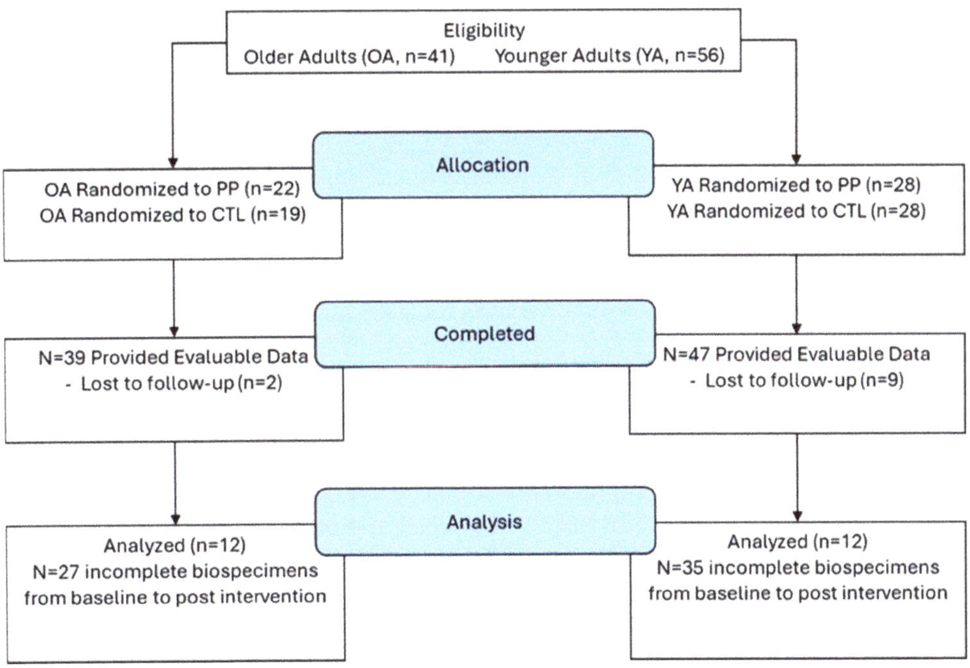

Figure 1. Study flow diagram.

Detailed methods of the original studies have been previously described [27,28]. Participants were recruited locally and at AU via flyers, emails, and direct contact, either face-to-face or over the phone. Both studies had identical eligibility criteria aside from age, which included (i) being 18–30 years old or 50–80 years old, (ii) body mass index (BMI) < 35 kg/m^2, (iii) not currently performing RT more than one time per week, (iv) no peanut allergy, (v) no metal implants that could affect X-ray procedures, (vi) minimal radiation exposure in the last six months, (vii) absence of obvious cardiovascular or metabolic disease, (viii) absence of conditions contraindicating participation in exercise program or donation of muscle biopsy, and (ix) exclusion of pregnant females. The eligible persons were informed of all study procedures and completed a medical history questionnaire prior to signing informed consent to participate.

2.2. Study Design

This is a brief overview of the procedures relevant to the data presented. Participants reported to AU School of Kinesiology for a pre-testing battery (PRE), which included urine specific gravity (USG) assessment for hydration and a rapid pregnancy test for female participants. Next, weight and height were assessed using digital column scales, right leg vastus lateralis (VL) thickness was measured using ultrasound, and body composition was obtained using a full-body dual-energy X-ray absorptiometry (DXA) scan. Venous blood was obtained from an arm vein in serum separator tubes (BD Vacutainer; Franklin Lakes, NJ, USA) and allowed to clot at room temperature prior to being centrifuged at $3500\times g$ for serum separation. The participants were provided 15–30 min education/training on recording dietary intake using a 24 h recall template. They were instructed to provide a three-day log of dietary intake, which was reviewed and verified with study staff at the following visit. They were also provided a stool specimen collection kit with a stool hat, a collection tube with a spoon connected to the lid, and instructions to immediately freeze the specimen after collection. The participants then performed 10 weeks of supervised full-body RT twice weekly, as described by Lamb et al. [28] and Sexton et al. [27]. All training sessions were supervised by the study personnel to ensure proper form and safety throughout the sessions. After completion of the 10-week RT program, the participants were provided with another set of three-day dietary intake forms and stool collection kits for post-intervention testing (POST), occurring 72 h after their last training session. POST replicated PRE procedures, which included USG, a pregnancy test in females, height and weight assessments, right leg VL thickness measurement using ultrasound, a DXA scan, a venous blood draw, and submission of food logs and stool samples. The following paragraphs provide more in-depth descriptions of the testing sessions.

2.3. Body Composition

Following an overnight fast, the participants submitted a urine sample for USG level measurement with a handheld refractometer (ATAGO; Bellevue, WA, USA). The participants were provided with water to drink if USG values were less than 1.020. Next, body weight (to the nearest 0.1 kg) and height (to the nearest 0.5 cm) were obtained (Seca 769; Hanover, MD, USA). Following these measurements, a single technician for all measures conducted DXA (Lunar Prodigy; GE Corporation, Fairfield, CT, USA), providing total lean soft tissue mass (LSTM) and fat mass (FM).

2.4. Ultrasound for Vastus Lateralis Thickness

Ultrasonography (Real-time B-mode; NextGen LOGIQe R8, GE Healthcare, Chicago, IL, USA) utilizing a multi-frequency linear-array transducer (L4-12T, 4-12 MHz, GE Healthcare, Chicago, IL, USA) captured images of the right mid-thigh vastus lateralis (VL). All ultrasound settings (frequency: 10 MHz, gain: 50 dB, dynamic range: 75), except for depth, were held constant across participants and time points. One image per participant at each time point was obtained. Following the study conclusion, the images were analyzed using the freely available ImageJ software (https://imagej.nih.gov/ij/, National Institutes of Health, Bethesda, MD, USA). VL thickness was measured using the straight-line function and defined as the distance between the subcutaneous adipose tissue–vastus lateralis interface and deep aponeurosis.

2.5. Supervised RT Program

The participants completed supervised, progressive RT twice weekly for 10 weeks, where detailed instructions were provided on proper posture, form, technique, and body positioning to ensure safety. The training protocol required a minimum of 48 h in between sessions to allow for appropriate recovery. Each training session was preceded by 10 bodyweight squats and 25 jumping jacks, and warm-up sets as follows: one set of 10 reps at 50% of working weight, one set of 5 reps at 75% of working weight, and one set of 3 reps at 90% of working weight. Younger participants performed either 4 sets of 10 reps (high volume) or 5 sets of 6 reps (high load) at working weight depending on the week. The older participants performed 3 sets of 10–12 reps at working weight. Following each set, the rating of perceived exhaustion (RPE) was recorded to ensure that appropriate loads were implemented throughout. An RPE below 7 resulted in a slight increase in working weight on the next set, and an RPE at 10 or incomplete set resulted in a slight decrease in working weight on the next set.

2.6. Dietary Analysis

The participants were instructed to complete three days of dietary intake forms prior to and following the 10-week training intervention, which included all food and beverages on two weekdays and one weekend day. The participants were encouraged to maintain their normal dietary intake. As previously discussed, half of the participants consumed defatted-peanut powder supplements (PPS); the outcomes did not differ between the PPS and control groups. The Nutrition Data System for Research (NDSR; NDSR 2022; University of Minnesota) software was utilized by the study personnel to analyze all young participants' food logs. The study personnel entered recalls into the Automated Self-Administered 24-h Dietary Assessment (ASA24; National Cancer Institute, Bethesda, MD, USA) tool to analyze all older participants' food logs.

2.7. Fecal Microbiome Analysis

Stool samples were collected using a commode specimen collection kit and sterile collection tubes. The participants were instructed to seal and store samples in the freezer prior to submission at the next visit. Upon receipt, the samples were stored at −80 °C prior to processing. Fecal microbial DNA was isolated using commercially available kits (Zymo, Irvine, CA, USA). DNA samples were prepared, and polymerase chain reaction (PCR) amplified 250 base pair variable region 4 of 16S rRNA. The PCR amplicon library was sequenced on Miseq (Illumina, San Diego, CA, USA) [29,30]. Further detailed processing steps have been previously described [23]. The Quantitative Insight into Microbial Ecology (QIIME) 2 pipeline [31] grouped the demultiplexed FASTQ files and UCLUST clustered sequences into PyNAST-generated Amplicon Sequence Variants (ASVs) with DADA2, ensuring a 97% similarity threshold [32–34]. Thereafter, taxonomic assignments were issued using the SILVA database [35]. ASVs with an average abundance >0.005% were processed and grouped by taxonomy.

2.8. Fecal and Serum SCFA Analysis

Fecal and serum samples were shipped on dry ice to a commercial vendor (Microbiome Insights, Richmond, BC, Canada) for SCFA analysis. Briefly, SCFAs were quantified using gas chromatography (Thermo Trace 1310) coupled with a flame ionization detector (Thermo Fisher Scientific, Waltham, MA, USA), as previously described [36]. Aliquots of stool samples were homogenized using MP Bio FastPrep post-suspension in MilliQ-grade water at 4.0 m/s for 1 min. Next, the samples were acidified by adding 5M HCl to the fecal suspensions until they reached a final pH of 2.0. The suspensions were incubated for 10 min and then centrifuged at 10,000 rpm. Supernatants were spiked with 2-ethylbturyic acid until a final concentration of 1 mM was reached. SCFAs were detected from the supernatants by direct injection into the Thermo TG-WAXMS A GC Column (30 m, 0.32 mm, 0.25 μm). Standard solutions of individual SCFAs were injected and used for calibration. Serum SCFAs were also analyzed using a similar process, as previously described [37].

2.9. Serum Biomarkers

The serum samples were stored and removed from −80 °C to determine concentrations of intestinal fatty acid-binding protein (FABP), leucine-rich alpha-2-glycoprotein 1 (LRG-1), and lipopolysaccharide-binding protein (LBP) using enzyme-linked immunosorbent assay (ELISA) kits according to the manufacturer's instructions (AFG Bioscience, Wood Dale, IL USA; catalog #'s: EK710951, EK710885, EK241481). All three assays followed similar protocols, which ended with determining absorbance readings at 450 nm using a microplate spectrophotometer (Biotek Synergy H1 hybrid reader; Agilent, Santa Clara, CA, USA). Sample absorbance readings were compared to standard curve absorbance readings, and the values were provided in serum concentration units. The three kits performed adequately, as determined by unknown absorbance values falling within the linear range of the standard curves and coefficient of variation values for duplicates being less than 25% (FABP = 22.8%, LBP = 12.3%, LRG-1 = 18.5%).

2.10. Statistics

Statistical analysis was conducted on non-microbiome data using Graphpad Prism v10.0, and microbiome data were analyzed using RStudio Team (2023) (Integrated Development for R. RStudio v2023.06, PBC, Boston, MA, USA). Repeated measures two-way (group × time; G × T) analysis of variance (ANOVA) tests were performed for all longitudinal measures. For microbiome data, false discovery rate (FDR)-corrected Kruskal–Wallis ANOVAs compared the relative abundance of all ASVs between both groups at both time points. Alpha diversity was measured using ASV counts, PD whole tree phylogeny, Simpson index, and Shannon index. Beta diversity was measured using the Bray–Curtis dissimilarity, unweighted Unifrac distance, and weighted Unifrac distance metrics. Change scores for select dependent variables were calculated by subtracting PRE values from POST values. Spearman correlations were then conducted on select change scores to explore the relationships between changes in muscle hypertrophy outcomes versus changes in dietary nutrients, fecal microbiome diversity, fecal SCFAs, and serum markers. Correlations were performed for each age cohort individually, as well as for all participants. Statistical significance for two-way ANOVAs was established as $p < 0.05$, and significance was adjusted to $0.05/576 = p < 0.000087$ for correlation analyses to account for the high number of associations.

3. Results

3.1. Participant Characteristics and RT Outcomes

Table 1 presents the baseline characteristics and training adaptations in both the younger and older groups. Significant main effects of time, but no significant interactions, were evident for DXA LSTM and VL thickness, indicating that training increased muscle mass regardless of age group. There were no significant main effects or G × T interactions for total calories, carbohydrate, and fat intake. However, protein and fiber intake increased in both the older and young participants.

Table 1. Participant characteristics, training outcomes, and self-reported food intakes.

Variable	Younger (n = 12)	Older (n = 12)	*p*-Values
Age (years)	22 ± 2	59 ± 5	$p < 0.001$
Sex	2 males/10 females	4 males/8 females	
Body mass (kg)			Group $p < 0.001$
PRE	68.0 ± 10.3	96.1 ± 13.6	Time $p = 0.028$
POST	69.1 ± 11.2	97.4 ± 15.1	G × T $p = 0.807$
DXA LSTM (kg)			Group $p = 0.009$
PRE	45.0 ± 7.2	54.8 ± 8.9	Time $p < 0.001$
POST	46.6 ± 7.6	56.0 ± 8.9	G × T $p = 0.454$
VL thickness (cm)			Group $p = 0.007$
PRE	2.32 ± 0.32	1.93 ± 0.50	Time $p = 0.013$
POST	2.54 ± 0.33	2.04 ± 0.34	G × T $p = 0.364$
Energy intake (kcal/d)			Group $p = 0.146$
PRE	1409.8 ± 431.5	1763.7 ± 566.6	Time $p = 0.804$
POST	1438.6 ± 369.2	1705.1 ± 597.5	G × T $p = 0.470$
Fat intake (g/d)			Group $p = 0.337$
PRE	64.9 ± 17.7	73.1 ± 24.2	Time $p = 0.144$
POST	58.4 ± 21.6	67.4 ± 26.1	G × T $p = 0.921$
Protein intake (g/d)			Group $p = 0.010$
PRE	54.2 ± 18.6	87.8 ± 31.8	Time $p = 0.003$
POST	75.7 ± 17.4	107.9 ± 46.3	G × T $p = 0.909$
Carbohydrate intake (g/d)			Group $p = 0.355$
PRE	151.9 ± 75.6	189.4 ± 80.1	Time $p = 0.331$
POST	154.6 ± 43.9	168.6 ± 63.9	G × T $p = 0.213$
Fiber intake (g/d)			Group $p = 0.621$
PRE	13.9 ± 6.9	14.2 ± 5.9	Time $p < 0.001$
POST	21.8 ± 5.5	18.5 ± 10.9	G × T $p = 0.208$
Sugar intake (g/d)			Group $p = 0.098$
PRE	54.4 ± 47.2	75.8 ± 44.4	Time $p = 0.352$
POST	43.3 ± 17.9	71.9 ± 37.4	G × T $p = 0.647$

Legend: Data are mean ± standard deviation values, with significant main effects of age group, time, and the group × time (G × T) interaction *p*-values being presented. Note: Age was analyzed using an independent samples *t*-test. Abbreviations: DXA LSTM, lean/soft tissue mass determined using dual-energy X-ray absorptiometry; VL, vastus lateralis.

3.2. Fecal Microbiota Between Age Groups with Resistance Training

Alpha diversity metrics (observed species and whole tree phylogeny) did not exhibit significant main or interaction effects (Figure 2a,b). The Firmicutes/Bacteroidetes (F/B) ratio increased, exhibiting a significant main effect of time (POST > PRE, $p = 0.040$), but no significant age or interaction effects (Figure 2c).

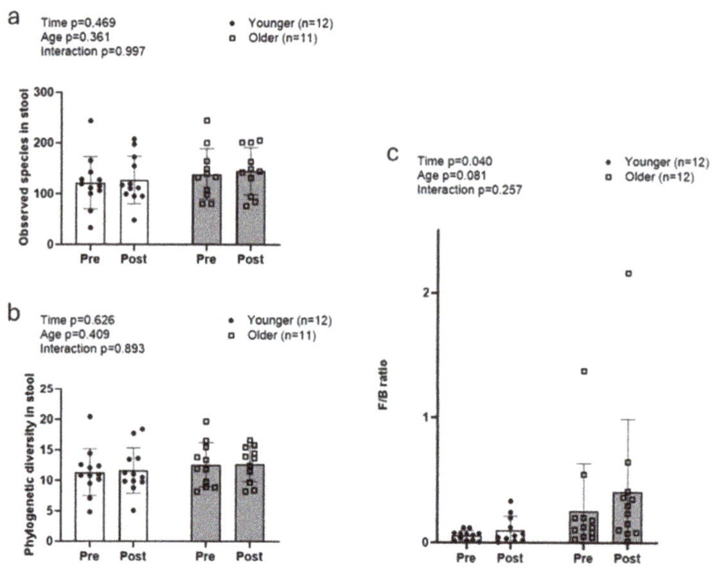

Figure 2. Changes in fecal microbiome alpha diversity with resistance training. Data in this figure indicate that there were no significant changes observed with fecal alpha diversity, including observed species (**a**) and whole tree phylogeny (**b**) in both older and younger participants. However, the Firmicutes/Bacteroidetes ratio (**c**) significantly increased in both groups.

3.3. Beta Diversity Between Age Groups with Resistance Training

Though alpha diversity did not differ between groups, younger and older samples did exhibit microbial population differences between the groups (Figure 3). Beta diversity analyses using Bray–Curtis and weighted Unifrac metrics indicated significant differences between younger and older groups ($p < 0.001$ for both), but no differences in composition from PRE to POST ($p > 0.05$ for all).

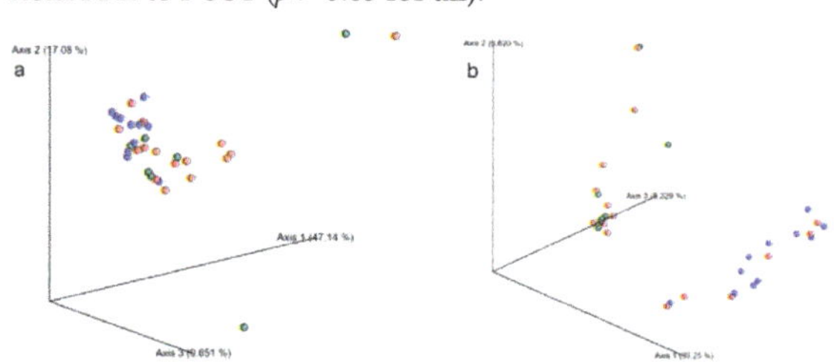

Figure 3. Changes in fecal microbiome beta diversity with resistance training. The average microbiome of young participants was significantly different from the older participants according to (**a**) Bray–Curtis ($p < 0.001$) and (**b**) weighted Unifrac ($p < 0.001$) metrics. Ten weeks of RT did not alter the microbiome composition in either group. Older PRE: red dots; older POST: blue dots; younger PRE: orange dots; younger POST: green.

3.4. Serum and Fecal SCFAs Between Age Groups with Resistance Training

Acetic acid was the only SCFA detected in serum in both older and younger participants, with no significant main effects or G × T interaction (Figure 4a). Seven SCFAs were detected in stool samples and included the three highly enriched acetic acid (Figure 4c), propionic acid (Figure 4d), and butyric acid (Figure 4e), as well as the less enriched isobutyric, isovaleric, valeric, and hexanoic acids. No significant main effects or G × T interactions were observed for the seven individual fecal SCFAs or total stool SCFA concentrations (Figure 4b).

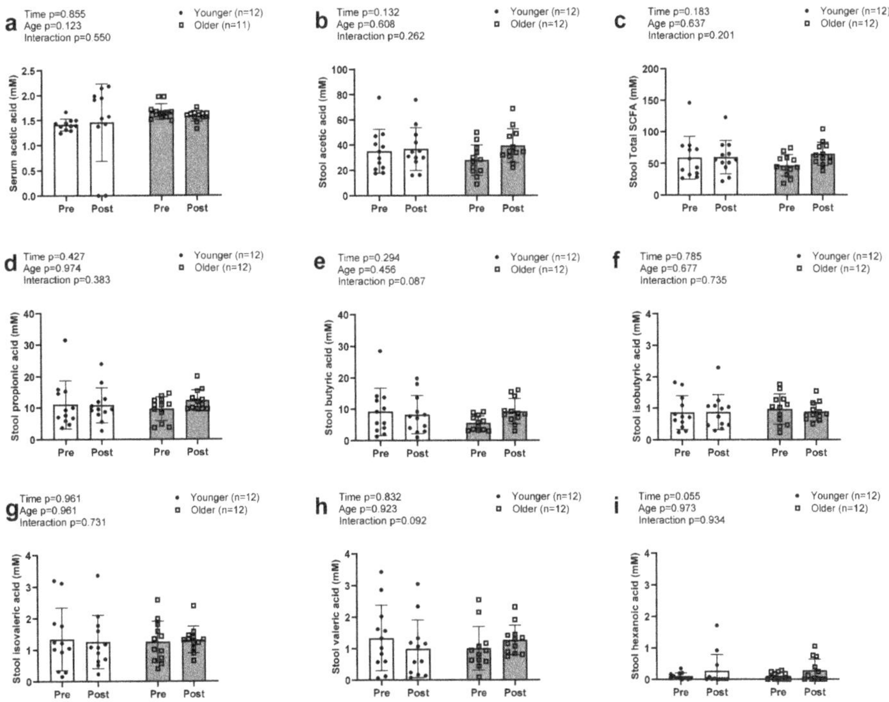

Figure 4. Changes in serum and stool short chain fatty acids with resistance training. Legend: Data in this figure indicates that only acetic acid (**a**) was found in the serum sample and there was no alteration observed between groups. Total SCFAs in the stool sample (**b**) were also not altered between groups. No changes in individual stool SCFAs, including acetic (**c**), propionic (**d**), butyric (**e**), isobutyric (**f**), isovaleric (**g**), and valeric acid (**h**), were observed. However, there was a trend towards a significant increase in hexanoic acids (**i**) in both groups.

3.5. Serum Biomarkers of Intestinal Barrier Function

No main effects or interactions were evident for FABP2 or LBP (Figure 5a,b). Serum LRG levels decreased from PRE to POST intervention in both groups (Figure 5c, $p = 0.007$). There was also an observed main effect of group, with older participants exhibiting lower values compared to younger individuals ($p = 0.015$); however, there was no G × T interaction ($p = 0.551$).

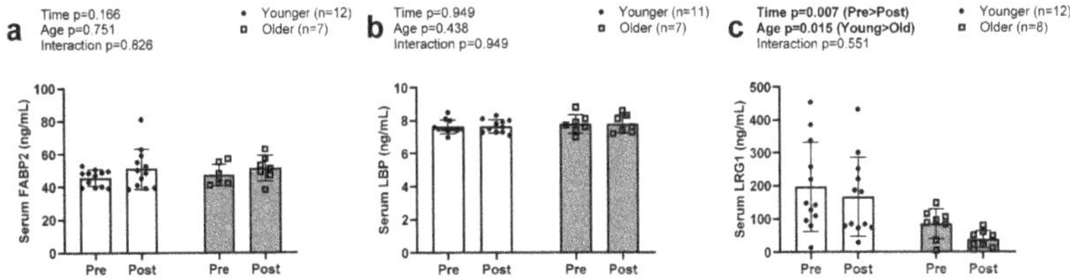

Figure 5. Serum FABP2, LBP, and LRG1 at PRE and POST in older and younger participants. Data in this figure indicate that serum FABP2 (**a**) and serum LBP (**b**) were not significantly altered in either older or younger participants. However, serum LRG1 (**c**) significantly decreased in both groups. Abbreviations: FABP2, fatty acid binding protein; LBP, lipopolysaccharide binding protein; LRG1, leucine-rich alpha-2-glycoprotein 1.

3.6. Correlations Among Dietary Intake, Fecal/Serum Measures, and Resistance Training Adaptations

Spearman correlations were performed among POST-PRE change scores for key dependent variables in the younger, older, and all participants (i.e., diet composition, fecal/serum SCFAs, fecal microbiome, and serum biomarkers; Figure 6). After adjusting for multiple comparisons, no correlations were statistically significant. However, the following exploratory findings are noteworthy: Lean muscle mass alterations were associated with changes in alpha diversity, and a stronger relationship was observed in younger compared to older adults. Dietary fat in younger adults and dietary sugar in older adults had the strongest associations with alpha diversity. Surprisingly, no relationships were observed between dietary or lean mass changes and serum and stool SCFAs. Serum biomarkers were most strongly associated with measures in older but not younger adults, with inverse relationships observed between LRG-1 and VL thickness, total dietary calories, and fat. Dietary carbohydrate, but not fiber, was inversely associated with LBP, whereas fiber was inversely associated with FABP2 (in older but not younger adults).

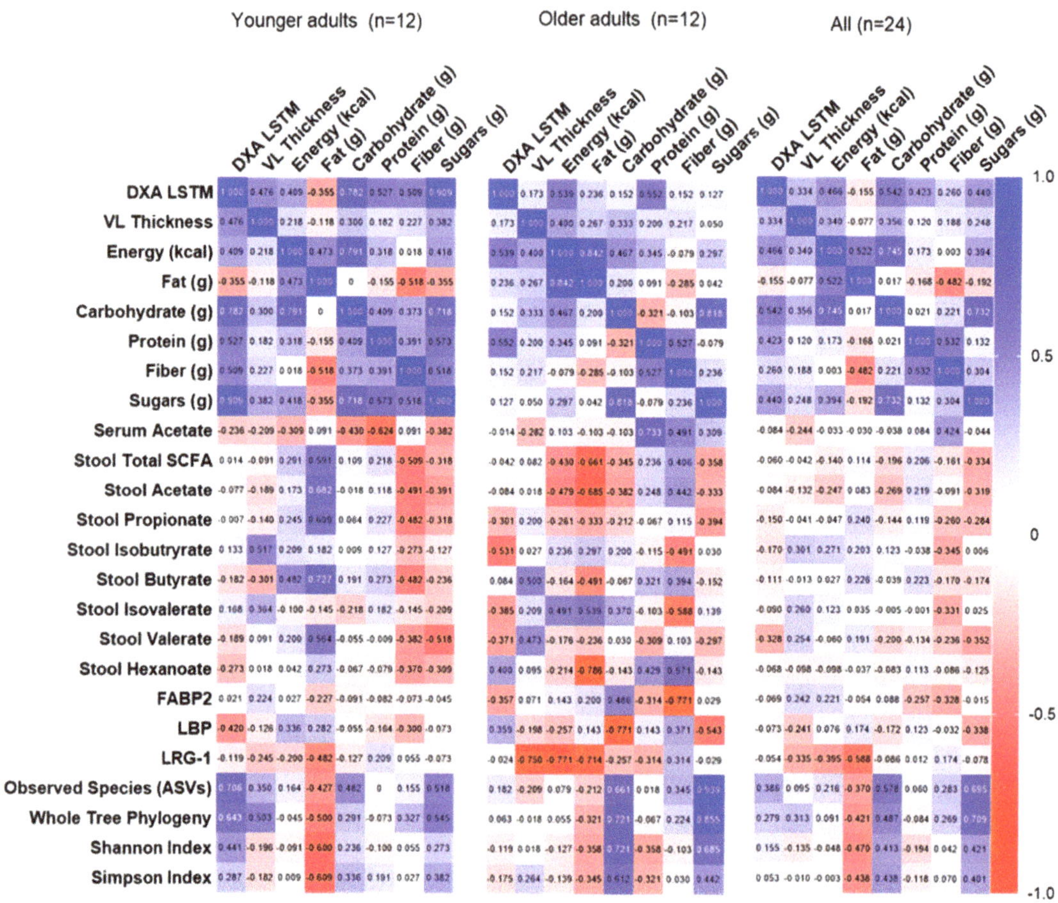

Figure 6. Correlations among changes in primary and secondary outcomes. Data are Spearman rho values. No correlations were significant after adjusting for multiple comparisons; $0.05/576 = p < 0.000087$. Abbreviations: DXA LSTM, lean/soft tissue mass determined using dual-energy X-ray absorptiometry; obs. species, observed species; SCFA, short chain fatty acids.

4. Discussion

This is the first known study to determine the effects of 10 weeks of RT on fecal microbiome, serum and fecal SCFAs, and gut-associated biomarkers in younger and older untrained adults. We observed an increase in LBM and VL thickness in both groups after the 10 weeks, which validated the effectiveness of the training program. The younger cohort presented a greater microbiome diversity than older individuals which did not change with RT. While many training studies have utilized ET interventions in younger adults, there are several studies that have now employed older participants and/or incorporated RT interventions. Taniguchi et al. [38] performed a five-week ET intervention in healthy elderly men and reported that the training program did not change alpha or beta diversity. Alternatively, Bycura et al. [25] examined the effects of the gut microbiome using both 8 weeks of ET and RT interventions in healthy college-aged adults. They found that changes in microbiota differed between training interventions. Although no significant changes in gut microbiota were observed overall, beta diversity analyses revealed notable shifts during the first few weeks of ET. However, post-intervention, these changes slightly regressed, with the microbiota composition resembling the baseline more closely. Similarly, a 6-week ET intervention in obese and lean young adults conducted by Allen et al. [22] supports the notion that beta-diversity changes are dependent on BMI. Additionally, following the 6-week sedentary washout period, the authors reported that changes in the microbiota had reverted to PRE-intervention levels.

Cullen at al. [11] conducted a 6-week resistance training intervention in healthy young sedentary adults and found that RT elicited mixed changes in alpha and beta diversity measures. Our data and previous data utilizing RT interventions collectively suggest that microbiome diversity is not appreciably altered with RT. Nonetheless, the reasons why ET greatly impacts microbiota composition compared to RT should be further investigated.

In our study, RT produced no significant changes in the seven detectable fecal SCFAs and one detectable serum SCFA. These findings are contrary to preclinical rodent studies suggesting the potential involvement of SCFAs in mitigating exercise adaptations. For instance, Huang et al. [39] treated mice with acetate, propionate, and butyrate for four weeks to investigate endurance capacity. They also reported that a higher concentration of SCFAs improved average running time compared to the control. Okamoto et al. [40] also investigated the effects of SCFAs on endurance training outcomes. The authors administered either a low or high microbiome-accessible carbohydrate (LMC or HMC) diet to 10-week-old mice for 6 weeks. They found that the LMC diet group had lower SCFA concentrations and slower treadmill running times compared to the HMC diet group.

The differences in diet composition and SCFA production are consistent with the study by Eveleens Maarse and colleagues [41], who supplemented older adults with a fiber-rich dietary mixture of acacia gum and carrot powder (30 g/day) and observed an increase in fecal SCFAs in the intervention group versus placebo. Estaki et al. investigated the effects of SCFAs on aerobic capacity in humans. They concluded that healthy young adults with higher SCFA concentrations had a higher VO_2 peak [42]. These studies suggest that changes in SCFA correlate with changes in exercise performance. However, our training involved resistance exercises rather than endurance exercises, which could explain the differences in the previously discussed results.

Given our investigation of the gut microbiome and SCFAs with RT interventions, it was ideal to assess biomarkers of intestinal barrier integrity. Although serum LBP was unchanged, we observed a trend toward increased serum FABP2 following RT. Numao et al. [43] reported similar findings, as they also observed an increase in FABP after low- and moderate-intensity exercise in healthy men. However, the authors utilized an aerobic training intervention. Additionally, we observed a significant decrease in LRG1 levels with RT intervention. Elevated levels of LRG1 in the bloodstream are often associated with inflammatory diseases, cancer, and cardiovascular disorders, making LRG1 a potential biomarker for disease activity [44–46]. Our findings suggest that RT could improve intestinal barrier integrity, and this should be further explored.

Limitations

Though this study provides new evidence for the gut–muscle axis in humans, it does have limitations. First, our sample was fairly homogeneous, as there were 63% white participants and 75% female participants. It would be valuable to investigate whether race or gender is a factor in gut microbiota composition and whether SCFAs change with training. Another limitation is that the older cohort had significantly greater total body mass, which is typically associated with dysbiosis [47]. While our sample included participants in an effective RT program, there was no control group that did not train, and our sample (n = 24) was relatively small. Importantly, the relative training volume was not equal for the two cohorts compared. We also did not request that participants collect stool samples at the same time of day, which may have affected fecal microbiome composition [48]. Another important limitation of our study was the lack of dietary guidance; the variance in fiber alone constitutes a major confounding factor that could have influenced these results. Future investigations should include personalized dietary interventions that allow standardization of dietary intakes, perhaps during a run-in period prior to RT. Finally, while we educated participants on completing accurate diet logs, self-reporting was a major limitation for our diet analysis [49].

5. Conclusions

This is the first known study to investigate the effects of RT on the fecal microbiome and SCFAs in humans. Alpha diversity and beta diversity analyses indicate that 10 weeks of RT did not change the overall microbiome composition of untrained adults, though younger and older participant cohorts had differing compositions across time. Fecal and serum SCFAs were not significantly altered after 10 weeks of the RT program. Additionally, fecal SCFAs did not translate to serum SCFAs, potentially due to utilization by colonocytes or maintenance of intestinal epithelium integrity. Although these results are preliminary, we posit that RT adaptations in humans are likely mitigated by factors other than the fecal microbiome or its metabolites.

Author Contributions: Conceptualization, A.A.-B., K.C.Y., C.B.M., K.W.H., M.D.R. and A.D.F.; data curation, S.L., K.S.S., M.A.S., C.L.S., D.A.L., M.D.R. and A.D.F.; formal analysis, W.V.D.P., D.A.L., M.D.R. and A.D.F.; funding acquisition, K.C.Y., K.W.H., M.D.R. and A.D.F.; investigation, A.A.-B., K.S.S., W.V.D.P., C.L.S., C.B.M., M.D.R. and A.D.F.; methodology, W.V.D.P., K.C.Y., M.D.R. and A.D.F.; project administration, M.A.S., K.C.Y., M.D.R. and A.D.F.; resources, M.D.R. and A.D.F.; supervision, K.S.S., C.L.S., D.A.L. and A.D.F.; visualization, M.D.R. and A.D.F.; writing—original draft, A.A.-B.; writing—review and editing, A.A.-B., S.L., K.S.S., W.V.D.P., M.A.S., C.L.S., D.A.L., K.C.Y., C.B.M., K.W.H., M.D.R. and A.D.F. All authors have read and agreed to the published version of the manuscript.

Funding: The original studies were supported through funding from the Peanut Institute (Albany, GA, USA), awarded to A.D.F. and M.D.R. Discretionary funding from A.D.F. and M.D.R. was used to perform fecal and serum analyses.

Institutional Review Board Statement: Both studies were conducted in accordance with the Declaration of Helsinki and under a single approved protocol by the Auburn University Institutional Review Board (IRB) (Protocol # 19-249 MR 1907). Both studies were pre-registered clinical trials (NCT04015479 registered 11 July 2019 [28]; NCT04707963 registered 13 January 2021 [27]).

Informed Consent Statement: Informed consent was obtained from all subjects involved in the study.

Data Availability Statement: Data can be obtained from the corresponding author upon reasonable request.

Acknowledgments: The authors appreciate prior laboratory members for assisting with resistance training and testing procedures.

Conflicts of Interest: The authors declare no conflicts of interest. The funders had no role in the design of the study; in the collection, analyses, or interpretation of data; in the writing of the manuscript; or in the decision to publish the results. The study performed is not related to K.S.S.'s current affiliation with Ocean Spray Cranberries.

Abbreviations

The following abbreviations are used in this manuscript:

ASV	Amplicon Sequence Variant
BMI	Body Mass Index
DXA	Dual-Energy X-ray Absorptiometry
ET	Endurance Training
FABP	Fatty Acid Binding Protein
F/B	Firmicutes to Bacteroidetes
FDR	False Discovery Rate
GC	Gas Chromatography
G × T	Group × Time
HMC	High Microbiome-Accessible Carbohydrate
IRB	Institutional Review Board
LBP	Lipopolysaccharide Binding Protein
LBM	Lean Body Mass
LMC	Low Microbiome-accessible Carbohydrate
LRG1	Leucine-Rich Alpha-2 Glycoprotein 1
LSTM	Lean Soft Tissue Mass
NDSR	Nutrition Data System for Research
OTU	Operational Taxonomic Unit
PCR	Polymerase Chain Reaction
PRE	Pre-intervention
POST	Post-intervention
RPE	Rating of Perceived Exertion
RT	Resistance Training
SCFA	Short-Chain Fatty Acid
USG	Urine Specific Gravity
VL	Vastus Lateralis

References

1. Ogunrinola, G.A.; Oyewale, J.O.; Oshamika, O.O.; Olasehinde, G.I. The Human Microbiome and Its Impacts on Health. *Int. J. Microbiol.* **2020**, *2020*, 8045646. [CrossRef]
2. Yoo, J.Y.; Groer, M.; Dutra, S.V.O.; Sarkar, A.; McSkimming, D.I. Correction: Yoo, J.Y., et al. Gut Microbiota and Immune System Interactions. *Microorganisms* **2020**, *8*, 2046. [CrossRef]
3. Carmody, R.N.; Gerber, G.K.; Luevano, J.M., Jr.; Gatti, D.M.; Somes, L.; Svenson, K.L.; Turnbaugh, P.J. Diet dominates host genotype in shaping the murine gut microbiota. *Cell Host Microbe* **2015**, *17*, 72–84. [CrossRef] [PubMed]
4. Maurice, C.F.; Haiser, H.J.; Turnbaugh, P.J. Xenobiotics shape the physiology and gene expression of the active human gut microbiome. *Cell* **2013**, *152*, 39–50. [CrossRef] [PubMed]
5. Howard, B.M.; Kornblith, L.Z.; Christie, S.A.; Conroy, A.S.; Nelson, M.F.; Campion, E.M.; Callcut, R.A.; Calfee, C.S.; Lamere, B.J.; Fadrosh, D.W.; et al. Characterizing the gut microbiome in trauma: Significant changes in microbial diversity occur early after severe injury. *Trauma Surg. Acute Care Open* **2017**, *2*, e000108. [CrossRef]

6. Sittipo, P.; Shim, J.W.; Lee, Y.K. Microbial Metabolites Determine Host Health and the Status of Some Diseases. *Int. J. Mol. Sci.* **2019**, *20*, 5296. [CrossRef]
7. Bäckhed, F.; Manchester, J.K.; Semenkovich, C.F.; Gordon, J.I. Mechanisms underlying the resistance to diet-induced obesity in germ-free mice. *Proc. Natl. Acad. Sci. USA* **2007**, *104*, 979–984. [CrossRef]
8. Chen, Y.M.; Wei, L.; Chiu, Y.S.; Hsu, Y.J.; Tsai, T.Y.; Wang, M.F.; Huang, C.C. Lactobacillus plantarum TWK10 Supplementation Improves Exercise Performance and Increases Muscle Mass in Mice. *Nutrients* **2016**, *8*, 205. [CrossRef]
9. Yan, H.; Diao, H.; Xiao, Y.; Li, W.; Yu, B.; He, J.; Yu, J.; Zheng, P.; Mao, X.; Luo, Y.; et al. Gut microbiota can transfer fiber characteristics and lipid metabolic profiles of skeletal muscle from pigs to germ-free mice. *Sci. Rep.* **2016**, *6*, 31786. [CrossRef]
10. Fernández, J.; Fernández-Sanjurjo, M.; Iglesias-Gutiérrez, E.; Martínez-Camblor, P.; Villar, C.J.; Tomás-Zapico, C.; Fernández-García, B.; Lombó, F. Resistance and Endurance Exercise Training Induce Differential Changes in Gut Microbiota Composition in Murine Models. *Front. Physiol.* **2021**, *12*, 748854. [CrossRef]
11. Cullen, J.M.A.; Shahzad, S.; Kanaley, J.A.; Ericsson, A.C.; Dhillon, J. The effects of 6 wk of resistance training on the gut microbiome and cardiometabolic health in young adults with overweight and obesity. *J. Appl. Physiol.* **2024**, *136*, 349–361. [CrossRef] [PubMed]
12. Silva, Y.P.; Bernardi, A.; Frozza, R.L. The Role of Short-Chain Fatty Acids From Gut Microbiota in Gut-Brain Communication. *Front. Endocrinol.* **2020**, *11*, 25. [CrossRef]
13. Remely, M.; Hippe, B.; Geretschlaeger, I.; Stegmayer, S.; Hoefinger, I.; Haslberger, A. Increased gut microbiota diversity and abundance of Faecalibacterium prausnitzii and Akkermansia after fasting: A pilot study. *Wien. Klin. Wochenschr.* **2015**, *127*, 394–398. [CrossRef] [PubMed]
14. Louis, P.; Flint, H.J. Formation of propionate and butyrate by the human colonic microbiota. *Environ. Microbiol.* **2017**, *19*, 29–41. [CrossRef]
15. Liu, H.; Wang, J.; He, T.; Becker, S.; Zhang, G.; Li, D.; Ma, X. Butyrate: A Double-Edged Sword for Health? *Adv. Nutr.* **2018**, *9*, 21–29. [CrossRef] [PubMed]
16. Frampton, J.; Murphy, K.G.; Frost, G.; Chambers, E.S. Short-chain fatty acids as potential regulators of skeletal muscle metabolism and function. *Nat. Metab.* **2020**, *2*, 840–848. [CrossRef]
17. Tang, G.; Du, Y.; Guan, H.; Jia, J.; Zhu, N.; Shi, Y.; Rong, S.; Yuan, W. Butyrate ameliorates skeletal muscle atrophy in diabetic nephropathy by enhancing gut barrier function and FFA2-mediated PI3K/Akt/mTOR signals. *Br. J. Pharmacol.* **2022**, *179*, 159–178. [CrossRef]
18. Lahiri, S.; Kim, H.; Garcia-Perez, I.; Reza, M.M.; Martin, K.A.; Kundu, P.; Cox, L.M.; Selkrig, J.; Posma, J.M.; Zhang, H.; et al. The gut microbiota influences skeletal muscle mass and function in mice. *Sci. Transl. Med.* **2019**, *11*, eaan5662. [CrossRef]
19. Yu, C.; Liu, S.; Chen, L.; Shen, J.; Niu, Y.; Wang, T.; Zhang, W.; Fu, L. Effect of exercise and butyrate supplementation on microbiota composition and lipid metabolism. *J. Endocrinol.* **2019**, *243*, 125–135. [CrossRef]
20. Yang, L.; Lin, H.; Lin, W.; Xu, X. Exercise Ameliorates Insulin Resistance of Type 2 Diabetes through Motivating Short-Chain Fatty Acid-Mediated Skeletal Muscle Cell Autophagy. *Biology* **2020**, *9*, 203. [CrossRef]
21. Erlandson, K.M.; Liu, J.; Johnson, R.; Dillon, S.; Jankowski, C.M.; Kroehl, M.; Robertson, C.E.; Frank, D.N.; Tuncil, Y.; Higgins, J.; et al. An exercise intervention alters stool microbiota and metabolites among older, sedentary adults. *Ther. Adv. Infect. Dis.* **2021**, *8*, 20499361211027067. [CrossRef] [PubMed]
22. Allen, J.M.; Mailing, L.J.; Niemiro, G.M.; Moore, R.; Cook, M.D.; White, B.A.; Holscher, H.D.; Woods, J.A. Exercise Alters Gut Microbiota Composition and Function in Lean and Obese Humans. *Med. Sci. Sports Exerc.* **2018**, *50*, 747–757. [CrossRef]
23. Moore, J.H.; Smith, K.S.; Chen, D.; Lamb, D.A.; Smith, M.A.; Osburn, S.C.; Ruple, B.A.; Morrow, C.D.; Huggins, K.W.; McDonald, J.R.; et al. Exploring the Effects of Six Weeks of Resistance Training on the Fecal Microbiome of Older Adult Males: Secondary Analysis of a Peanut Protein Supplemented Randomized Controlled Trial. *Sports* **2022**, *10*, 65. [CrossRef] [PubMed]
24. Cronin, O.; Barton, W.; Skuse, P.; Penney, N.C.; Garcia-Perez, I.; Murphy, E.F.; Woods, T.; Nugent, H.; Fanning, A.; Melgar, S.; et al. A Prospective Metagenomic and Metabolomic Analysis of the Impact of Exercise and/or Whey Protein Supplementation on the Gut Microbiome of Sedentary Adults. *mSystems* **2018**, *3*, e00044-18. [CrossRef]
25. Bycura, D.; Santos, A.C.; Shiffer, A.; Kyman, S.; Winfree, K.; Sutliffe, J.; Pearson, T.; Sonderegger, D.; Cope, E.; Caporaso, J.G. Impact of Different Exercise Modalities on the Human Gut Microbiome. *Sports* **2021**, *9*, 14. [CrossRef] [PubMed]
26. Aya, V.; Jimenez, P.; Muñoz, E.; Ramírez, J.D. Effects of exercise and physical activity on gut microbiota composition and function in older adults: A systematic review. *BMC Geriatr.* **2023**, *23*, 364. [CrossRef]
27. Sexton, C.L.; Smith, M.A.; Smith, K.S.; Osburn, S.C.; Godwin, J.S.; Ruple, B.A.; Hendricks, A.M.; Mobley, C.B.; Goodlett, M.D.; Frugé, A.D.; et al. Effects of Peanut Protein Supplementation on Resistance Training Adaptations in Younger Adults. *Nutrients* **2021**, *13*, 3981. [CrossRef]

28. Lamb, D.A.; Moore, J.H.; Smith, M.A.; Vann, C.G.; Osburn, S.C.; Ruple, B.A.; Fox, C.D.; Smith, K.S.; Altonji, O.M.; Power, Z.M.; et al. The effects of resistance training with or without peanut protein supplementation on skeletal muscle and strength adaptations in older individuals. *J. Int. Soc. Sports Nutr.* **2020**, *17*, 66. [CrossRef]
29. Kumar, R.; Eipers, P.; Little, R.B.; Crowley, M.; Crossman, D.K.; Lefkowitz, E.J.; Morrow, C.D. Getting started with microbiome analysis: Sample acquisition to bioinformatics. *Curr. Protoc. Hum. Genet.* **2014**, *82*, 18.8.1–18.8.29. [CrossRef]
30. Frugé, A.D.; Van der Pol, W.; Rogers, L.Q.; Morrow, C.D.; Tsuruta, Y.; Demark-Wahnefried, W. Fecal Akkermansia muciniphila Is Associated with Body Composition and Microbiota Diversity in Overweight and Obese Women with Breast Cancer Participating in a Presurgical Weight Loss Trial. *J. Acad. Nutr. Diet.* **2020**, *120*, 650–659. [CrossRef]
31. Bolyen, E.; Rideout, J.R.; Dillon, M.R.; Bokulich, N.A.; Abnet, C.C.; Al-Ghalith, G.A.; Alexander, H.; Alm, E.J.; Arumugam, M.; Asnicar, F.; et al. Reproducible, interactive, scalable and extensible microbiome data science using QIIME 2. *Nat. Biotechnol.* **2019**, *37*, 852–857. [CrossRef]
32. Van Der Pol, W.J.; Kumar, R.; Morrow, C.D.; Blanchard, E.E.; Taylor, C.M.; Martin, D.H.; Lefkowitz, E.J.; Muzny, C.A. In Silico and Experimental Evaluation of Primer Sets for Species-Level Resolution of the Vaginal Microbiota Using 16S Ribosomal RNA Gene Sequencing. *J. Infect. Dis.* **2019**, *219*, 305–314. [CrossRef] [PubMed]
33. Callahan, B.J.; McMurdie, P.J.; Rosen, M.J.; Han, A.W.; Johnson, A.J.; Holmes, S.P. DADA2: High-resolution sample inference from Illumina amplicon data. *Nat. Methods* **2016**, *13*, 581–583. [CrossRef]
34. Estaki, M.; Jiang, L.; Bokulich, N.A.; McDonald, D.; González, A.; Kosciolek, T.; Martino, C.; Zhu, Q.; Birmingham, A.; Vázquez-Baeza, Y.; et al. QIIME 2 Enables Comprehensive End-to-End Analysis of Diverse Microbiome Data and Comparative Studies with Publicly Available Data. *Curr. Protoc. Bioinform.* **2020**, *70*, e100. [CrossRef] [PubMed]
35. Quast, C.; Pruesse, E.; Yilmaz, P.; Gerken, J.; Schweer, T.; Yarza, P.; Peplies, J.; Glöckner, F.O. The SILVA ribosomal RNA gene database project: Improved data processing and web-based tools. *Nucleic Acids Res.* **2013**, *41*, D590–D596. [CrossRef]
36. Zhao, G.; Nyman, M.; Jönsson, J.A. Rapid determination of short-chain fatty acids in colonic contents and faeces of humans and rats by acidified water-extraction and direct-injection gas chromatography. *Biomed. Chromatogr. BMC* **2006**, *20*, 674–682. [CrossRef] [PubMed]
37. Zhao, G.; Liu, J.F.; Nyman, M.; Jönsson, J.A. Determination of short-chain fatty acids in serum by hollow fiber supported liquid membrane extraction coupled with gas chromatography. *J. Chromatogr. B Anal. Technol. Biomed. Life Sci.* **2007**, *846*, 202–208. [CrossRef]
38. Taniguchi, H.; Tanisawa, K.; Sun, X.; Kubo, T.; Hoshino, Y.; Hosokawa, M.; Takeyama, H.; Higuchi, M. Effects of short-term endurance exercise on gut microbiota in elderly men. *Physiol. Rep.* **2018**, *6*, e13935. [CrossRef]
39. Huang, L.; Li, T.; Zhou, M.; Deng, M.; Zhang, L.; Yi, L.; Zhu, J.; Zhu, X.; Mi, M. Hypoxia Improves Endurance Performance by Enhancing Short Chain Fatty Acids Production via Gut Microbiota Remodeling. *Front. Microbiol.* **2022**, *12*, 820691. [CrossRef]
40. Okamoto, T.; Morino, K.; Ugi, S.; Nakagawa, F.; Lemecha, M.; Ida, S.; Ohashi, N.; Sato, D.; Fujita, Y.; Maegawa, H. Microbiome potentiates endurance exercise through intestinal acetate production. *Am. J. Physiol. Endocrinol. Metab.* **2019**, *316*, E956–E966. [CrossRef]
41. Eveleens Maarse, B.C.; Eggink, H.M.; Warnke, I.; Bijlsma, S.; van den Broek, T.J.; Oosterman, J.E.; Caspers, M.P.M.; Sybesma, W.; Gal, P.; van Kraaij, S.J.W.; et al. Impact of fibre supplementation on microbiome and resilience in healthy participants: A randomized, placebo-controlled clinical trial. *Nutr. Metab. Cardiovasc. Dis. NMCD* **2024**, *34*, 1416–1426. [CrossRef] [PubMed]
42. Estaki, M.; Pither, J.; Baumeister, P.; Little, J.P.; Gill, S.K.; Ghosh, S.; Ahmadi-Vand, Z.; Marsden, K.R.; Gibson, D.L. Cardiorespiratory fitness as a predictor of intestinal microbial diversity and distinct metagenomic functions. *Microbiome* **2016**, *4*, 42. [CrossRef]
43. Numao, S.; Uchida, R.; Kurosaki, T.; Nakagaichi, M. Correction: Circulating Fatty Acid-binding Protein 4 Response to Acute Aerobic Exercise in Healthy Men. *Int. J. Sports Med.* **2023**, *44*, e1. [CrossRef] [PubMed]
44. Shinzaki, S.; Matsuoka, K.; Iijima, H.; Mizuno, S.; Serada, S.; Fujimoto, M.; Arai, N.; Koyama, N.; Morii, E.; Watanabe, M.; et al. Leucine-rich Alpha-2 Glycoprotein is a Serum Biomarker of Mucosal Healing in Ulcerative Colitis. *J. Crohn's Colitis* **2017**, *11*, 84–91. [CrossRef]
45. Wang, Y.; Shan, Q.; Hou, G.; Zhang, J.; Bai, J.; Lv, X.; Xie, Y.; Zhu, H.; Su, S.; Li, Y.; et al. Discovery of potential colorectal cancer serum biomarkers through quantitative proteomics on the colonic tissue interstitial fluids from the AOM-DSS mouse model. *J. Proteom.* **2016**, *132*, 31–40. [CrossRef]
46. Yasutomi, E.; Inokuchi, T.; Hiraoka, S.; Takei, K.; Igawa, S.; Yamamoto, S.; Ohmori, M.; Oka, S.; Yamasaki, Y.; Kinugasa, H.; et al. Leucine-rich alpha-2 glycoprotein as a marker of mucosal healing in inflammatory bowel disease. *Sci. Rep.* **2021**, *11*, 11086. [CrossRef]
47. Shen, J.; Obin, M.S.; Zhao, L. The gut microbiota, obesity and insulin resistance. *Mol. Asp. Med.* **2013**, *34*, 39–58. [CrossRef]

48. Bell, D.S.H. Changes seen in gut bacteria content and distribution with obesity: Causation or association? *Postgrad. Med.* **2015**, *127*, 863–868. [CrossRef]
49. De Keyzer, W.; Huybrechts, I.; De Vriendt, V.; Vandevijvere, S.; Slimani, N.; Van Oyen, H.; De Henauw, S. Repeated 24-hour recalls versus dietary records for estimating nutrient intakes in a national food consumption survey. *Food Nutr. Res.* **2011**, *55*, 7307. [CrossRef]

sports MDPI

Article

Quantifying Long-Term Adaptations in Performance Variables in Adolescent Athletes: A 1.5 Year Longitudinal Training Study Utilising a Standardised, Progressive, Blocked Linear Periodisation Resistance Training Program

Michael A. Carron [1,2] and Vincent J. Dalbo [1,2,*]

[1] School of Health, Medical and Applied Sciences, Central Queensland University, Rockhampton 4702, Australia; m.carron@cqu.edu.au
[2] Health, Education, Lifestyle, and Performance (HELP) Laboratory, St Brendan's College, Yeppoon 4703, Australia
* Correspondence: v.dalbo@cqu.edu.au

Abstract: We examined the effects of resistance training over 1.5 years (two seasons). Body mass, strength, power, and aerobic capacity were assessed during the first 1.5 years of a standardised, progressive, blocked linear periodisation training program in adolescent males with no prior history of resistance training (N = 11, 16.4 ± 0.5 years). Testing occurred during the start of pre-season (SPS), end of pre-season (EPS), and end of season (EOS) during the first and second year of resistance training. Changes over time were assessed with within-group ANOVAs and follow-up independent *t*-tests. Differences in relative change that occurred during the first and second year of training for each variable were assessed with dependent *t*-tests. Body mass changed over time ($p < 0.001$, $n^2p = 0.794$). Body mass increased from SPS to EPS ($p = 0.008$, *Large*) and EPS to EOS ($p = 0.019$, *Large*) in year 1, and from EOS in year 1 to SPS in year 2 ($p < 0.001$, *Large*). Bench press ($p < 0.001$, $n^2p = 0.806$), squat ($p < 0.001$, $n^2p = 0.670$), and medicine ball throw ($p < 0.001$, $n^2p = 0.350$) changed over time. Bench press (Year 1: $p < 0.001$, *Large*; Year 2: $p < 0.001$, *Large*), squat (Year 1: $p < 0.001$, *Large*; Year 2: $p < 0.001$, *Large*), and medicine ball throw (Year 1: $p = 0.007$, *Large*; Year 2: $p = 0.026$, *Large*) increased from SPS to EPS in year 1 and year 2. Bench press ($p = 0.010$, *Large*) and squat ($p = 0.004$, *Large*) increased more from SPS to EPS during year 1 than year 2. By quantifying diminished returns, our study offers practitioners novel information, helping practitioners manage expectations, avoid excessive training and support long-term adolescent development.

Keywords: youth; strength training; strength and conditioning; gym; fitness

1. Introduction

As recently as the early 1970s, gym-based training was believed to hinder on-field player performance. This view began to change when Boyd Epley was hired as the first full-time strength and conditioning coach at the University of Nebraska in 1969 and was able to help improve the performance of their football team through gym-based exercise [1]. Since that time, there has been great interest in the ability of resistance training to improve the health and performance of adolescent (<18 years), college-age (18–35 years), middle-aged (>35–64 years) and older individuals (≥65 years). Indeed, the positive effects of resistance training are so pervasive that most adolescents who partake in sport during high school engage in a strength and conditioning program to reduce their injury risk and enhance their performance [2]. In an attempt to develop an optimal strength and conditioning program, practitioners are encouraged to develop an annual plan (i.e., macrocycle) that is composed of smaller blocks of training, termed mesocycles (i.e., a cycle of training that may last weeks to months), which are composed of smaller blocks of training, termed microcycles (i.e., the structure of training during the hypertrophy cycle of training; it can be structured in weekly or daily blocks).

Despite the belief that structured, progressive resistance training programs will yield optimal performance outcomes, most published research has quantified the effects of resistance training on muscle strength and other performance outcomes over a single phase or mesocycle [3–7]. As such, most resistance training programs are conducted over periods of twelve weeks or less [3–7] and are designed to represent a single mesocycle. However, a well-established negative correlation exists between training experience and the rate of progression, whereby the more trained an individual becomes, the more slowly their performance improves [8]. The reduced rate of progression with enhanced training experience is the result of diminished physiological adaptations occurring as an individual moves closer to their genetic potential [9], and this phenomenon has been termed the ceiling effect. The ceiling effect is widely accepted, but we are only aware of a few studies that have specifically sought to quantify the decreased rate of progression that occurs following chronic resistance training ≥1 year [8,10–12]. Importantly, the studies that we are aware of [8,10–12] were conducted retrospectively, and only one study [10] employed a standardised resistance training protocol. As a result, research is needed to quantify the effects of standardised, progressive resistance training protocols on performance outcomes to establish expected rates of progression among adolescent athletes longitudinally. Furthermore, research is needed to quantify the degree of diminishing returns among adolescent athletes to fill the gap concerning the expected longitudinal returns from periodisation programming, to assist coaches in optimising workloads, managing expectations, and supporting long-term athlete development. Consequently, we quantified the physiological adaptations that occur in adolescents with no prior history of resistance training over their first 1.5 years of following a standardised, progressive, linear periodisation program designed for adolescent rugby league athlete development.

2. Methods

A longitudinal experimental design was utilized to monitor physiological adaptions that occur in response to a standardised, progressive, blocked linear periodisation training program occurring over two seasons. Data were collected over a period of 1.5 years (i.e., March 2023 to September 2024) in adolescent, male athletes with no previous history of resistance training. Outcome variables for the study were as follows: body mass, one-repetition maximum (1RM), barbell bench press (bench press), 1RM barbell back squat (squat), medicine ball throw (MBT), counter-movement jump (CMJ) and multi-stage fitness test (MSFT).

2.1. Participants

All participants were recruited from the same schoolboy rugby league team prior to the commencement of the 2023 season, and their training and performance was monitored from February 2023 to September 2024, which corresponded with the start of training for the 2023 rugby league season and the conclusion of the 2024 rugby league season. To be included in the study, participants had to have no prior history of resistance training, had to qualify for the first-grade rugby league team during the 2023 season and had to be in grade 11 or 12. Athletes were excluded from the study if they were in grade 12 (i.e., seniors) as it would not have been possible to monitor their performance during the following season due to graduation.

The study started with 25 potential participants (e.g., boys who qualified for the first-grade rugby team and volunteered to participate in the study) but ended with 11 participants. Potential participants were excluded due to having prior resistance training experience ($n = 1$), not being selected to the first-grade rugby team during the 2023 season (n = 2) or being a senior during the 2023 season (n = 6). Of the 16 participants meeting the inclusion criteria, 5 participants were lost due to incomplete data from testing occasions (i.e., did not complete more than one entire testing session, including gym- and field-based tests). As a result, 11 participants were observed across the 1.5-year testing period (age: 16.4 ± 0.5 years; age range: 16–17 years). Notably, 4 participants concurrently partook in an external rugby league academy program, which exposed them to additional gym-based and field-based training. Written assent was obtained from each participant, and written consent was obtained from the legal guardian of each participant prior to the commencement of the study. All study procedures were approved by the Human Research Ethics Committee (#0000023904).

2.2. On-Field Training Program

Throughout each macrocycle, on-field training occurred on Monday and Wednesday from the start of the pre-season to the end of the season. Each Monday session consisted of an additional 15 min video analysis and team meeting session, prior to on-field training. Each on-field training session typically consisted of conditioning (i.e., bouts of sprinting over 10-, 20- and 40-m distances with rest intervals ranging from 15 to 60 s), conditioning drills including small-sided games in conjunction with bouts of high-intensity interval training (i.e., running) or coach-led field training consisting of skill performance (e.g., tackle simulation, passing and kicking), drills (e.g., set plays), game-based conditioning (i.e., aerobic capacity) and opposed sessions (i.e., practice/friendly games). On-field training programs were revised for individual athletes if an injury was present. Each on-field session typically lasted 45 min in duration in the pre-season and 30 min while in season, and no on-field training sessions occurred during the off-season.

2.3. Resistance Training Program

Weekly gym-based training was composed of an upper-body lift on Monday, a lower-body lift on Wednesday and a whole-body lift on Friday. Each gym-based exercise session started with a 15 min warm-up. The warm-up consisted of light aerobic cycling activity (5 min), various mobility exercises targeting major functional movements with dynamic stretches targeting the lower and upper-body (4 min), movement-preparatory exercises with body weight or resistance bands (e.g., banded squats, lunges, chest presses and rows, 4 min) and passing a football repeatedly across 10 m intervals while moving at different intensities (2 min).

The upper-body lift consisted of the selection of a primary exercise followed by four supplementary exercises and one trunk exercise. The lower-body lift consisted of the selection of a primary exercise followed by four supplementary exercises and one trunk exercise. The whole-body lift consisted of two primary exercises (i.e., one upper-body primary exercise and one lower-body primary exercise) followed by four supplementary exercises (i.e., two upper-body supplementary exercises and two lower-body supplementary exercises) and one trunk exercise. Table 1 presents the list of primary and supplementary exercises that were utilized for upper-body, lower-body, and whole-body exercises. The resistance training program followed the principles of a traditional linear blocked periodization program (i.e., macrocycle) with a progression in load of 3% to 5% when applicable (i.e., when athletes were able to complete the prescribed sets, repetitions and load). When power was an aim of the mesocycle (e.g., during pre-season), one supplementary exercise was removed from the training program and three plyometric exercises for the upper-body or lower body were included in the training program depending on the focus of the specific training session (e.g., if the upper-body was being trained, the three plyometric exercises selected would be upper-body plyometric exercises). During the power phase of the mesocycle for whole-body days, one upper (all performed bilaterally) and two lower plyometric exercises were selected (i.e., one bilateral and one unilateral exercise).

Table 1. Primary and secondary exercises used throughout the 1.5 year (two-season) resistance training program.

	Upper-Body			*Lower-Body*			*Full-Body*	*Plyometrics*		*Trunk*
Classification	**Overhead**	**Anterior**	**Posterior**	**Anterior**	**Posterior**	**Hip/Glute**		**Upper-Body**	**Lower-Body**	
Primary										
	Push Jerk	BB Bench Press	BB Bent Over Rows	Front Squat	Trap Bar Deadlift	Hip Thrust	Clean			
	DB Push Press	BB Incline Bench Press	Seated Row	Back Squat	Romanian Deadlift		Power Clean			
	BB Push Press	BB Decline Bench Press	DB Rows	Overhead Squat			Hang Clean			
	BB Overhead						Full Clean			
Secondary										
	Seated DB Overhead Press	DB Bench	Chest Supported Rows		SL Deadlift	Hip Hinge	Clean Pull	Clap Push-up	Alternating Bounds	Sit-ups
	Standing DB Overhead	Incline Bench	Landmine row	Box Squat	DB Deadlift	Back Elevated Hip Up	Clean Shrug	Med Ball Chest Pass	Tuck Jumps	Barbell Rollouts
	DB Cuban Press	Incline DB Bench	BB Inverted Row	Overhead Squat	Band Deadlift	SL Hip Ups	DB Cleans	MB OH Forward Pass		Copenhagen
	Neutral Grip DB Overhead	Dips	Band Rows	Goblet Squat	Below Knee Rack Pull	Band Hip Extensions	KB Cleans	Wall Ball	Broad Jumps	Hanging Leg Raises
	Y-raise, W-raise, T-raise	Band Bench	Straight Arm Pulldown	Hack squat	Above Knee Rack Pull	Hip Adduction	Famers Walk	Med Ball Rotational Throws	Depth Drops	Cable Chop
	Side Delt Raises	Push-ups	Reverse Fly	High Box Squat	SL DB Romanian Deadlift	Hip Abduction		Med Ball Ground Slam	Depth Jumps w/ Bound	Band Rotation Fend
	Rear Delt Raises	Elevated Push-ups	Pullups	Deep Box Squat	DB Romanian Deadlift	Hip Flexion		Lying Medball Chest Pass	Hurdle Hops	

Table 1. *Cont.*

		Upper-Body		*Lower-Body*			*Full-Body*	*Plyometrics*		*Trunk*
Classification	**Overhead**	**Anterior**	**Posterior**	**Anterior**	**Posterior**	**Hip/Glute**		**Upper-Body**	**Lower-Body**	
Primary										
	Face Pulls	Foot Elevated Push-ups	Lat Pulldowns	Band Squat	Reverse Hypers				Lateral Bounds	Planks
	Internal and external Shoulder Rotations	DB Flies	Band Pulldowns	Body weight Squat	Landmine Romanian Deadlift				SL Box Jumps	3 Way Plank
		DB Incline Flies	Chin-ups	5 second Pause Squat	Band Leg Curls				Lateral Bounds	Russian Twists
		Band Push-ups	Inverted Row		Nordic Hamstring Curls				Seated Jump	V-shape Sit-ups
		DB Push-ups			Band Good Morning				Vertical Jumps	Toes to Bar
					Sled Pull				Calf Hops	SA Farmer Walk
					Sled Push				Split Squat Jump	
					BB Lunges				MB Rotational Throws	
					Walking DB Lunges				KB Swings	
					Walking BB Lunges				SL Vertical Jump	
					SL Box Squat				Split Squat Jumps	
					SL Squat					
					SL Hip Lift				SL Hurdle Jumps	
					Lateral Lunges					
					DB Split Squat					
					DB Step Up					
					BB Step Up					
					Power Step Up					
					Leg Extension					

Notes: One primary lift was selected for a session subject to the objective of the session (i.e., one lower-body primary lift was selected on lower-body training days), followed by four secondary lifts and one trunk exercise. For example, on a lower-body day, one may select a back squat from the primary list, followed by a single leg RDL, DB split squat, Nordics, and sled push from the secondary list, followed by barbell rollouts from the trunk list. For full-body days, in general, one upper-body and one lower-body exercise would be selected from the list of primary exercises and two upper-body and two lower-body exercises would be selected from the list of secondary exercises. One trunk exercise was included for upper-body, lower-body, and full-body days. Where the emphasis was on power development, three additional plyometric movements were included during each session. Abbreviations: BB, barbell; DB, dumbbell; RDL, Romanian deadlift; KD, kettlebell; SA, single arm; SL, single leg; MB, medicine ball.

2.4. Two-Year Macrocycle

Our 1.5 year resistance training program was composed of two one-year-long macrocycles focused on preparing the participants to compete in a first-grade rugby league competition. Each year-long macrocycle employed a gradual increase in training intensity with a decrease in training volume over the course of the seasonal phases, while utilising a blocked strategy consisting of mesocycles with an emphasis on improving specific physical qualities (i.e., strength and power) to support rugby league performance. Our standardised, progressive, linear, blocked periodisation program (Figure 1) was composed of 10 mesocycles across the two-season training period (preparation phase, pre-season phase, competition phase, transition phase/recovery phase and off-season phase; these 5 phases occurred during each year of training). Each of the 5 repeated mesocycles was broken down into microcycles, which were also repeated during each year of training.

2023 Macrocycle (Annual Plan)												
Week of Year	1-6	7-13	14,15	16	17-20	21	22-34			35	36-39	40-52
Phase of Training	Off season	Preparation phase	Transition/ Recovery	Test	Pre-season	Test	Competition			Test	Transition/ Recovery	Off season
Mesocycle: Primary Objective(s)	Familiarisation, safety and technical focus	Optimize technical proficiencies, familiarisation with assessments	De-load (school holiday)	-	Strength - Power	-	Strength	Power	Maintenance	-	Rehabilitation Maintain physical status Recover physiologically	Recovery Basic physical maintenance
Mesocycle Secondary Objective(s)	-	Aerobic capacity	-		Aerobic capacity		Muscular endurance	Speed	-		-	-
2024 Macrocycle (Annual Plan)												
Week of Year	1-6	7-13	14,15	16	17-20	21	22-34			35		
Phase of Training	Off season	Preparation phase	Transition/ Recovery	Test	Pre-season	Test	Competition			Test		
Mesocycle: Primary Objective(s)	Familiarisation, safety and technical focus	Optimize technical proficiencies, familiarisation with assessments	De-load (school holiday)	-	Strength - Power	-	Strength	Power	Maintenance	-		
Mesocycle Secondary Objective(s)	-	Aerobic capacity	-		Aerobic capacity		Muscular endurance	Speed	-			

Figure 1. The 1.5 year (two-season) linear blocked periodisation program.

2.5. Off-Season, Preparation and Transition Phases of Training

The start of each calendar year commenced with participants in the off-season (weeks 1–6), in which no on-field or resistance training was prescribed. During weeks 7–13, participants engaged in the preparation phase of training, which was composed of two on-field sessions per week and three resistance training sessions per week, which were broken down into upper-body training on Monday, lower-body training on Wednesday and full-body training on Friday. Resistance training sessions lasted 45 min and were focused on teaching proper technique and developing skeletal muscle as a result. A self-selected load was used in this study to prioritise technical competency and ensure safety among untrained individuals during the preparatory phase of training, given that untrained participants often are not competent enough to perform strength assessments (e.g., 1RM testing) to derive data or possess the motor control required for maximal loading. Therefore, allowing participants to self-select their load during the preparatory phase of training enabled participants to work at an intensity appropriate to their ability while minimising the injury risk. Participants were required to perform warm-up sets with the bar before adding a self-determined amount of load under guided instruction, placing an emphasis on technique. Participants were informed to cease performing the exercise when they believed that they could only complete 1–2 more repetitions with the load. Moreover, athletes were familiarised with all testing protocols. Weeks 14–15 served as a transition/recovery phase as the athletes were away for school holidays, and no on-field or resistance training sessions were prescribed during this time.

2.6. Start of Pre-Season Testing and Pre-Season Phase

Week 16 served as baseline testing, so no on-field or resistance training sessions were scheduled during this week, and participants were instructed to refrain from vigorous activity for 48 h prior to testing, which occurred on Wednesday and Friday. Weeks 17–20 served as the pre-season phase which was composed of two on-field sessions per week and three resistance training sessions per week. The resistance training sessions were broken down into upper-body training on Monday, lower-body training on Wednesday, and full-body training on Friday. Resistance training sessions lasted 45 min and were focused on strength. As a result, 5 sets were typically performed per lift at 85% 1RM for primary exercises and 3 sets were typically performed per lift at 85% 1RM for secondary exercises.

2.7. End of Pre-Season Testing

Week 21 served as follow-up testing (end-pre-season), so no on-field or resistance training sessions were scheduled during this week, and participants were instructed to refrain from vigorous activity for 48 h prior to testing, which occurred on Wednesday and Friday.

2.8. In-Season Phase

Weeks 22–34 served as the in-season phase, which was composed of two on-field sessions per week and two resistance training sessions per week, which were broken down into upper-body training on Monday and full-body training on Friday, except for weeks containing a game, which comprised of full-body training on Monday and Friday. Resistance training sessions for weeks 22–26 lasted 30 min and were focused on maintaining skeletal muscle and strength for the initial four-week mesocycle; as a result, five sets were typically performed per lift at 85% 1RM for primary exercises, and three sets were typically performed per lift at 85% 1RM for secondary exercises. Resistance training sessions lasted 30 min and were focused on power for the second four-week mesocycle for weeks 26–30. As a result, three sets were typically performed per lift at 80% 1RM for primary exercises, and three sets were typically performed per lift at 75% 1RM for secondary exercises. For plyometric-based activities, athletes were instructed to perform movements at 80–100% maximal violation[3]. Resistance training sessions for weeks 30–34 lasted 30 min and were focused on maintaining performance (maintenance); they consisted of one team-based rehabilitation session and one strength session to maintain skeletal muscle. As a result, five sets were typically performed per lift at 85% 1RM for primary exercises, and three sets were typically performed at 85% 1RM for secondary exercises.

2.9. End-of-Season Testing and Off-Season

Week 35 served as end-of-season testing; no on-field or resistance training sessions were scheduled during this week, and participants were instructed to refrain from vigorous activity for 48 h prior to testing, which occurred on Wednesday and Friday. Weeks 36–40 served as a transition/recovery period as the athletes were away for school holidays, and no on-field or resistance training sessions were prescribed during this time. The end of each calendar year concluded with participants in the off-season (weeks 40–52), in which no on-field or resistance training was prescribed.

2.10. Testing Protocol for Outcome Variables

The testing of performance outcomes comprised six tests, implemented during the pre-season, end of pre-season and end-of-season phases of training. The administration of the six tests was conducted in accordance with an established methodology [13]. All tests included in the protocol have been reported to be reliable [14] and can be utilized to monitor potential changes over time [15]. Athletes were instructed to refrain from vigorous activity, consume their typical diets and undertake their normal daily schedules (i.e., sleep, hydration and school participation) for 48 h prior to each testing session [16]. Prior to the first testing session of each season, all participants were familiarized with each test throughout the duration of the preparation phase (i.e., weeks 7–13), in which participants received verbal instruction, visual demonstrations and practice attempts on all tests on at least two occasions. Participants were only allowed to partake in the 1RM lifts after gaining clearance from the strength and conditioning coach, who held a Master's degree in strength and conditioning. For all tests, verbal encouragement was provided by the experimenter, and athletes were tested during the same time of day.

2.11. Body Mass

Body mass was measured using electronic scales (SECA 813, SECA Corp) with athletes wearing normal rugby league attire (i.e., shirt and shorts), without footwear or socks. The body mass assessment protocol utilized has been reported to be reliable in adolescents (coefficient of variation (CV) = 0.63%; interclass correlation coefficient (ICC) = 0.999) [14].

2.12. One-Repetition-Maximum Barbell Bench Press

Maximal upper-body strength was assessed using the 1RM barbell bench press. Testing was performed in accordance with the procedures outline by the National Strength and Conditioning Association (NSCA) [17]. Specifically, a 1RM bench press had to be obtained in a maximum of five attempts, and a minimum of 180 s of seated rest was provided between attempts [17]. All attempts were completed using a 2.13 m Olympic bar (20 kg). The bench press was assessed with hands pronated using a hook grip and athletes maintaining a supine position on a flat bench. The 1RM barbell bench press assessment protocol utilized has been reported to be reliable in adolescents (CV = 1.08%, ICC = 0.988) [14].

2.13. One-Repetition-Maximum Barbell Back Squat

Maximal lower-body strength was assessed using the 1RM barbell back squat. Testing was performed in accordance with the procedures outline by the NSCA [17]. Specifically, the 1RM squat had to be obtained in a maximum of five attempts, and a minimum of 180 s of seated rest was provided between attempts [17]. All attempts were completed using a 2.13 m Olympic bar (20 kg). The back squat was performed with self-selected footing using a high bar position and a pronated hook grip. For a squat attempt to be counted as successful, athletes had to reach a depth where their thighs were parallel to the floor. The 1RM barbell back squat assessment protocol utilized has been reported to be reliable in adolescents (CV = 1.12%, ICC = 0.985) [14].

2.14. Medicine Ball Throw

Maximal upper-body power was assessed with the MBT. The MBT required participants to throw a 2 kg medicine ball (Celsius; Australia) horizontally to achieve the maximum distance (m) possible. Athletes were seated (side saddle) on a flat bench placed flush against a wall. Throughout the duration of the MBT attempt, athletes were required to have their scapula (i.e., shoulder blades) in contact with the wall, remain seated with knees flexed to 90° and have their feet in full contact with the floor. Participants were required to grip the medicine ball in both hands, bring the medicine ball to their chest and push the medicine ball away from their chest with both hands, throwing the medicine ball as far as possible. A measuring tape was fastened to the floor at the wall positioned directly below the athlete when sitting on the bench, with the distance measured in a direct line from the wall to the initial floor marking (indicating the landing of the ball, which was covered in chalk) to the nearest 1 cm. The experimenter positioned the measuring tape in line with the closest point of contact from the ball to the participant. The MBT assessment protocol utilized has been reported to be reliable in adolescents (CV = 3.72%, ICC 0.733) [14].

2.15. Counter-Movement Jump

The CMJ required participants to stand erect with both arms fully extended overhead; while in this position, the experimenter adjusted the height of the yardstick device (Swift; Lismore, Australia) to ensure that the first vane was at fingertips reach for each participant. In one fluid motion, athletes squatted to a depth of their choice while swinging their arms below their waist and jumped vertically as high as possible utilizing an arm swing. To obtain the vertical jump height, athletes were required to displace a vane on the yardstick device. Athletes completed three attempts, with 60 s of passive standing rest between attempts. For all attempts, the CMJ height was measured to the nearest 1 cm, with the best attempt recorded for analysis. The CMJ assessment protocol utilized has been reported to be reliable in adolescents (CV = 4.02%, and ICC = 0.874) [14].

2.16. Multi-Stage Fitness Test

Aerobic capacity was estimated in one attempt using the MSFT, following established procedures [18]. The MSFT involves repeated 20-m shuttle runs with progressive increases in speed dictated by audio cues. The MSFT was concluded when participants either voluntarily stopped or failed to cover the requisite distance as signalled by audio cues across two successive shuttles. Maximal oxygen uptake (VO2max [mL/kg/min]) was estimated from the last successful shuttle completed during the MSFT using a valid equation [18]. The MSFT assessment protocol utilized has been reported to be reliable in adolescents (CV = 3.04% and ICC = 0.840) [14].

3. Statistical Analysis

Normality and homogeneity of variance for each outcome variable were confirmed using the Shapiro–Wilk ($p > 0.05$) and Levene's tests ($p > 0.05$), respectively (Jamovi software; version 2.3.28; the Jamovi project). As a result, parametric statistics were utilized for each statistical analysis, and data are reported as the mean ± standard deviation (SD). Prior to data collection, it was determined that each statistical analysis would be conducted to test for repeatability, with *a priori* alpha level of <0.05 needing to be met for a finding to be deemed significant; meaningfulness was determined utilizing an appropriate effect size statistic. As the significance and meaningfulness of a finding may provide conflicting results, it was determined prior to data collection that all statistical decisions (e.g., whether to break down a model such as a within-group ANOVA with separate dependent *t*-tests) were made based on significance. The collected data are presented in two phases to provide a comprehensive analysis of the performance adaptations that occurred in response to the 1.5 year-long resistance training protocol.

During phase one, separate within-group ANOVAs (6 timepoints) were performed for each dependent variable to analyse the effects of the 1.5-year resistance training protocol on each dependent variable over time. The effect size of each within-group ANOVA was quantified using the partial eta-squared (n^2p), with the effect size magnitudes interpreted as follows: *small* = 0.01, *moderate* = 0.06 or *large* = 0.14 [19]. If a significant effect was found to occur for a within-group ANOVA, follow-up dependent *t*-tests were conducted. To reduce the probability of making a type I error, the follow-up dependent tests compared each timepoint to the successive timepoint (i.e., timepoint 1 was compared to timepoint 2, timepoint 2 was compared to timepoint 3, etc.). A standardised Hedge's *g* (g) was utilized as the effect size to quantify whether meaningful differences occurred between timepoints due to the small sample size [20] and was reported with 95% confidence intervals (95% CI). The magnitude of the effect size of Hedges' *g* was determined as *trivial*: <0.20, *small*: 0.20–0.49, *medium*: 0.50–0.79 or *large*: ≥0.80; however, if the 95% CI overlapped with 0, the magnitude of the effect was defined as *trivial* regardless of the effect size. The Jamovi software (version 2.3.28; the Jamovi project) was used to analyse the within-group ANOVAs, n^2p and subsequent dependent *t*-tests. The standardised Hedge's *g* and the respective 95% CIs were quantified manually using Microsoft Excel (version 15, Microsoft Corp; Redmond, WA, USA) as follows.

Step 1: Quantify Standardised Cohen's d [20].

Cohen's *d* = (Timepoint A Mean–Timepoint B Mean)/Pooled Standard Deviation.

We utilized (Post-Test Timepoint–Pre-Test Timepoint)/Pooled Standard Deviation.

Step 2: Quantify Standardised Hedges' *g* [20].

Hedges' *g* = *d**(1-(3/(4*(Number of Pairs-1)-1))),

where d = Cohen's d.

Step 3: Quantify 95% Confidence Interval for Standardised Hedges' *g*.

95% CI for Hedges' *g* = $g \pm (t_{\alpha/2} * SE_g)$,

where *g* = the effect size of the standardised Hedges' *g*;

$t_{\alpha/2}$ = the critical value from a dependent-samples t-distribution table [21]*;

SE_g = the standard error of Hedges' *g* quantified as

SE_g = √((1/Number of Pairs) + (g^2/(2*Number of Pairs)))).

Note: The t-critical value is predicated on the number of paired samples and was adjusted to account for missing data when applicable. * Where n = 11, df = n − 1 and t-critical = $t_{2.201}$; where n = 10, df = n − 1 and t-critical = $t_{2.228}$ [21].

During phase two, we converted the raw values utilized in phase one of the study into change values to quantify potential differences in relative change that occurred in the first year of training compared to the second year of training. Differences in relative change were quantified as subsequent timepoint-previous timepoint. As a result, we have two timepoints for year 1 of training and two timepoints for year 2 of training. Timepoint 1 for each year of training was quantified as: end of pre-season-start of pre-season. Timepoint 2 for each year was quantified as end of season-end of pre-season. After quantifying the differences in relative change for each year and timepoint, separate dependent *t*-tests were used to detect potential repeatable differences that occurred in the relative change for each outcome variable in participants during their first year of training compared to their second year of training (Jamovi software, version 2.3.28; the Jamovi project). The standardised Hedges' *g* (*g*) with 95% CIs was utilized as the effect size measure to quantify potential differences between timepoints (i.e., end of pre-season–start of pre-season year 1–end of pre-season–start of pre-season year 2)/pooled standard deviation)). The standardised Hedges' *g* and the 95% CIs were quantified manually using Microsoft Excel (Microsoft Excel, version 15, Microsoft Corp; Redmond, WA, USA).

4. Results

4.1. Phase One: Athlete Progression over the First 1.5 Years of Resistance Training

Results from phase one of the study are presented in Table 2. The results from the within-group ANOVA revealed a significant, *large* change in body mass over time ($p < 0.001$, $n^2p = 0.794$). Follow-up dependent *t*-tests revealed a significant, *large* increase in body mass from the start of pre-season to the end of pre-season during the first year of training ($p = 0.008$, $g = 0.91$, 95% CI = 0.11 to 1.71); a significant, *medium* increase from the end of pre-season and end of season in the first year of training ($p = 0.019$, $g = 0.77$, 95% CI = 0.01 to 0.54); and a significant, *large* increase from the end of season in the first year of training to the start of pre-season in the second year of training ($p < 0.001$, $g = 2.37$, 95% CI = 1.03 to 3.71).

Results from the within-group ANOVA revealed a significant, *large* change in the 1RM bench press over time ($p < 0.001$, $n^2p = 0.806$). Follow-up dependent *t*-tests revealed a significant, *large* increase in the 1RM bench press from the start of pre-season to the end of pre-season during the first year of training ($p < 0.001$, $g = 1.72$, 95% CI = 0.65 to 2.80) and second year of training ($p < 0.001$, $g = 1.85$, 95% CI = 0.72 to 2.97).

Results from the within-group ANOVA revealed a significant, *large* change in the 1RM back squat over time ($p < 0.001$, $n^2p = 0.670$). Follow-up dependent *t*-tests revealed a significant, *large* increase in the 1RM squat from the start of pre-season to the end of pre-season during the first year of training ($p < 0.001$, $g = 1.92$, 95% CI = 0.77 to 3.08) and second year of training ($p < 0.001$, $g = 1.38$, 95% CI = 0.43 to 2.33).

Results from the within-group ANOVA revealed a significant, *large* change in the MBT over time ($p = <0.001$, $n^2p = 0.350$). Follow-up dependent *t*-tests revealed a significant, *large* increase in MBT from the start of pre-season to the end of pre-season during the first year of training ($p = 0.007$, $g = 0.94$, 95% CI = 0.14 to 1.77) and a significant, *trivial* increase in the second year of training ($p = 0.026$, $g = 0.73$, 95% CI = −0.03 to 1.48).

Results from the within-group ANOVA revealed a non-significant, *moderate* change in the CMJ over time ($p < 0.279$, $n^2p = 0.115$). Results from the within-group ANOVA revealed a non-significant, *moderate* change in the MSFT over time ($p = 0.825$, $n^2p = 0.173$).

Table 2. Means and standard deviations of changes in physical qualities that occurred across the 1.5 year resistance training program.

Test	N	Pre-Season	End Pre-Season	End Season	Pre-Season	End Pre-Season	End Season	Sig (ANOVA)	Partial ETA-Squared (n^2p)
Body mass (kg)	11	75.6 ± 8.7	77.8 ± 7.7	79.1 ± 7.7	83.0 ± 7.9	83.6 ± 6.8	84.4 ± 6.9	<0.001 †	0.794 (*Large*)
		* $p = 0.008$, (g = 0.91, 95% CI = 0.11 to 1.71)‡	* $p = 0.019$, (g = 0.77, 95% CI = 0.01 to 0.54) ‡	* $p < 0.001$, (g = 2.37, 95% CI = 1.03 to 3.71)‡					
Bench press (kg)	11	81.8 ± 11.9	98.6 ± 11.2	97.7 ± 10.1	98.2 ± 9.0	108.2 ± 9.3	106.0 ± 9.9	<0.001 †	0.806 (*Large*)
		* $p < 0.001$, (g = 1.72, 95% CI = 0.65 to 2.80)‡			* $p < 0.001$, (g = 1.85, 95% CI = 0.72 to 2.97)‡				
Back squat (kg)	11	104.1 ± 16.9	123.2 ± 15.4	122.3 ± 13.3	120.5 ± 11.3	128.2 ± 13.3	129.5 ± 10.8	<0.001 †	0.670 (*Large*)
		* $p < 0.001$, (g = 1.92, 95% CI = 0.77 to 3.08)‡			* $p = <0.001$, (g = 1.38, 95% CI = 0.43 to 2.33)‡				
MBT (m)	11	6.7 ± 0.8	7.2 ± 0.8	6.7 ± 0.7	6.7 ± 0.7	7.3 ± 0.8	7.2 ± 0.8	<0.001 †	0.350 (*Large*)
		* $p = 0.007$, (g = 0.94, 95% CI = 0.14 to 1.77)‡			* $p = 0.026$, (g = 0.73, 95% CI = -0.03 to 1.48)‡				
CMJ (cm)	11	59.5 ± 6.6	60.6 ± 2.9	60.5 ± 5.3	60.0 ± 2.9	61.9 ± 3.6	61.0 ± 3.5	0.279	0.115 (*Moderate*)
MSFT (mL/kg/min)	11	45.0 ± 3.7	46.5 ± 4.4	46.2 ± 5.3	45.0 ± 3.4	48.1 ± 3.5	47.6 ± 3.1	0.825	0.173 (*Large*)

Notes: † denotes a significant effect for the within-group ANOVA ($p < 0.05$). * denotes a significant difference between timepoints determined by separate dependent *t*-tests ($p < 0.05$). ‡ denotes a meaningful difference between timepoints (effect size magnitude ≥ small).

4.2. Phase Two: Comparison of the Relative Change That Occurs During the First and Second Year of Resistance Training

A comparison of the relative change that occurred in each outcome variable across the pre-season and in-season phases of training during the first and second year of resistance training is presented in Figure 2. A non-significant, *trivial* effect was revealed for body mass at timepoint 1 (p = 0.088, g = −0.53, 95% CI = −1.24 to 0.19) and timepoint 2 (p = 0.314, g = −0.30, 95% CI = −0.97 to 0.38). A significant, *large* difference was revealed for the 1RM bench press at timepoint 1 as participants experienced a larger increase in strength during their first year of resistance training (p = 0.010, g = −0.88, 95% CI = −1.67 to −0.09), while a non-significant, *trivial* difference was revealed between years of training at timepoint 2 (p = 0.64, g = −0.13, 95% CI = −0.84 to 0.58). A significant, *large* difference was revealed for the 1RM back squat at timepoint 1 as individuals experienced a larger increase in strength during their first year of resistance training (p = 0.004, g = −1.05, 95% CI = −1.89 to −0.21), while a non-significant, *trivial* difference was revealed between years of training at timepoint 2 (p = 0.461, g = 0.21, 95% CI =−0.46 to 0.89). A non-significant, *trivial* effect was found for the MBT at timepoint 1 (p = 0.88, g = 0.04, 95% CI = −0.62 to 0.71) and timepoint 2 (p = 0.12, g = 0.47, 95% CI = −0.23 to 1.18). A non-significant, *trivial* effect was found for the CMJ at timepoint 1 (p = 0.66, g = 0.13, 95% CI = −0.54 to 0.79) and timepoint 2 (p = 0.57, g = −0.17, 95% CI = −0.83 to 0.50). A non-significant, *trivial* effect was found for the MSFT at timepoint 1 (p = 0.71, g = −0.11, 95% CI = −0.77 to 0.56) and timepoint 2 (p = 0.76, g = −0.09, 95% CI = −0.75 to 0.58).

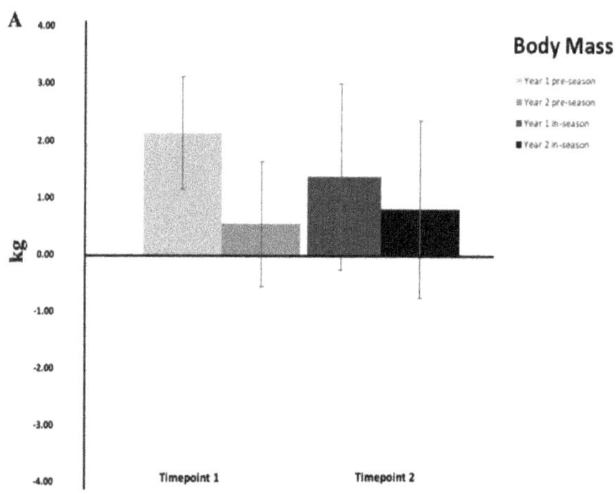

Figure 2. *Cont.*

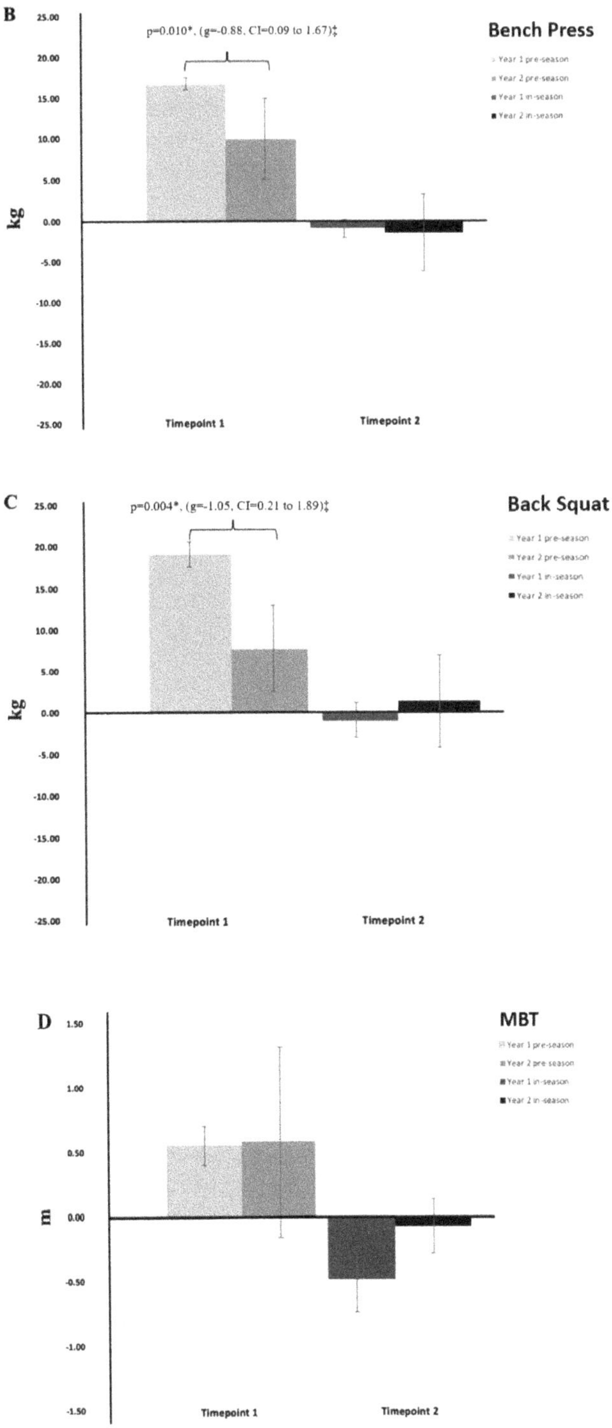

Figure 2. *Cont.*

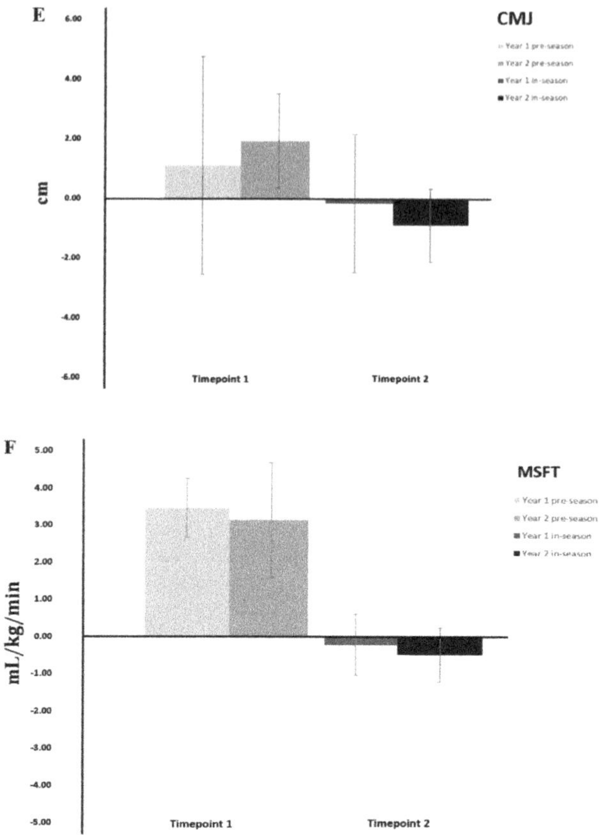

Figure 2. Differences in relative change that occurred during timepoint 1 (change from start of pre-season to start of in-season) and timepoint 2 (change from start of in-season to end of season) during the first and second year of resistance training. Notes: (**A**) Body mass (kg); (**B**) 1RM bench press (kg); (**C**) 1RM back squat (kg); (**D**) medicine ball throw (m); (**E**) counter-movement jump (cm); (**F**) multi-stage fitness test (mL/kg/min). * denotes a significant difference between timepoints determined by separate dependent *t*-tests. ‡ denotes a meaningful difference between timepoints (effect size magnitude $\geq$ small).

5. Discussion

Nearly all studies examining the effects resistance training on physiological adaptations occur over training durations of $\leq$12 weeks [3–7] and are typically structured to assess adaptations that occur over a single phase or mesocycle of training. Consequently, there is a paucity of research examining adaptations that occur in response to resistance training over durations of >12 weeks, and even less research exists that examines adaptations that occur in response to resistance training over multiple phases or mesocycles of training. As a result, we quantified the effects of the first 1.5 years of a standardised, progressive, blocked, linear periodisation resistance training program in adolescents with no prior history of resistance training. We quantified the overall effects of the 1.5 year standardised, progressive, blocked, linear periodisation resistance training program on each outcome variable over time with the use of separate within-group one-way ANOVAs, and we quantified the differences in relative change that occurred in each outcome variable during the first year and second year of resistance training with separate dependent *t*-tests to directly assess the ceiling effect. We found significant, large increases to occur in body mass at each timepoint for the first

12 months of training (year 1 start of pre-season to year 2 start of pre-season). Significant, large increases in bench press, squat and MBT occurred from the start of pre-season to end of pre-season during the first and second years of resistance training, with relative change during the first year of training being significantly larger than in the second year of training for bench press and back squat, but with a non-significant, trivial difference occurring for the relative change in the CMJ.

5.1. Body Mass

Participants experienced a significant, *large* increase in body mass over the 1.5 year study (baseline: 75.6 ± 8.7 kg; end of study: 84.4 ± 6.9 kg). Participants experienced significant, large increases in body mass from the start of pre-season to the end of pre-season, from the end of pre-season to end of season and from the end of season to start of pre-season the following year, representing the first 12 months of training. At which point, body mass remained statistically unchanged from the start of pre-season in year 2 to the end of season in year 2, representing the final 6 months of training. The large increase in body mass during the first 12 months of training (start of pre-season year 1 to start of pre-season year 2) followed by the stabilization of body mass in the subsequent six months of training (start of pre-season year 2 to end of season year 2), despite participants following a standardised, progressive, blocked, linear periodisation resistance training program, suggests that skeletal muscle accumulation is a meaningful contributor to the increases in body mass and strength that occur upon the onset of resistance training. Our hypothesis is consistent with research demonstrating molecular pathways regulating skeletal muscle growth are activated during the first bout of resistance exercise [22–24]. Further, Defreitas et al. [25] reported a significant increase in skeletal muscle cross-sectional area of the midpoint of the thigh between the greater trochanter and lateral epicondyle to occur in previously untrained college-age males following two resistance training sessions, assessed with a peripheral quantitate computed tomographic (pQCT) imaging device. The authors [25] acknowledged muscular edema may have contributed to the initial finding of increased muscle cross-sectional area after two resistance training sessions but were confident muscle cross-sectional area significantly increased following three to four weeks of resistance training (~9–12 resistance training sessions), as the increase in muscle cross-sectional area after 3–4 weeks of resistance training corresponded with the first significant increase in isometric maximal voluntary contraction, which occurred in week 4. We also found the largest performance increases to occur in bench press and back squat during the start of pre-season to the end of pre-season in year one, which is strongly suggestive of the accretion of skeletal muscle mass and neural adaptations.

Our findings regarding changes in body mass are in agreement with the work of Waldron et al. [26], who reported body mass to significantly increase in adolescent rugby league athletes (age: 15–17 years) assessed at the pre-season across three seasons (year 1: 81.9 ± 9.1 kg; year 2: 86.1 ± 6.0 kg, year 3: 86.3 ± 9.4 kg). Till et al. [27] also reported younger (under 14 years of age) rugby league athletes to experience a greater percent change in body mass when assessed pre- and post-season (7.4 ± 4.3%), compared to older rugby league athletes (under 16 s: 5.2 ± 5.0%; under 18 s: 2.5 ± 4.7%; under 20 s: 1.2 ± 3.3%). While Till et al. [27] did not speculate as to why the diminished increases in body mass occurred with advancing age, their findings may have been the result of younger age groups being less trained and thus more responsive to resistance training stimuli. Furthermore, given the sample population was in the developmental phase of puberty, we recognise that, in part, some of the observed changes in body mass may be attributed to maturation.

5.2. Maximal Muscular Strength

Participants experienced a significant, *large* increase in muscular strength across our 1.5-year training study, as indicated by improvements in the 1RM bench press (baseline: 81.8 ± 11.9 kg; end of study: 106.0 ± 9.9 kg) and 1RM back squat (baseline: 104.1 ± 16.9 kg, end of study: 129.5 ± 10.8 kg). The largest improvements in the 1RM bench press and 1RM back squat occurred from the start of pre-season to the end of pre-season during the first and second year of resistance training, with the largest increases in strength occurring during the start of pre-season to end of pre-season in the first year of training. Moreover, neuromuscular efficiency likely increased [28], and individuals would have become more biomechanically efficient at performing lifts over time [29], with greater improvements likely to be experienced during the early phases of training/learning. The emphasis of the resistance training program from the start of pre-season to the end of pre-season was also structured to emphasise strength adaptations, and is consistent with reported findings of a previous systematic review and meta-analysis [30].

Maximal upper-body (i.e., bench press) and lower-body (i.e., back squat) strength was maintained during the season (i.e., end of pre-season to the end of season) during each year of training. We expected this result as the in-season phase of training was designed to maintain performance gains achieved during the pre-season phase of training, as the focus of training shifted to focus on on-field performance. Our finding of strength being maintained during the in-season phase of training in agreement with other research conducted in adolescent rugby league athletes [15,30].

Bench press and back squat 1RM remained unchanged from the end of season in year 1 to the start of pre-season in year 2. This could have been due to several factors. Firstly, at the start of the study participants were 16.4 ± 0.5 years of age. As a result, during the off-season, the loss of training gains could have been offset by the gains in strength incurred from maturation. Secondly, athletes were not instructed to perform resistance training during the off-season, but they were not precluded from strength training. Thus, some participants may have improved their strength by resistance training in the off-season, which could have offset potential decrements in strength experienced by participants who did not resistance train during the off-season. Thirdly, the start of pre-season testing occurred during week 16 of the season; as a result, all participants were exposed to seven weeks of resistance training prior to the strength testing in year 2. Testing occurred in this manner to ensure participants' safety, but it is possible participants regressed during the off-season and regained their lost strength during the initial preparation phase of training that occurred prior to the start of pre-season testing.

Results from our study clearly support evidence of the ceiling effect. Specifically, we found improvements in 1RM bench press and 1RM back squat strength to significantly and meaningfully slow from the first year to the second year of training, as assessed by the relative change from the start of pre-season to end of pre-season. Specifically, improvements in 1RM bench press strength during the second year of training were −0.88 (95% CI: −1.67 to −0.09) standard deviations below the improvements made during the first year of training. The effects were even more pronounced in 1RM back squat, as improvements made during the second year of training were −1.05 (95% CI: −1.89 to −0.21) standard deviations below the improvements made during the first year of training. Although research examining chronic adaptations is limited, Baker et al.[10] reported younger sub-elite (19.0 ± 0.6 years) male rugby league athletes to experience larger increases in strength, assessed via 1RM bench press, when compared to older elite (21.3 ± 1.4 years) male rugby league athletes. Furthermore, Appleby et al. [12] examined changes in strength among adult rugby union athletes (24.4 ± 3.4 years) across two years. The authors [12] reported 1RM bench press and back squat strength performances increased by 6.5% and 11.5%, respectively, following 2 years of training. Moreover, Appleby and colleagues [12] reported that the magnitude of improvements was negatively associated with initial strength data, meaning individuals who started the study with higher levels of strength experienced lower increases in strength over the course of the study. However, testing only occurred during the pre-season period, and the authors did not account for the seasonal fluctuations in training programs and changes in game-based demands, which influence test performance outcomes. Crucially, our study is the first to quantify the rate of diminishing returns in adolescent athletes over an extended 1.5-year resistance training program. To the best of our knowledge, previous studies have typically examined short timeframes (<1 year) [3–7], making our investigation a valuable contribution to the current understanding of long-term athletic development. Our study provides a practical framework that practitioners may apply to monitor and assess training responses in their own athletes. Measuring the rate of diminishing returns relative to an athlete's training status (e.g., training age) offers valuable insights into the effectiveness of a given program. As athletes become more trained, performance improvements naturally slow, and, by identifying this early, coaches can avoid unnecessarily increasing training volume in the pursuit of unrealistic improvements. By quantifying the rate of diminishing returns, our findings may better inform practitioners regarding program design and could have positive implications for long-term player development.

5.3. Maximal Muscular Power

Participants experienced a significant, *large* increase in upper-body muscular power across our 1.5 year training study, as indicated by improvements in the MBT (baseline: 6.7 ± 0.8 m; end of study: 7.2 ± 0.8 m). The increases in upper-body muscular power may be attributed to concomitant increases in upper-body muscular strength (i.e., 1RM bench press) given significant increases 1RM bench press and MBT each occurred from the start of pre-season to end of pre-season during the first and second year of training. The significant and meaningful improvements in upper-body muscular power and strength corresponded with increases in body mass during the first year of training. Accordingly, we posit a significant and meaningful increase in body mass was primarily composed of increases in lean body mass, given corresponding increases in muscle strength (i.e., upper and lower-body) and upper-body muscular power occurred at this time. Our findings corroborate the findings of Baker [11], who reported a 22% improvement in upper-body muscle power assessed via bench press throw to occur over a 10 year period of time in professional rugby league athletes (N = 6, age at start of study: 19.3 ± 1.6 years), with progression slowing over time.

In contrast, participants experienced a non-significant, *moderate* increase in CMJ performance (baseline: 59.5 ± 6.6 cm; end of season: 61.0 ± 3.5 cm) across our 1.5 year training study. A non-significant finding for lower-body muscular power is surprising, but body mass of the participants increased from 75.6 ± 8.7 kg at the start of the study to 84.4 ± 6.9 kg by the end of the study, meaning participants had to vertically displace significantly greater body mass during successive testing sessions, particularly when compared to the first testing session. CMJ is frequently used to assess lower-body power in research [13], but further consideration may be required when using the CMJ to assess lower-body power in participants with differing body masses or for studies in which the body mass of participants is expected to significantly and/or meaningfully change over time, as improvements in absolute lower-body power can be masked by increases in body weight when assessing lower-body power via the CMJ height. Accordingly, the CMJ is a suitable measure of relative lower-body power, but absolute lower-body power is a valuable measure for practitioners (particularly those who coach athletes in non-weight-dependent sports, such as rugby league) and researchers.

6. Limitations

When possible, we recommend the use of a larger sample size, as the predictability of statistical tests improve and reduced likelihood of making a type II error [31]. Specifically, p-values become lower and 95% CIs become tighter for the same test outcomes with a larger compared to a smaller sample size. However, longitudinal study designs present challenges, evident by the paucity of research examining training adaptations that occur in interventions of >12 weeks. Further, many studies of longer durations that have examined training adaptations do not report enough information about the training protocol for the study to be replicated. The periodisation and progression of our training program can be replicated in future practice and research, but the exact sessional program implemented (i.e., session exercise selection) cannot be replicated as the exercises performed for each session are not provided, which is a limitation of the present study. Moreover, we acknowledge load was prescribed at a percentage of the 1RM, and the explicit load (kg) was not prescribed or reported for each participant, precluding an examination of total load performed. Indeed, this would require participants to log a diary of exercises performed, loads and the completion of repetitions and sets for the entire duration of the study; we recommend future research consider these limitations in the study designs. In this regard, to build upon our findings, researchers should consider the use of training diaries to enable the comparison of total load prescribed versus total load lifted, which may help researchers to better understand the effects of load on physiological adaptations. Despite our best efforts, we recognise four participants in our study were concurrently enrolled in an external rugby league academy, which exposed them to additional on-field and off-field training over the 1.5 year training period. Participants were also instructed to refrain from lifting during the off-season, but some athletes were likely to have resistance trained during this period of time.

7. Conclusions

We quantified physiological adaptations that occurred in adolescents with no prior history of resistance training over their first 1.5 years of following a standardised, progressive, blocked, linear periodisation program designed for adolescent rugby league athlete development. We found the majority of adaptation in body mass to occur during the first 12 months of training. Moreover, increases in body mass corresponded with an increase in 1RM bench press, back squat and MBT; therefore, we posit the body mass adaptation was the result of the accretion of lean body mass, demonstrating the highly responsive nature of the body to adapt to novel training stimuli. Additionally, our findings demonstrate the degree at which returns diminish, given improvements in 1RM bench press and squat were −0.88 and −1.05 standard deviations lower from the start of pre-season to end of pre-season in the second year of training compared to the first year of training.

Generally, the current understanding of the physiological response to resistance training is based on results obtained from acute (≤12 weeks) training studies designed to mimic a single phase or mesocycle of training. However, very few studies report chronic adaptions that occur in response to standardised, progressive, blocked, linear periodisation programs, despite evidence that physiological adaptation in response to training decreases over time. We found that untrained adolescents yielded positive physiological adaptations in response to a standardised, progressive, blocked, linear periodisation program across multiple seasons, with the rates of progression slowing over time. It is broadly acknowledged that rates of progression slow over time, and future research is needed to quantify the expected rate of progression to determine whether training programs yield results that are superior or inferior to the expected rates of improvement given the training status of participants in the study or members of the team. Moreover, researchers should examine how advanced training statuses influence the expression of pathways regulating skeletal muscle growth so that training programs to optimize human development can be based on science rather than intuition.

Key points

1. Diminished returns occur in adolescents (16 $\pm$ 0.5 years) following a standardised, progressive, blocked linear periodisation resistance training program within their first 1.5 years of training.
2. The majority of physiological adaptations in body mass (84%) and strength (1RM bench press: 68%, back squat: 65%) occurred during the first 12 months of training.
3. Improvements in strength adaptations were lower by -0.88 (95% CI = -1.67 to -0.09) and -1.05 (95% CI = -1.89 to -0.21) standard deviations for the 1RM bench press and back squat, respectively, from the start of pre-season to end of pre-season in the second year of training compared to the first year of training.

Author Contributions: Conceptualization, M.A.C. and V.J.D.; methodology, M.A.C. and V.J.D.; formal analysis, M.A.C. and V.J.D.; investigation, M.A.C. and V.J.D.; data curation, M.A.C.; writing—original draft preparation, M.A.C.; writing—review and editing, M.A.C. and V.J.D.; project administration, M.A.C. and V.J.D. All authors have read and agreed to the published version of the manuscript.

Funding: No funding.

Institutional Review Board Statement: Our research and authorship team included two males, one junior and one senior investigator from multiple disciplines and of different ethnicities; one was Western European and one was North American. The study population included a spectrum of ages, genders and demographics. In reviewing the current physical activity recommendations set by governing bodies and independent groups, we included the literature and discussed pertinent issues irrespective of the sample description.

Informed Consent Statement: Informed consent was obtained from all subjects involved in the study.

Data Availability Statement: Data supporting the findings for this study are available upon reasonable request from the corresponding author.

Conflicts of Interest: The authors report that there are no competing interests to declare.

References

1. Shurley, J.P.; Todd, J.S. "The strength of Nebraska": Boyd Epley, Husker Power, and the formation of the strength coaching profession. *J. Strength Cond. Res.* **2012**, *26*, 3177–3188. [CrossRef] [PubMed]
2. Faigenbaum, A.D.; Myer, G.D. Resistance training among young athletes: Safety, efficacy and injury prevention effects. *Br. J. Sports Med.* **2010**, *44*, 56–63. [CrossRef] [PubMed]
3. Lorez, D.; Morrison, S. Current concepts in periodization of strength and conditioning for the sports physical therapist. *Int. J. Sports Phys. Ther.* **2015**, *10*, 734–747.
4. Zachary, M.T. Impact of resistance training on sports performance and muscular adaptations. *Int. J. Sports Exerc. Med.* **2022**, *8*, 218. [CrossRef]
5. Gentil, P.; Fisher, J.; Steele, J. A review of the acute effects and long-term adaptations of single- and multi-joint exercises during. *Sports Med.* **2017**, *47*, 843–855. [CrossRef]
6. Behringer, M.; Vom Heede, A.; Matthews, M.; Mester, J. Effects of strength training on motor performance skills in children and adolescents: A meta-analysis. *Pediatr. Exerc. Sci.* **2011**, *23*, 186–206. [CrossRef]
7. Harries, S.K.; Lubans, D.R.; Callister, R. Resistance training to improve power and sports performance in adolescent athletes: A systematic review and meta-analysis. *J. Sci. Med. Sport* **2012**, *15*, 532–540. [CrossRef]
8. Latella, C.; Teo, W.P.; Spathis, J.; van den Hoek, D. Long-Term strength adaptation: A 15-year analysis of powerlifting athletes. *J. Strength Cond. Res.* **2020**, *34*, 2412–2418. [CrossRef]

9. Verkhoshansky, Y.; Siff, M. *Supertraining*, 6th ed.; Expanded Version; Verkhoshansky.com: Rome, Italy, 2009.
10. Baker, D.G.; Newton, R.U. Adaptations in upper-body maximal strength and power output resulting from long-term resistance training in experienced strength-power athletes. *J. Strength Cond. Res.* **2006**, *20*, 541–546.
11. Baker, D.G. 10-year changes in upper body strength and power in elite professional rugby league players--the effect of training age, stage, and content. *J. Strength Cond. Res.* **2013**, *27*, 285–292. [CrossRef]
12. Appleby, B.; Newton, R.U.; Cormie, P. Changes in strength over a 2-year period in professional rugby union players. *J. Strength Cond. Res.* **2012**, *26*, 2538–2546. [CrossRef] [PubMed]
13. Carron, M.A.; Scanlan, A.T.; Power, C.J.; Doering, T.M. What tests are used to assess the physical qualities of male, adolescent rugby league players? a systematic review of testing protocols and reported data across adolescent age groups. *Sports Med. Open* **2023**, *9*, 106. [CrossRef] [PubMed]
14. Carron, M.A.; Scanlan, A.T.; Doering, T.M. The retest reliability of common tests to assess physical qualities in adolescent rugby league players. *Pediatr. Exerc. Sci.* **2024**, *1*, 1–8. [CrossRef]
15. Carron, M.A.; Scanlan, A.T.; Doering, T.M. Quantifying the training loads and corresponding changes in physical qualities among adolescent, schoolboy rugby league players. *Sports* **2024**, *12*, 251. [CrossRef]
16. Gabbett, T.; Kelly, J.; Sheppard, J. Speed, change of direction speed, and reactive agility of rugby league players. *J. Strength Cond. Res.* **2008**, *22*, 174–181. [CrossRef]
17. Miller, T. *NSCA's Guide to Tests and Assessments*; Human Kinetics Publishing: Champaigne, IL, USA, 2012.
18. Ramsbottom, R.; Brewer, J.; Williams, C. A progressive shuttle run test to estimate maximal oxygen uptake. *Br. J. Sports Med.* **1988**, *22*, 141–144. [CrossRef]
19. Richardson, J.T.E. Eta squared and partial eta squared as measures of effect size in educational research. *Educ. Res. Rev.* **2011**, *6*, 135–147. [CrossRef]
20. Cohen, J. *Statistical Power Analysis for the Behavioral Sciences*, 2nd ed.; Routledge: Oxfordshire, UK, 1988.
21. Beyer, W.H. *Handbook of Tables for Probability and Statistics*, 2nd ed.; e-Book; CRC Press: Boca Raton, FL, USA, 2019.
22. McIntosh, M.C.; Sexton, C.L.; Godwin, J.S.; Ruple, B.A.; Michel, J.M.; Plotkin, D.L.; Ziegenfuss, T.N.; Lopez, H.L.; Smith, R.; Dwaraka, V.B.; et al. Different resistance exercise loading paradigms similarly affect skeletal muscle gene expression patterns of myostatin-related targets and mtorc1 signaling markers. *Cells* **2023**, *12*, 898. [CrossRef]
23. Roberts, M.D.; Dalbo, V.J.; Hassell, S.E.; Kerksick, C.M. The expression of androgen-regulated genes before and after a resistance exercise bout in younger and older men. *J. Strength Cond. Res.* **2009**, *23*, 1060–1067. [CrossRef]
24. Dalbo, V.J.; Roberts, M.D.; Sunderland, K.L.; Poole, C.N.; Stout, J.R.; Beck, T.W.; Bemben, M.; Kerksick, C.M. Acute loading and aging effects on myostatin pathway biomarkers in human skeletal muscle after three sequential bouts of resistance exercise. *J. Gerontol. A Biol. Sci. Med. Sci.* **2011**, *66*, 855–865. [CrossRef]
25. DeFreitas, J.M.; Beck, T.W.; Stock, M.S.; Dillon, M.A.; Kasishke, P.R., II. An examination of the time course of training-induced skeletal muscle hypertrophy. *Eur. J. Appl. Physiol.* **2011**, *111*, 2785–2790. [CrossRef] [PubMed]
26. Waldron, M.; Worsfold, P.; Twist, C.; Lamb, K. Changes in anthropometry and performance, and their interrelationships, across three seasons in elite youth rugby league players. *J. Strength Cond. Res.* **2014**, *28*, 3128–3136. [CrossRef] [PubMed]
27. Till, K.; Jones, B.; Emmonds, S.; Tester, E.; Fahey, J.; Cooke, C. Seasonal changes in anthropometric and physical characteristics within English academy rugby league players. *J. Strength Cond. Res.* **2014**, *28*, 2689–2696. [CrossRef]
28. Trezise, J.; Blazevich, A.J. Anatomical and neuromuscular determinants of strength change in previously untrained men following heavy strength training. *Front. Physiol.* **2019**, *10*, 1001. [CrossRef]
29. Maden-Wilkinson, T.M.; Balshaw, T.G.; Massey, G.J.; Folland, J.P. What makes long-term resistance-trained individuals so strong? A comparison of skeletal muscle morphology, architecture, and joint mechanics. *J. Appl. Physiol.* **2020**, *128*, 1000–1011. [CrossRef]
30. Redman, K. Seasonal changes in strength and power in elite rugby league: A systematic review and meta-analysis. *Br. J. Sports Med.* **2015**, *49*, 14–19. [CrossRef]
31. Shreffler, J.; Huecker, M.R. Type I and Type II errors and statistical power. In *StatPearls (Internet)*; StatPearls Publishing: Treasure Island, FL, USA, 2023.

sports

MDPI

Article

Acute Effects of Beetroot Supplementation on Resistance Exercise Performance in Physically Active Men

Maitê Yorioka Rodrigues [1,*], Monica Yuri Takito [2], Gabriel Albanese Kafouri [1], Rebeca Soares Pires [1], Felipe Gasperini Mello [1], Reza Zare [3], Sthefano Ventura Hernandez [4], Katie M. Heinrich [5] and Emerson Franchini [2]

1 School of Physical Education and Sport, University of São Paulo, São Paulo 05508-030, Brazil; gabrielkafouri@usp.br (G.A.K.); felipe.gaspermello@gmail.com (F.G.M.)
2 Laboratory of Energetic Determinants of Sport Performance, School of Physical Education and Sport, University of São Paulo, São Paulo 05508-030, Brazil
3 SRH Campus Hamburg, Berlin University of Applied Sciences, 20095 Hamburg, Germany
4 School of Medicine and Health Sciences, Tecnológico de Monterrey Campus Guadalajara, Zapopan 45201, Mexico
5 Department of Kinesiology, College of Health and Human Sciences, Kansas State University, Manhattan, KS 66506, USA; kmhphd@ksu.edu
* Correspondence: maite.rodrigues@usp.br

Abstract

The objective of this study was to investigate the effect of nitrate (NO_3^-) supplementation on exercise performance in multiple sets of bench press (BP) and leg press (LP) at 80% of one-repetition maximum (1RM), to determine whether it would be beneficial towards the number of repetitions to failure (RTF). A total of 18 trained male subjects (25 ± 3 years old) completed two sessions of repeated number of maximum repetition (NMR) tests in BP and LP to assess RTF, power output, heart rate (HR), rating of perceived exertion (RPE) 2 h after NO_3^- or placebo intake. Comparisons between dependent variables were conducted using a two-factor analysis of variance (ANOVA) with repeated measures, examining the factors of condition and sets. The results for RTF showed only a main effect of set for BP and LP. No significant differences were found between conditions for total RTF. Our results showed that the NO_3^- supplementation had no significant effect on RTF, mean power, peak power, HR, and RPE when compared to placebo conditions. Results demonstrated that for physically active male individuals with experience in strength training, NO_3^- supplementation did not affect strength endurance performance.

Keywords: dietary nitrate; strength endurance; leg press; bench press

1. Introduction

Practitioners frequently use dietary supplements to enhance performance, particularly to increase total training volume by improving both repetition capacity and recovery between sets [1]. Over the past decades, researchers have investigated the ergogenic effects of dietary nitrate (NO_3^-)—commonly found in beetroot—across various exercise modalities, reporting positive outcomes in submaximal continuous efforts as well as high-intensity exercise protocols [2], including single- and multiple-bout strength exercises [3]. When training within specific intensity zones aimed at developing strength endurance, hypertrophy, or maximal strength, one widely recommended strategy involves the use of higher loads, typically around 80% of one-repetition maximum (1RM) [4–6]. However, despite this recommendation, there remains no scientific consensus regarding the most effective approach for optimizing these adaptations [7]. The expected mechanism underlying the effects of NO_3^- involves its role as a precursor of nitric oxide (NO). Through the enterosalivary pathway, NO_3^- is reduced to nitrite (NO_2^-) and subsequently to NO, increasing its bioavailability [8]. Elevated NO levels may influence oxygen consumption [9–12] and ATP expenditure [2,13], modulate excitation–contraction coupling [14,15], and promote vasodilation [16]. These physiological responses can enhance fatigue resistance during repeated muscle contractions [15,17], attenuate metabolic perturbations [2,18], and augment force production [19–21], thereby reducing the overall energetic cost of exercise. In recognition of this evidence, NO_3^- is listed by the International Olympic Committee as an effective dietary supplement [1]. Given these properties, nitrate supplementation may provide acute performance benefits in strength training contexts for both recreational practitioners and athletes. Empirical evidence supports these potential benefits. For example, studies by Coggan et al. [19,20] demonstrated that acute NO_3^- supplementation increased peak power during knee extension in untrained men and women ($p < 0.05$), with a significant correlation between peak power and plasma NO_2^- concentration ($r = 0.60$; $p < 0.01$) [19]. However, no improvements were observed in muscle function during 50 consecutive knee extensions [20]. Complementing these findings, a recent systematic review [22] reported that NO_3^- supplementation significantly increased the number of repetitions to failure (RTF) compared with placebo, both in bench press (BP) and back squat exercises. In addition, significant improvements were observed in peak power and mean power during back squat performance [22]. Despite these promising findings, the current evidence remains limited and inconclusive, particularly regarding high-intensity, multi-joint strength-endurance exercises [22]. This lack of consensus is reflected in the heterogeneity of results observed across acute supplementation protocols, which typically range from ~300 to 800 mg of NO_3^-. Results have been demonstrated for a spectrum of dosage administration, mostly for 400 mg and 800 mg [22]. Importantly, current data do not support a clear dose–response relationship for strength performance, suggesting that increasing nitrate intake does not necessarily enhance neuromuscular outcomes [23]. Even though the focus of the present study was the acute effects of NO_3^- supplementation, studies indicated that chronic doses have the potential to increase exercise tolerance and resistance training performance [24,25]. Moreover, inter-individual variability further complicates interpretation, as responsiveness to nitrate supplementation appears to be influenced by baseline NO status, oral microbiome composition, habitual dietary nitrate intake, and training background [3,26]. Additionally, positive effects are more frequently observed in isolated or single-joint exercise models, whereas findings in multi-joint, high-load exercises such as the BP and back squat are less consistent [14,19,20]. Thus, the primary aim of this study was to investigate the effect of NO_3^- supplementation on performance in multiple sets of BP and leg press (LP) at 80% of 1RM. The hypothesis was that NO_3^- supplementation is beneficial in maintaining performance and increasing the RTF throughout the sets, specifically, in the last sets of the strength exercises.

2. Materials and Methods

A total of 19 males (mean ± SD: 86 ± 17 kg; 179 ± 7 cm; 25 ± 3 years old) with experience in strength training (5 ± 2 years) were recruited via posters, social media, and institutional university email. All tests were performed after the consent form was explained and signed. Participants were eligible for inclusion if they met the following criteria: (a) males aged between 18 and 35 years old; (b) a minimum of 6 months of strength training experience; (c) free from neuromuscular problems. Participants were excluded if they were unable to execute the tests in the allotted time or made use of illegal performance-enhancement drugs (e.g., anabolic steroids).

https://doi.org/10.3390/sports14030094

The sample size was calculated using four factors: (a) number of maximum repetitions at 80% of 1RM, 9 ± 2 repetitions for BP and 13 ± 4 repetitions for LP [27]; (b) in a study, Panissa et al. [28], observed a drop of 30%, 40% and 40% of repetitions for the second, third and fourth sets of a half squat exercise in relation to the first set, with half squat exercise, and, therefore, the total number of repetitions was 56 ± for LP and 34 ± for BP; (c) the mean difference between NO_3^- supplementation and placebo reported in the last set (mean difference 3.1 ± 4.8 repetitions) in a study by Williams et al. [29], with 3 sets at 70% of 1RM; and (d) the total number of repetitions in each exercise was considered the dependent variable, with 80% power and alpha $p < 0.05$. This calculation indicated the necessity of 17 participants. Even though 19 participants were recruited, only 18 remained until the last tests (one participant dropped out for personal reasons unrelated to the study) (Figure 1).

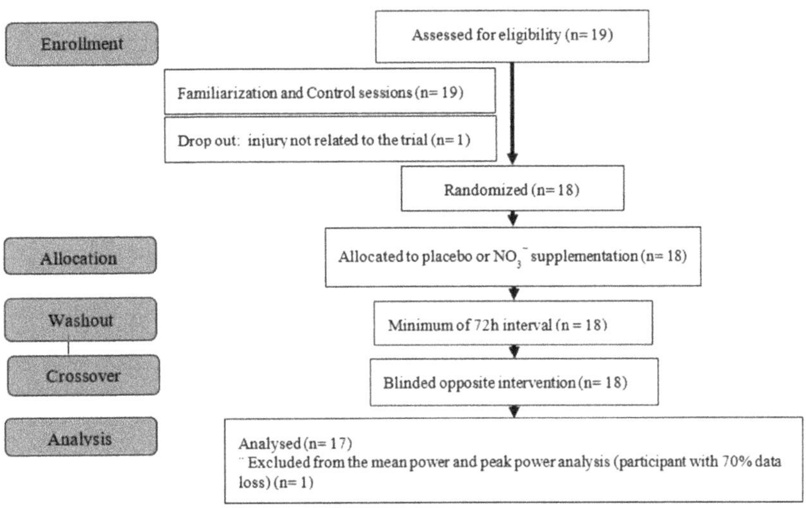

Figure 1. CONSORT flow chart.

The present study was conducted as a double-blind, crossover, randomized, placebo-controlled trial. The participants first completed a familiarization session, which consisted of a 1RM test in BP and LP, followed by repeated maximum repetition tests (NMR) for both exercises (Figure 2). All participants and assessors were blinded throughout data collection and processing. In a subsequent session, designated as a control session, on a different day, participants underwent the same procedures as the familiarization. After randomization, participants were invited to engage in two additional sessions, one preceded by the ingestion of NO_3^- (beetroot powder) and another preceded by the ingestion of a placebo. All sessions were conducted with a minimum of 72 h washout period between them. The subjective measurements of perceived exertion (Borg and OMNI), Perceived Recovery Status (PRS), and heart rate (HR) were assessed throughout all sessions.

https://doi.org/10.3390/sports14030094

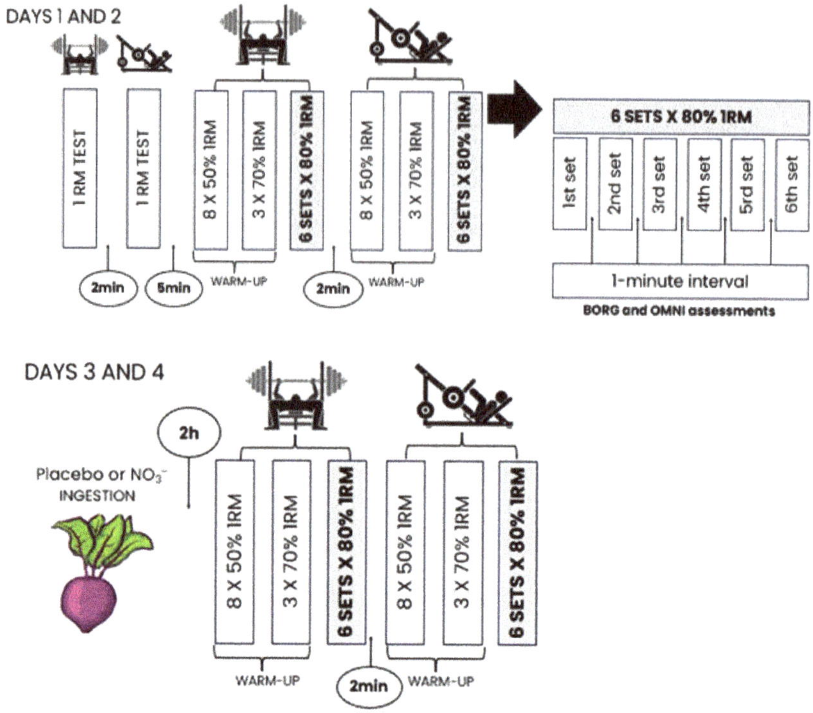

Figure 2. Experimental design.

The 1RM test began with a general warm-up, consisting of 5 min on an ergometric bicycle, followed by 2 sets of BP or LP. In the first set, participants performed 8 repetitions at 50% of 1RM (estimated). For the second set, they did 3 repetitions at 70% of 1RM (estimated), with a 2 min interval between sets. After the specific warm-up, participants rested for 2 min and then performed up to 5 tries, with 3 to 5 min of rest between tries to establish their 1RM value [28]. This value represented the greatest mass lifted in each exercise with proper execution, as indicated by De Souza, Tricoli, and Franchini [30].

For the NMR test, participants started with a general warm-up, identical to the description above for the 1RM test. They then executed 6 sets of each exercise at 80% of 1RM, with 1 min rest intervals between sets and 2 min rest between exercises. The 1 min break was adopted in accordance with Schoenfeld et al.'s [7] work challenging common practices for strength training and Salles et al.'s [31] work on rest intervals for strength endurance. While Schoenfeld et al. [7] discuss the lack of strong evidence for the typical recommendations within the repetition continuum, Salles et al. [31] emphasize how shorter rest intervals benefit localized muscular and aerobic endurance (resulting in greater oxygen consumption), and that "extremely short intervals may allow for greater maintenance of relative force levels" (pg. 775). Suffice to say that for the proper maintenance of repetitions, longer rest intervals would be advised; however, our objective was to elicit performance decrements so that the effects of nitrate supplementation would be evident. Execution velocity was self-selected, similar to normal training sessions and in other studies [28,30,32]. At the end of each set, subjective assessments were taken (Borg and OMNI). During all sets, velocity was monitored by a linear encoder (Vitruve encoder; Madrid, Spain), to enable calculation of mean power and peak power completed in each experimental session. To ensure participants were in similar conditions before each experimental session, a recovery scale

https://doi.org/10.3390/sports14030094

(PRS) was used. To secure proper technique and a full range of motion in the BP exercise, all repetitions were visually controlled, accounting for full elbow extension at the start of each repetition and the lowering of the bar to the chest. The repetition was completed when the elbows returned to full extension. For the LP exercise, participants were positioned on the machine with both feet on the platform, and after unlocking the machine, they lowered the platform until their knees reached a 90-degree angle. The repetition was completed when the knees returned to full extension. The position of the platform was measured using a tape beside the machine's track, and a plastic marker was placed to indicate the 90-degree angle, ensuring proper form for each repetition.

The NO_3^- supplementation followed procedures by Williams et al. [29]: 20 g of beetroot powder (Dobro BT 400 NIT, Dobro, São Paulo, Brazil) mixed with 100 mL of tea (Orange and strawberry caffeine-free iced tea, Leão, São Paulo, Brazil) or placebo (Orange and strawberry caffeine-free iced tea, Leão, São Paulo, Brazil) 2 h before each exercise session. The beetroot powder was standardized to provide approximately 400 mg of NO_3^- per dose (20 g of powder), while the placebo provided none to insignificant amounts of NO_3^-. The dosage was selected based on the prior literature, specifically the systematic review and meta-analysis by Tan et al. [22], in which 3 of 6 studies using this dosage reported significant effects on RTF for either BP or back squat. Participants were advised to consume the totality of the liquid and to plug their noses while doing so, and ingestion was administered through a black squeeze bottle. Dietary instructions were to consume the same foods and beverages on the day of the experimental sessions. Drinks were distributed to all participants by a third party, not involved in the testing, and the order of distribution was only revealed to the researchers after the completion of the data collection.

A list of food sources that can contain a considerable amount of NO_3^- was given to the participants, with instructions to avoid them 24 h prior to their arrival at the laboratory (beetroot, celery, arugula, lettuce, spinach, turnip, endive, parsley, cabbage, leek, etc.). Beverages containing caffeine, as well as fruits and vegetables rich in NO_3^-, were forbidden 72 h before tests due to their ergogenic potential. On the day of the tests, water was provided ad libitum during the rest periods between tests.

The HR was assessed using a sensor (Polar sensor H10; Polar Electro Brazil Comercio, Cajamar, Almería, Spain) attached to the subject's chest. Immediately after each set, HR information was registered in a data collection sheet.

The Borg scale of perceived exertion [33], the OMNI picture system of perceived exertion [34], and the PRS [35] were used to extract subjective assessments between sets (Borg and OMNI) and between sessions (PRS). The rate of perceived exertion (RPE) was recorded after each set during the 1 min interval of the NMR test. Participants were presented with two separate sheets displaying the Borg and OMNI scales and asked to report the number corresponding to their perceived exertion. The perceived recovery was assessed at the beginning of each session, starting from session one, in the same way as the perceived exertion. The three scales were previously explained to each subject, and all information was registered in a data collection sheet.

Data were reported as mean $\pm$ standard deviation. Comparisons between dependent variables were conducted using a two-factor analysis of variance (ANOVA) with repeated measures, examining the factors of condition and sets. Mauchly's test of sphericity was applied, and when assumptions were violated, Greenhouse–Geisser corrections were implemented to meet the requirements of repeated measures ANOVA. Post hoc analyses were conducted using the Bonferroni adjustment. The effect size was calculated using eta partial squared, and interpretation was made using Cohen's proposal [36]. The initial data analysis was performed by a professor who was blinded to the group allocation to minimize potential bias and ensure objectivity in the evaluation of the results.

https://doi.org/10.3390/sports14030094

Considering the data from the familiarization and from the control condition, the intraclass correlation coefficient (ICC), typical error (TE), coefficient of variation (CV), and smallest worthwhile change (SWC) were calculated to determine reliability, and the 95% confidence interval (95%CI) was also calculated. For the NMR test, reliability was conducted like the 1RM tests, but we also calculated the SWC for various effect sizes (0.2, 0.6, and 1.2) by multiplying these values by the between-subject standard deviation (SD), following Cohen's principle. The usefulness of each variable in both studies was then evaluated by comparing the SWC score to the typical error (TE) [37]. When the TE exceeded the SWC, the variable's evaluation was classified as "marginal". If the TE was comparable to the SWC, it was rated as "medium", whereas a TE smaller than the SWC resulted in a "good" evaluation for detecting small (0.2), medium (0.6), and large (1.2) differences. Additionally, the MDC (minimum detectable change) was calculated using the formula TE $\times$ 1.96 $\times$ $\sqrt{2}$ and interpreted as the smallest change in a variable that allows us to confidently identify a true change [38].

3. Results

3.1. Reliability Analysis

In the NMR test, in BP, the following values were found (mean value and 95%CI): ICC = 0.890 (0.697, 0.960); TE = 3.0 (1.6, 4.4) reps; and CV = 15.97 (8.37, 23.55) %. The SWC was 1.3 (0.7, 2.0), 4.0 (2.1, 5.9), and 7.9 (4.2, 11.7) reps for 0.2, 0.6, and 1.2, respectively, presenting a good probability for detecting medium changes. The MDC was 8.3 (4.3, 12.2) reps. For the LP, these values were: ICC = 0.686 (0.134, 0.886); TE = 6.5 (3.4, 9.6) reps; and CV = 21.3 (11.18, 31.43) %. The SWC was 1.9 (1.0, 2.7), 5.6 (2.9, 8.2), and 11.1 (5.8, 31.4) reps, for 0.2, 0.6, and 1.2, respectively, presenting a good probability for detecting close to medium changes. The MDC was 18.0 (9.4, 26.5) reps. For the 1RM test, in BP, the following values were found (mean value and 95%CI): ICC = 0.990 (0.972, 0.996); TE = 3.3 (1.7, 4.8) kg; and CV = 3.52 (1.85, 5.19)%. For the LP, these values were: ICC = 0.978 (0.940, 0.992); TE = 17.8 (9.4, 26.3) kg; and CV = 4.54 (2.38, 6.70)%.

At the end of the testing period, participants were asked to identify which session they believed they had consumed the supplement or the placebo, and 50.0% correctly identified what they had ingested, which is exactly the proportion expected in a guess based purely on chance (50%).

3.2. Data Loss

During the tests, ongoing data checks revealed an 8.1% data loss from the encoder (for total RTF in control, placebo, and supplemented conditions, with 90.2% of this problem concentrated in the leg press exercise, and a similar loss for each condition. This affected only the mean power and peak power variables, due to the encoder's incapability to detect movements under 0.04 m/s, especially in the last repetitions (1.4%) and due to errors in device manipulation (6.7%). One subject was removed from the mean power and peak power analysis because of a 71% loss in data from the leg press exercise (representing 36% of all data loss) (Figure 1). It is important to point out that a few participants in different sessions, for the last four sets, could not execute a single repetition (failure to complete one repetition in the set; in these cases, zero was inserted), and that was accounted for in the means and SDs for all variables. Repeating testing sessions in which greater data loss occurred would be advised to minimize data loss, as well as making use of two encoders simultaneously.

https://doi.org/10.3390/sports14030094

3.3. Heart Rate

For the HR responses (BP: control = 125 ± 12 bpm; placebo = 126 ± 15 bpm; NO_3^- = 124 ± 15 bpm; LP: control = 141 ± 15 bpm; placebo = 144 ± 18 bpm; and NO_3^- = 143 ± 16 bpm) to the BP and LP exercises, no statistically significant effects or interactions were observed ($p > 0.096$).

3.4. Borg's RPE and OMNI Responses

Borg's RPE ($F_{1.48,75.69} = 56.58$, $p < 0.001$, $\eta_p^2 = 0.526$, large) and OMNI ($F_{1.67,85.47} = 58.71$, $p < 0.001$, $\eta_p^2 = 0.535$, large) responses significantly differed across the sets (Figure 3) for BP and for LP (Borg's: $F_{1.46,74.59} = 54.36$, $p < 0.001$, $\eta_p^2 = 0.516$, large; OMNI: $F_{1.60,81.73} = 45.99$, $p < 0.001$, $\eta_p^2 = 0.474$, large).

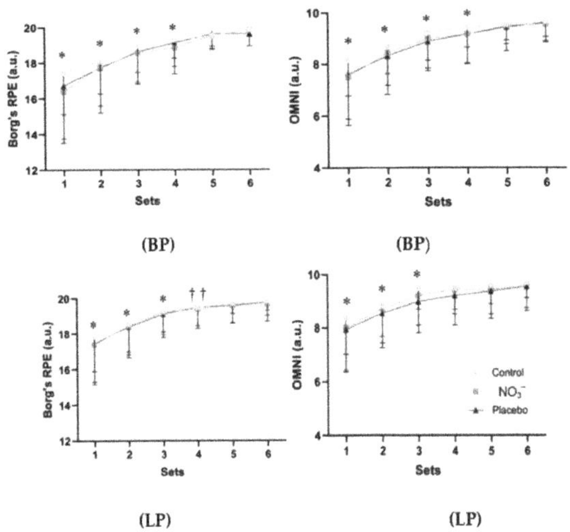

Figure 3. Ratings of perceived (RPE) exertion responses using Borg 6–20 and OMNI scales during six sets of bench press (BP) and leg press (LP) exercises at 80% of 1RM in the control, placebo, or nitrate supplementation (NO_3^-) conditions. Data are presented as mean ± SD. *, significantly lower than all subsequent sets ($p < 0.05$). ††, significantly lower than the last set ($p < 0.01$).

3.5. Power Output

Results indicated a significant main effect of set in the BP exercise (Figure 4), for peak power ($F_{3.35,160.69} = 37.53$, $p < 0.001$, $\eta_p^2 = 0.439$, large) and for mean power ($F_{3.20,153.62} = 39.98$, $p < 0.001$, $\eta_p^2 = 0.454$, large), as well as for the LP exercise's peak power ($F_{3.22,138.67} = 11.31$, $p < 0.001$, $\eta_p^2 = 0.208$, large) and mean power ($F_{3.25,139.64} = 13.33$, $p < 0.001$, $\eta_p^2 = 0.237$, large). Figure 5 shows the average mean power and peak power in the BP and LP exercises for each condition. No significant differences were found between conditions ($p > 0.05$), except for the mean power in LP, which showed significantly higher values for the placebo condition when compared to the control condition ($p < 0.02$).

https://doi.org/10.3390/sports14030094

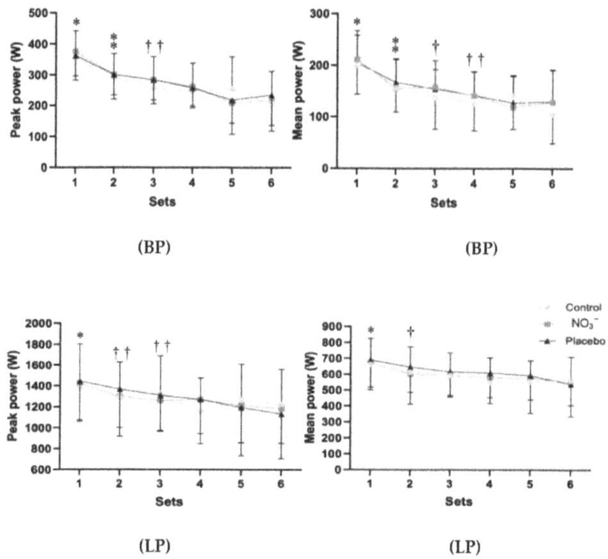

Figure 4. Peak and mean power in each of the six sets of bench press (BP) and leg press (LP) exercises at 80% of 1RM in the control, placebo, or nitrate supplementation (NO_3^-) conditions. Data are presented as mean ± SD. *, significantly higher than all subsequent sets ($p < 0.004$). **, significantly higher than the last 3 sets ($p < 0.003$). †, significantly higher than the last 2 sets ($p < 0.05$). ††, significantly higher than the last set ($p < 0.05$).

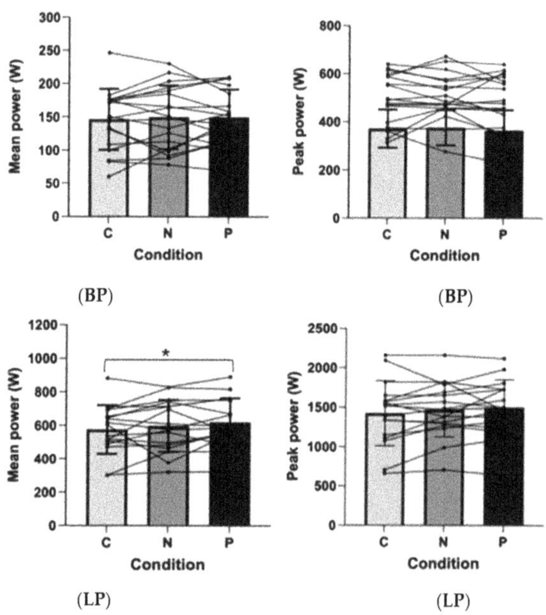

Figure 5. Mean power and peak power for the control (C), nitrate (N), and placebo (P) conditions in the bench press (BP) and leg press (LP) exercises at 80% of 1RM. Mean power for LP in the placebo condition was significantly higher than control ($p < 0.05$); For all others, no significant difference was found ($p > 0.05$). Data are presented as mean ± SD. *, significantly higher for the placebo condition compared with the control condition ($p < 0.05$).

https://doi.org/10.3390/sports14030094

3.6. Repetitions to Failure

The results for RTF (Figure 6) showed only a main effect of set for BP ($F_{2.32,118.34} = 287.68$, $p < 0.001$, $\eta_p^2 = 0.849$, large) and LP ($F_{2.32,115.25} = 86.95$, $p < 0.001$, $\eta_p^2 = 0.630$, large). Figure 7 shows the total number of RTF for the BP and LP exercises for each condition. No significant differences were found between conditions for total RTF ($p > 0.05$).

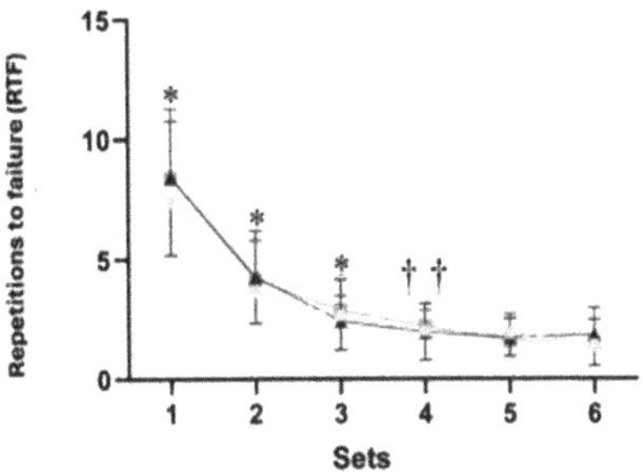

(BP)

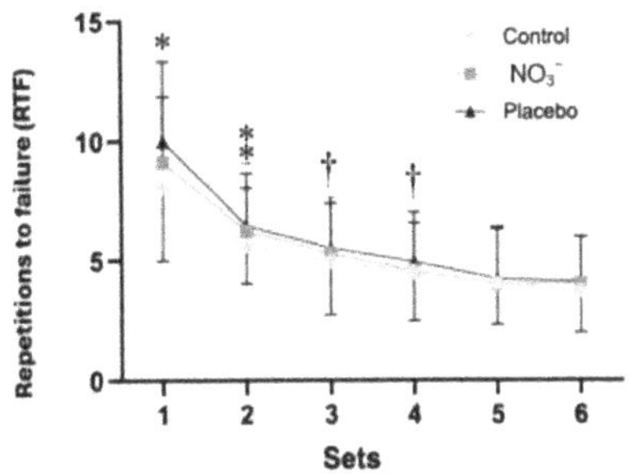

(LP)

Figure 6. Repetitions to failure (RTF) in each of the six sets of bench press (BP) and leg press (LP) exercises at 80% of 1RM in control, placebo, and nitrate supplementation (NO_3^-) conditions. Data are presented as mean ± SD. *, significantly higher than all subsequent sets ($p < 0.001$). $\overset{*}{*}$, significantly higher than the last 3 sets ($p < 0.001$). †, significantly higher than the last 2 sets ($p < 0.001$). ††, significantly higher than the last set ($p < 0.001$).

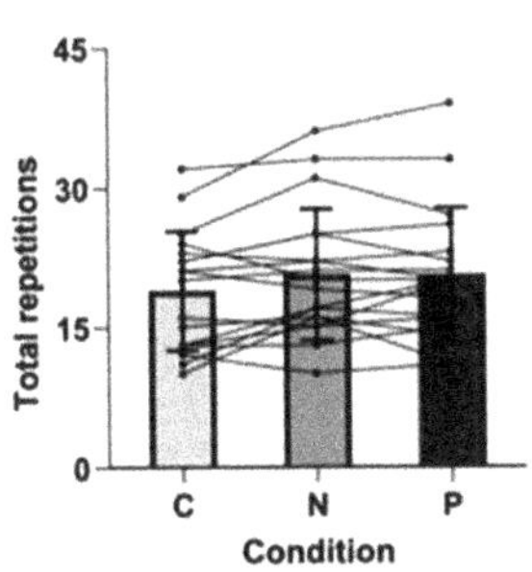

(BP)

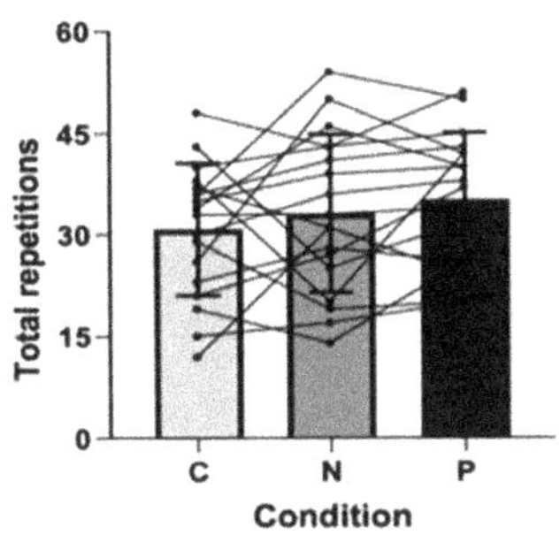

(LP)

Figure 7. Total repetitions to failure (RTF) for bench press (BP) and leg press (LP) in control (C), nitrate (N), and placebo (P) supplementation conditions at 80% of 1RM. No significant differences were found between conditions for total RTF ($p > 0.05$). Data are presented as mean ± SD.

https://doi.org/10.3390/sports14030094

4. Discussion

This study aimed to investigate whether the intake of 400 mg of NO_3^- supplementation could enhance strength-endurance performance during six sets of BP and LP at 80% of 1RM with one-minute rest intervals between sets. Contrary to our hypothesis, our results showed that supplementation did not enhance performance in terms of total RTF and power output. All variables presented a similar behavior between conditions throughout the sets, increasing (RPE) or decreasing (RTF, mean power, and peak power) from first to last set, apart from HR, suggesting that the cardiovascular demand was similar for each set, considering the one-minute interval rest period [39–41].

The NO_3^- supplementation effect on strength endurance relies on the premise that as energy storage gets lower, mostly from phosphocreatine (PCr) usage, the higher oxygen availability, provided by the nitric oxide production pathway, would facilitate PCr resynthesis throughout the six sets. Additionally, it could impact ATP turnover [2] and oxygen consumption efficiency [9–11], enhancing the possibility of increased RTF as compared to placebo. One possible explanation for the lack of significant effects in our study is that the one-minute rest interval may have been insufficient to fully resynthesize phosphocreatine (PCr), despite the potential for enhanced oxygen availability from the NO_3^- supplementation [42]. At higher intensities, muscle recruitment increases along with substrate depletion as a result of intense muscle contraction and accumulated fatigue, negatively impacting exercise performance. This impact could be attenuated, specifically related to subsequent bouts of maximal efforts, when preceded by rest intervals where PCr resynthesis allows recovery, given that PCr levels could be significantly reestablished between the first and the second minute of recovery [43]. Therefore, higher intensities can induce a greater disturbance in homeostasis, meaning the larger oxygen availability, induced by NO_3^- supplementation, could be redirected to reestablishing basal levels, possibly having no impact on between-sets recovery. The decrease in PCr concentration, significantly diminishing the muscle's capability to maintain performance, combined with increased RPE, could explain the behavior of the RTF, mean power, and peak power throughout the six sets, especially when comparing the first sets with the last ones.

The unique characteristics of our study, specifically the intensity (80% of 1RM) and volume (six sets), combined with the limited number of studies examining resistance exercise and NO_3^- supplementation, create challenges in comparing results across different research studies. Nevertheless, certain similarities allow for the formulation of inferences. The possible effect of NO on muscle force production was demonstrated by Bailey et al. [2] at high intensity work rates (30% maximum voluntary contraction) after 6 days of supplementation, by Whitfield et al. [21] and Haider and Folland [14] associated with low frequency stimulation after 7 days of supplementation, all on single joint exercises, involving chronic intervention and/or involuntary contraction. Focusing on power output, Tan et al. [17] observed no effect of 800 mg acute NO_3^- supplementation during a single set of BP and back squat exercises at 60% of 1RM. However, Tan et al. did report a significant difference in the RTF for the BP between placebo and supplemented conditions, a finding not observed in our study during the initial sets. The aforementioned study's results are consistent with those of two other studies, concerning the RTF in BP, which employed 70% [29] and 60% of 1RM [24], both with 2 min rest intervals. In contrast, Ranchal-Sanchez et al. [44] found no effects of 400 mg acute NO_3^- supplementation on RTF or power output in an incremental test for BP at 60%, 70%, and 80% of 1RM with three-minute rest intervals. In this study, the back squat performance showed increased RTF under the supplemented condition at 60% and 70% of 1RM. The discrepancies between our findings and those of these studies may be attributed to differences in exercise intensity (60% and 70% of 1RM), rest intervals (2–3 min), and the dosage of supplementation used (up to 800 mg of NO_3^-).

https://doi.org/10.3390/sports14030094

Our finding provides an important contribution to the current literature by helping to delineate the contexts in which NO_3^- supplementation is effective and where it may not be beneficial. Such evidence is critical for practitioners, coaches, and athletes when making evidence-based decisions about supplementation strategies. Based on this section's previous observation, we suggest that future research should consider longer rest intervals, particularly at higher intensities, to better assess the effects of NO_3^- supplementation, within this protocol. Additionally, it would be advised to test strength endurance aligned with high-intensity strength training protocols to better assess the supplementation effect in situations closer to practitioners' reality. Based on the current evidence, NO_3^- supplementation may be most relevant for strength-training contexts that prioritize fatigue resistance, power maintenance, or repeated submaximal efforts, particularly in single-joint or controlled exercise modalities [2,14,19,20]. Practitioners should be cautious when applying NO_3^- supplementation to high-intensity, multi-joint strength training performed at $\geq$80% of 1RM with short inter-set rest intervals, as performance benefits under these conditions are inconsistent. Additionally, increasing NO_3^- dosage does not appear to guarantee enhanced strength outcomes [23], highlighting the importance of individualized approaches that consider exercise selection, training intensity, recovery duration, and potential inter-individual responsiveness when integrating NO_3^- supplementation into training programs [45].

Although this was a randomized, double-blind, and placebo-controlled trial with blinding at multiple levels, from supplement administration to statistical analysis, some limitations were present. First, there was the impossibility of determining the optimal individual dose–response of the NO_3^- for each. Second, no control was implemented to prevent participants from self-pacing across the six sets, which may have led some participants to conserve effort to complete all sets. However, this behavior was not clearly detected during the investigation. Third, the control condition was not included in the randomization to establish some stability in the RTF throughout the six sets for the other two conditions. Fourth, given that the sample size of the present study did not allow the division of participants based on maximal strength performance, it is recommended that future studies address whether NO_3^- ingestion could affect individuals with different strength training statuses. Finally, exercise order was not randomized, which may have influenced performance outcomes.

5. Conclusions

Our results demonstrated that for physically active individuals with experience in strength training, 400 mg of NO_3^- supplementation did not significantly affect strength endurance after 2 h of intake in BP and LP exercises.

Author Contributions: Conceptualization, R.Z. and E.F.; methodology, M.Y.R., M.Y.T., R.Z. and E.F.; formal analysis, M.Y.R., M.Y.T. and E.F.; investigation, M.Y.R., M.Y.T., G.A.K. and R.S.P.; data curation, M.Y.R., M.Y.T. and E.F.; writing—original draft preparation, M.Y.R., G.A.K., R.S.P. and E.F.; writing—review and editing, M.Y.R., M.Y.T., F.G.M., K.M.H. and E.F.; visualization, M.Y.R.; supervision, E.F.; project administration, M.Y.R. and S.V.H. All authors have read and agreed to the published version of the manuscript.

Funding: This research received no external funding.

Institutional Review Board Statement: The research protocol received ethical approval from the Ethics Committee of the School of Physical Education, University of São Paulo (USP) (CAAE: 76911524.7.0000.5391; approval date: 12 March 2024). Ethical guidelines were diligently adhered to, with all procedures conducted in strict accordance with the principles stipulated in the Declaration of Helsinki.

https://doi.org/10.3390/sports14030094

Informed Consent Statement: Informed consent was obtained from all subjects involved in the study.

Data Availability Statement: The original data presented in the study are openly available in FigShare at https://doi.org/10.6084/m9.figshare.30411049.

Acknowledgments: The authors would like to thank the University of Cambridge ReachSci Society for their support and assistance (special thanks to Krisztián Iszak for providing the supplements). This project was an outcome of the Mini-PhD Programme 2024: Food Science & Nutrition.

Conflicts of Interest: The authors declare no conflicts of interest.

Abbreviations

The following abbreviations are used in this manuscript:

BP	Bench press
LP	Leg press
1RM	One-repetition maximum
RTFs	Repetitions to failure
NMR	Number of maximum repetitions
HR	Heart rate
RPE	Rate of perceived exertion
PRS	Perceived recovery status
ICC	Intraclass correlation coefficient
TE	Typical error
CV	Coefficient of variance
CI	Confidence interval
SWC	Smallest worthwhile change
MDC	Minimum detectable change
PCr	Phosphocreatine

References

1. Maughan, R.J.; Burke, L.M.; Dvorak, J.; Larson-Meyer, D.E.; Peeling, P.; Phillips, S.M.; Rawson, E.S.; Walsh, N.P.; Garthe, I.; Geyer, H.; et al. IOC Consensus Statement: Dietary Supplements and the High-Performance Athlete. *Br. J. Sports Med.* **2018**, *52*, 439–455. [CrossRef]
2. Bailey, S.J.; Fulford, J.; Vanhatalo, A.; Winyard, P.G.; Blackwell, J.R.; DiMenna, F.J.; Wilkerson, D.P.; Benjamin, N.; Jones, A.M. Dietary Nitrate Supplementation Enhances Muscle Contractile Efficiency During Knee-Extensor Exercise in Humans. *J. Appl. Physiol.* **2010**, *109*, 135–148. [CrossRef] [PubMed]
3. Jones, A.M.; Thompson, C.; Wylie, L.J.; Vanhatalo, A. Dietary Nitrate and Physical Performance. *Annu. Rev. Nutr.* **2018**, *38*, 303–328. [CrossRef] [PubMed]
4. Carvalho, L.; Junior, R.M.; Barreira, J.; Schoenfeld, B.J.; Orazem, J.; Barroso, R. Muscle Hypertrophy and Strength Gains after Resistance Training with Different Volume-Matched Loads: A Systematic Review and Meta-Analysis. *Appl. Physiol. Nutr. Metab.* **2022**, *47*, 357–368. [CrossRef] [PubMed]
5. Iversen, V.M.; Norum, M.; Schoenfeld, B.J.; Fimland, M.S. No Time to Lift? Designing Time-Efficient Training Programs for Strength and Hypertrophy: A Narrative Review. *Sports Med.* **2021**, *51*, 2079–2095. [CrossRef]
6. Grgic, J.; Schoenfeld, B.J.; Orazem, J.; Sabol, F. Effects of Resistance Training Performed to Repetition Failure or Non-Failure on Muscular Strength and Hypertrophy: A Systematic Review and Meta-Analysis. *J. Sport Health Sci.* **2022**, *11*, 202–211. [CrossRef]
7. Schoenfeld, B.J.; Grgic, J.; Van Every, D.W.; Plotkin, D.L. Loading Recommendations for Muscle Strength, Hypertrophy, and Local Endurance: A Re-Examination of the Repetition Continuum. *Sports* **2021**, *9*, 32. [CrossRef]
8. Lundberg, J.O.; Weitzberg, E.; Gladwin, M.T. The Nitrate-Nitrite-Nitric Oxide Pathway in Physiology and Therapeutics. *Nat. Rev. Drug Discov.* **2008**, *7*, 156–167. [CrossRef]
9. Bailey, S.J.; Winyard, P.; Vanhatalo, A.; Blackwell, J.R.; DiMenna, F.J.; Wilkerson, D.P.; Tarr, J.; Benjamin, N.; Jones, A.M. Dietary Nitrate Supplementation Reduces the O2 Cost of Low-Intensity Exercise and Enhances Tolerance to High-Intensity Exercise in Humans. *J. Appl. Physiol.* **2009**, *107*, 1144–1155. [CrossRef]

10. Vanhatalo, A.; Bailey, S.J.; Blackwell, J.R.; DiMenna, F.J.; Pavey, T.G.; Wilkerson, D.P.; Benjamin, N.; Winyard, P.G.; Jones, A.M. Acute and Chronic Effects of Dietary Nitrate Supplementation on Blood Pressure and the Physiological Responses to Moderate-Intensity and Incremental Exercise. *Am. J. Physiol.-Regul. Integr. Comp. Physiol.* **2010**, *299*, R1121–R1131. [CrossRef]
11. Whitfield, J.; Ludzki, A.; Heigenhauser, G.J.F.; Senden, J.M.G.; Verdijk, L.B.; van Loon, L.J.C.; Spriet, L.L.; Holloway, G.P. Beetroot Juice Supplementation Reduces Whole Body Oxygen Consumption but Does Not Improve Indices of Mitochondrial Efficiency in Human Skeletal Muscle. *J. Physiol.* **2016**, *594*, 421–435. [CrossRef]
12. Larsen, F.J.; Weitzberg, E.; Lundberg, J.O.; Ekblom, B. Effects of Dietary Nitrate on Oxygen Cost during Exercise. *Acta Physiol.* **2007**, *191*, 59–66. [CrossRef]
13. Fulford, J.; Winyard, P.G.; Vanhatalo, A.; Bailey, S.J.; Blackwell, J.R.; Jones, A.M. Influence of Dietary Nitrate Supplementation on Human Skeletal Muscle Metabolism and Force Production during Maximum Voluntary Contractions. *Pflügers Arch.-Eur. J. Physiol.* **2013**, *465*, 517–528. [CrossRef] [PubMed]
14. Haider, G.; Folland, J.P. Nitrate Supplementation Enhances the Contractile Properties of Human Skeletal Muscle. *Med. Sci. Sports Exerc.* **2014**, *46*, 2234. [CrossRef] [PubMed]
15. Stamler, J.S.; Meissner, G. Physiology of Nitric Oxide in Skeletal Muscle. *Physiol. Rev.* **2001**, *81*, 209–237. [CrossRef] [PubMed]
16. Bailey, S.J.; Vanhatalo, A.; Winyard, P.G.; Jones, A.M. The Nitrate-Nitrite-Nitric Oxide Pathway: Its Role in Human Exercise Physiology. *Eur. J. Sport Sci.* **2012**, *12*, 309–320. [CrossRef]
17. Tan, R.; Pennell, A.; Price, K.M.; Karl, S.T.; Seekamp-Hicks, N.G.; Paniagua, K.K.; Weiderman, G.D.; Powell, J.P.; Sharabidze, L.K.; Lincoln, I.G.; et al. Effects of Dietary Nitrate Supplementation on Performance and Muscle Oxygenation during Resistance Exercise in Men. *Nutrients* **2022**, *14*, 3703. [CrossRef]
18. Vanhatalo, A.; Fulford, J.; Bailey, S.J.; Blackwell, J.R.; Winyard, P.G.; Jones, A.M. Dietary Nitrate Reduces Muscle Metabolic Perturbation and Improves Exercise Tolerance in Hypoxia. *J. Physiol.* **2011**, *589*, 5517–5528. [CrossRef]
19. Coggan, A.R.; Broadstreet, S.R.; Mikhalkova, D.; Bole, I.; Leibowitz, J.L.; Kadkhodayan, A.; Park, S.; Thomas, D.P.; Thies, D.; Peterson, L.R. Dietary Nitrate-induced Increases in Human Muscle Power: High versus Low Responders. *Physiol. Rep.* **2018**, *6*, e13575. [CrossRef]
20. Coggan, A.R.; Leibowitz, J.L.; Kadkhodayan, A.; Thomas, D.T.; Ramamurthy, S.; Spearie, C.A.; Waller, S.; Farmer, M.; Peterson, L.R. Effect of Acute Dietary Nitrate Intake on Maximal Knee Extensor Speed and Power in Healthy Men and Women. *Nitric Oxide* **2015**, *48*, 16–21. [CrossRef]
21. Whitfield, J.; Gamu, D.; Heigenhauser, G.J.F.; Van Loon, L.J.C.; Spriet, L.L.; Tupling, A.R.; Holloway, G.P. Beetroot Juice Increases Human Muscle Force without Changing Ca2+-Handling Proteins. *Med. Sci. Sports Exerc.* **2017**, *49*, 2016. [CrossRef] [PubMed]
22. Tan, R.; Pennell, A.; Karl, S.T.; Cass, J.K.; Go, K.; Clifford, T.; Bailey, S.J.; Perkins Storm, C. Effects of Dietary Nitrate Supplementation on Back Squat and Bench Press Performance: A Systematic Review and Meta-Analysis. *Nutrients* **2023**, *15*, 2493. [CrossRef] [PubMed]
23. Tan, R.; Lincoln, I.G.; Paniagua, K.K.; Foster, J.M.; Wideen, L.E.; Gerardo, R.T.; Ornelas, N.J.; Tchaprazian, I.; Li, J.; Egiazarian, M.; et al. The Effect of Dietary Nitrate Supplementation on Resistance Exercise Performance: A Dose-Response Investigation. *Eur. J. Appl. Physiol.* **2025**, *125*, 2869–2883. [CrossRef] [PubMed]
24. Mosher, S.L.; Sparks, S.A.; Williams, E.L.; Bentley, D.J.; Mc Naughton, L.R. Ingestion of a Nitric Oxide Enhancing Supplement Improves Resistance Exercise Performance. *J. Strength Cond. Res.* **2016**, *30*, 3520–3524. [CrossRef]
25. Salem, A.; Ammar, A.; Kerkeni, M.; Ali Boujelbane, M.; Merve Uyar, A.; Moritz Köbel, L.; Selvaraj, S.; Zare, R.; Heinrich, K.M.; Jahrami, H.; et al. Acute Effects of Beetroot Juice vs. Creatine Supplementation on Maximal Strength, Autonomic Regulation, and Muscle Oxygenation during Incremental Resistance Exercise. *Biol. Sport* **2025**, *42*, 241–259. [CrossRef]
26. Senefeld, J.W.; Wiggins, C.C.; Regimbal, R.J.; Dominelli, P.B.; Baker, S.E.; Joyner, M.J. Ergogenic Effect of Nitrate Supplementation: A Systematic Review and Meta-Analysis. *Med. Sci. Sports Exerc.* **2020**, *52*, 2250–2261. [CrossRef]
27. Nuzzo, J.L.; Pinto, M.D.; Nosaka, K.; Steele, J. Maximal Number of Repetitions at Percentages of the One Repetition Maximum: A Meta-Regression and Moderator Analysis of Sex, Age, Training Status, and Exercise. *Sports Med.* **2024**, *54*, 303–321. [CrossRef]
28. Panissa, V.L.G.; Neto, R.A.; Julio, U.F.; Andreato, L.V.; e Silva, C.P.; Hardt, F.; Franchini, E. Maximum Number of Repetitions, Total Weight Lifted and Neuromuscular Fatigue in Individuals with Different Training Backgrounds. *Biol. Sport* **2013**, *30*, 131–136. [CrossRef]
29. Williams, T.D.; Martin, M.P.; Mintz, J.A.; Rogers, R.R.; Ballmann, C.G. Effect of Acute Beetroot Juice Supplementation on Bench Press Power, Velocity, and Repetition Volume. *J. Strength Cond. Res.* **2020**, *34*, 924–928. [CrossRef]
30. De Souza, E.O.; Tricoli, V.; Franchini, E.; Paulo, A.C.; Regazzini, M.; Ugrinowitsch, C. Acute Effect of Two Aerobic Exercise Modes on Maximum Strength and Strength Endurance. *J. Strength Cond. Res.* **2007**, *21*, 1286. [CrossRef]
31. Freitas de Salles, B.; Simao, R.; Miranda, F.; da Silva Novaes, J.; Lemos, A.; Willardson, J.M. Rest Interval between Sets in Strength Training. *Sports Med.* **2009**, *39*, 765–777. [CrossRef]

https://doi.org/10.3390/sports14030094

32. Panissa, V.L.G.; Tricoli, V.A.A.; Julio, U.F.; Ribeiro, N.; De Azevedo Neto, R.M.A.; Carmo, E.C.; Franchini, E. Acute Effect of High-Intensity Aerobic Exercise Performed on Treadmill and Cycle Ergometer on Strength Performance. *J. Strength Cond. Res.* **2015**, *29*, 1077–1082. [CrossRef] [PubMed]
33. Borg, G.A. Psychophysical Bases of Perceived Exertion. *Med. Sci. Sports Exerc.* **1982**, *14*, 377–381. [CrossRef] [PubMed]
34. Robertson, R.J.; Goss, F.L.; Rutkowski, J.; Lenz, B.; Dixon, C.; Timmer, J.; Frazee, K.; Dube, J.; Andreacci, J. Concurrent Validation of the OMNI Perceived Exertion Scale for Resistance Exercise. *Med. Sci. Sports Exerc.* **2003**, *35*, 333–341. [CrossRef] [PubMed]
35. Laurent, C.M.; Green, J.M.; Bishop, P.A.; Sjökvist, J.; Schumacker, R.E.; Richardson, M.T.; Curtner-Smith, M. A Practical Approach to Monitoring Recovery: Development of a Perceived Recovery Status Scale. *J. Strength Cond. Res.* **2011**, *25*, 620–628. [CrossRef]
36. Cohen, J. *Statistical Power Analysis for the Behavioral Sciences*, 2nd ed.; Lawrence Erlbaum Associates: Mahwah, NJ, USA, 1988; ISBN 978-0-8058-0283-2.
37. Hopkins, W.G.; Schabort, E.J.; Hawley, J.A. Reliability of Power in Physical Performance Tests. *Sports Med.* **2001**, *31*, 211–234. [CrossRef]
38. Hopkins, W.G. A New View of Statistics. Available online: https://www.sportsci.org/resource/stats/newview.html (accessed on 11 February 2024).
39. Yoon, C.; Kim, B.-M. Pilot Study on Exercise Performance Level and Physiological Response According to Rest Intervals between Sets during 65% 1RM Bench Press Exercise. *Appl. Sci.* **2023**, *13*, 7850. [CrossRef]
40. McCartney, N. Acute Responses to Resistance Training and Safety. *Med. Sci. Sports Exerc.* **1999**, *31*, 31–37. [CrossRef]
41. Apkarian, M.R. Acute Heart Rate Responses to Resistance Exercise at Different Cadences. *Int. J. Sports Exerc. Med.* **2019**, *5*, 143. [CrossRef]
42. Gonzalez, A.M.; Townsend, J.R.; Pinzone, A.G.; Hoffman, J.R. Supplementation with Nitric Oxide Precursors for Strength Performance: A Review of the Current Literature. *Nutrients* **2023**, *15*, 660. [CrossRef]
43. McMahon, S.; Jenkins, D. Factors Affecting the Rate of Phosphocreatine Resynthesis Following Intense Exercise. *Sports Med.* **2002**, *32*, 761–784. [CrossRef]
44. Ranchal-Sanchez, A.; Diaz-Bernier, V.M.; De La Florida-Villagran, C.A.; Llorente-Cantarero, F.J.; Campos-Perez, J.; Jurado-Castro, J.M. Acute Effects of Beetroot Juice Supplements on Resistance Training: A Randomized Double-Blind Crossover. *Nutrients* **2020**, *12*, 1912. [CrossRef]
45. Silva, K.V.C.; Costa, D.B.; Gomes, A.C.; Saunders, B.; Mota, J.F. Factors that Moderate the Effect of Nitrate Ingestion on Exercise Performance in Adults: A Systematic Review with Meta-Analyses and Meta-Regressions. *Adv. Nut.* **2022**, *13*, 1866–1881. [CrossRef]

https://doi.org/10.3390/sports14030094

sports

MDPI

Article

Mindfulness and Emotional Intelligence as Predictors of Psychological Well-Being in Athletes with Disabilities

Diana Reklaitiene [1] and Jolita Vveinhardt [2,*]

1 Department of Coaching Science, Lithuanian Sports University, 44221 Kaunas, Lithuania; diana.reklaitiene@lsu.lt
2 Institute of Sport Science and Innovations, Lithuanian Sports University, 44221 Kaunas, Lithuania
* Correspondence: jolita.vveinhardt@lsu.lt

Abstract

Although athletes who have disabilities face unique challenges, little is known about the interaction between mindfulness and emotional intelligence in the context of their psychological self-feeling. This study is among the first to systematically examine how mindfulness and emotional intelligence are related to stress, anxiety and depression in this population and to reveal the pathways through which the mediating effect of emotional intelligence manifests itself. A total of 95 athletes who have various types of disabilities were surveyed. The research instrument consisted of several scales: Depression, Anxiety, and Stress Scale (DASS-21), the Mindfulness Inventory for Sport (MIS), and the Emotional Intelligence Scale for Use in Sport (EIS). The data were analysed by employing descriptive statistical methods, performing correlation analysis, creating regression models, and through mediation analysis. Several significant trends were identified: professional athletes demonstrated higher mindfulness than amateurs, and higher education was associated with lower mindfulness and emotional intelligence. Mindfulness predicted better emotional competencies ($B = 0.511$, $p < 0.001$), which were related to lower levels of stress, anxiety, and depression ($B = -0.310$, $p = 0.001$), confirming a partial mediating effect ($B = -0.158$, 95% PI [-0.273; -0.065]). These findings add to the existing knowledge, demonstrating that in the context of sport for people with disabilities, mindfulness can improve mental health not only directly but also indirectly—through emotional intelligence. This study lays the foundation for individually tailored psychological interventions that would correspond to the specific needs of athletes who have disabilities.

Keywords: sport for people with disabilities; mindfulness; emotional intelligence; psychological self-feeling; psychological well-being

1. Introduction

Although the media and society are gradually paying attention to sports for people with disabilities, athletes themselves are usually viewed through the medical prism of health status [1]. Significantly less attention is paid to psychosocial aspects and individual emotional experiences, which, as Silva and Howe (2022) [2] point out, have a strong impact on the athlete's self-feeling and engagement in the social context. These aspects are particularly important, considering that physical disability is accompanied by pain, fatigue, and an increased risk of infectious diseases [3], reduced self-esteem [4], anxiety, and depressiveness [5,6].

 https://doi.org/10.3390/sports13110389

Symptoms of stress, anxiety, and depression, understood herein as indicators of psychological self-feeling, are not only widespread among athletes with disabilities but also related to specific physical and lifestyle factors. For example, Bentzen et al. (2025) [7] found that approximately one in two members of the Swedish Paralympic team had experienced anxiety and depression over a one-year period, particularly during periods when they were suffering from injuries, illnesses, or sleep disorders. Therefore, coaches, medical specialists, and sports psychologists should pay attention not only to the physical but also to the psychological self-feeling of athletes and develop long-term psychological support strategies tailored to their experiences and risk factors [6,7].

Research conducted over the past few years shows that emotional intelligence, understood as the ability to recognize, perceive, and manage emotions [8], and mindfulness techniques, encompassing meditation, practices of accepting the present situation and oneself, can be tools that help manage stress, anxiety, and symptoms of depression in individuals of different ages and health conditions [9,10]. However, the results are not unambiguous. Many previous studies have confirmed a positive relationship between mindfulness and emotional intelligence, especially the ability to regulate emotions [11], but more recent findings suggest that this relationship may vary depending on the context and personal characteristics. For example, Guo et al. (2023) [12] note that by reducing emotional arousal, mindfulness practices can weaken the relationship with empathy and prosocial behaviour, especially among individuals with high intelligence. This suggests that the impact of mindfulness practice on emotional expression and interpersonal relationships may be contextual. Although previous research has shown that in the context of people with disabilities, emotional intelligence can act as an internal resource that helps relieve stress [13], there is still a lack of empirically grounded results demonstrating how emotional intelligence acts as an intermediate mechanism between mindfulness and psychological self-feeling indicators, such as symptoms of stress, anxiety, and depression. Greater clarity would contribute to enhancing the psychological well-being of athletes with disabilities, which includes not only the absence of psychological difficulties but also such aspects of positive self-feeling as self-esteem, life satisfaction, a sense of meaningfulness, the ability to cope with stress, maintain emotional balance, experience inner satisfaction, and constructively act in the social environment [3,4].

Although mindfulness interventions are increasingly being used to improve athletes' psychological self-feeling, a share of research reveals more than just positive effects. Schindler et al. (2019) [14] emphasize that in certain cases, such practices can weaken moral responsibility or even encourage unethical behaviour. There have also been cases where meditation has been associated with negative phenomena: distorted self-perception, affective disorders, depressiveness, hallucinations, or false memories [15]. Such evidence suggests that the effects of mindfulness are not unambiguous and may depend on individual or contextual factors.

In the context of sport, mindfulness is most often associated with relieving psychological stress. For example, Tingaz et al. (2023) [16] found that mindfulness was negatively associated with depression, anxiety, and stress and had a positive effect on athletic performance. However, a meta-analysis performed by Kanaujia et al. (2023) in [17] showed that changes in anxiety levels were not statistically significant. Such mixed findings suggest that the effectiveness of mindfulness may depend on the nature and duration of practicing it, the sports branch, and the specific characteristics of participants. For example, de Jesus et al. (2025) [18] found that mindfulness could be beneficial for athletes with disabilities, but there were individual differences in applying this practice, and physical difficulties arose when implementing interventions. In addition, a study by Macdougall et al. (2019) [19] demonstrated that although mindfulness intervention was acceptable and safe, some effectiveness indicators (e.g., social well-being) remained unconvincing. This is particularly important when it comes to the individual needs of athletes who have disabilities, seeking more durable effects and broader applicability. Therefore, larger-scale, more tailored studies, which would take into account the specific aspects of this population, are needed.

Given the ambiguous results of previous research and the specific needs of athletes who have disabilities, this study aims to explore the links between mindfulness and emotional intelligence with stress, anxiety, and depression among athletes who have disabilities. In this context, three questions are raised: (Q1) How is mindfulness related to emotional intelligence? (Q2) What factors predict the level of mindfulness and emotional intelligence in the population of athletes with disabilities? (Q3) Does emotional intelligence act as a mediator explaining the effect of mindfulness on psychological self-feeling? All this allows not only to evaluate links between the variables under study but also to reveal possible mechanisms through which mindfulness practices or emotional intelligence contribute to the well-being of athletes who have disabilities.

2. Conceptual Framework

2.1. Mindfulness and Personal Well-Being

Mindfulness, which has become popular in the West in recent decades, is understood as a practice that allows an individual to observe, non-judgmentally accept, and reflect on personal experiences [10,20]. Mindfulness has gained popularity largely due to standardized mindfulness-based interventions that integrate the essence of traditional Eastern mindfulness practices with contemporary psychological practices to improve psychological functioning and self-feeling [20].

Three components of mindfulness-based practice include avoiding judgment of personal experiences, cultivating awareness, and focusing on the present moment [10]. That is, it enables the person to observe and reflect on his/her physical, emotional, and cognitive state without automatic judgment. The positive outcomes of this practice include reduced levels of anxiety, depression, and stress, reduced pain, and vulnerability to mental illness [11]. However, the impact of this practice on athletes is not unambiguous. The findings of a meta-analysis by Wang et al. (2023) [21] show that the level of athletic performance and awareness improved but no significant effect on athletes' health was found.

2.2. The Structure of Emotional Intelligence

Emotional intelligence is defined as a set of skills that help to evaluate, express, and effectively regulate one's own and other people's emotions and use them for motivation, planning, and achievement [22]. In a later work, Mayer et al. (2016) [23] expand the conception of emotional intelligence as a kind of form of "hot" cognition, related to emotions and values, but distinguish it from other related constructs such as personal intelligence and social intelligence. Emotional intelligence is understood as the ability to perceive, understand, manage, and use emotions in solving problems, while personal intelligence encompasses broader self-knowledge, the ability to accurately describe one's intrinsic world and its characteristics.

According to Olderbak et al. (2018) [24], the most commonly applied theoretical four-branch model proposed by Mayer and Salovey (1997) [25] consists of perceiving emotion, facilitating thought using emotion, understanding emotions, and managing emotions [23,24]. These branches reflect progressive skills ranging from the ability to recognize one's own and other people's emotions to the conscious regulation of these emotions.

2.3. The Mediating Role of Emotional Intelligence

Considering that mindfulness helps create emotional distance and reduces affective arousal [26,27] and that emotional intelligence enhances the perception and control of emotions [23,24], it is likely that emotional intelligence can explain how mindfulness affects psychological self-feeling. This way, emotional intelligence would act as a mediating factor, transforming the effect of mindfulness into better self-feeling.

Mediation models are often used in behavioural sciences to find mechanisms that help explain indirect relationships [28]. In this study, it is assumed that mindfulness (X) affects psychological self-feeling (Y—stress, anxiety, and depression) both directly and indirectly through emotional intelligence (M). The mediating role of emotional intelligence between mindfulness, stress, anxiety, and depression has previously been confirmed in other populations [29], but this model has not been tested in the context of sport for people with disabilities. That is, it remains unclear whether it applies to people with disabilities, whose psychological self-feeling is affected by specific factors of stress, stigma, and physical limitations. For this reason, it is worth examining whether emotional intelligence actually mediates between mindfulness and psychological self-feeling in this specific group.

3. Methodology

3.1. Participants

Since there is no unified sports register in Lithuania, it is quite difficult to determine the population of athletes who have disabilities. There is also a lack of official statistics of people who have disabilities by the type of disability (hearing, visual, mental, or physical) [30]. Some data on the population can be obtained indirectly. In 2025, the list of members and candidates for sports teams of the Lithuanian Sport Federation for the Disabled included 94 individuals, and it was also planned that in 2025, about 900 athletes would participate in various championships [31].

In total, there are three organizations uniting athletes with disabilities and conducting competitions and sports activities in Lithuania: the Lithuanian Sport Federation for the Disabled, the Lithuanian Blind Sports Federation, and the Lithuanian Deaf Sport Committee. We reviewed the websites of these organizations and the Lithuanian Paralympic Committee but did not find any recent official information about the number of participants. Thus, before conducting the study, we asked the leaders of these organizations about the adult athletes currently belonging to their organization and participating in competitions. There were about 80 athletes in the Deaf Sport Committee; 25 in the Blind Sports Federation; and about 40 athletes in the Lithuanian Sport Federation for the Disabled.

Questionnaires were prepared and distributed during two Lithuanian championships (different sports branches hold different championships). After the championships, 150 questionnaires were distributed to all athletes who had taken part in them. A total of 94 properly completed questionnaires were returned. Criteria for inclusion in the study were as follows: adult (at least 18 years old, a person able to give informed consent) participating in at least national championship level competitions, disability–blindness, deafness, or physical disability. Participants were divided into four age groups: 18–25, 26–35, 36–45, and 46–65 years old.

Assistance in completing the questionnaire was provided to deaf people, to whom questions were read and the chosen answers were marked. Everyone could choose a trusted person from their circle. The assistance did not change the content or meaning of the questions, and it is therefore considered that it did not affect the reliability of the results.

Since the population of athletes with disabilities is relatively small, the sample size is considered sufficient, taking into account several circumstances. As noted by Pensgaard and Sørensen (2002) [32], one of the main methodological challenges in research on athletes who have disabilities is the limited number of potential participants; therefore, researchers often work with samples that are close to the entire population. For example, a similar sample size was used in Martin's (2008) [33] study, which involved 92 wheelchair basketball players, to analyse the relationship between self-efficacy and psychological self-feeling. In addition, according to Cohen's (1992) [34] recommendations, for a multivariate regression analysis with eight independent variables, aiming for a medium effect size ($f^2 \approx 0.15$) and statistical power ≥ 0.80, approximately 92 participants are sufficient. Therefore, the sample size of this study ($n = 95$) is considered sufficient to reliably identify significant relationships even in a small population under study.

3.2. Measure

The survey employed three adapted psychometric scales: the Depression, Anxiety and Stress Scale (DASS) [35], the Mindfulness Inventory for Sport (MIS) [36], and the Emotional Intelligence Scale for Use in Sport (EIS) [37].

The DASS scale assessed the intensity of three components—stress, anxiety, and depression—and an overall indicator of psychological self-feeling.

The MIS scale was adapted to the context of sport and encompassed three components of mindfulness: awareness, non-judgmental, and refocusing.

The EIS scale measured five dimensions of emotional intelligence: appraisal of others' emotions, appraisal of own emotions, regulation, social skills, and utilization of emotions.

All statements were rated on a five-point Likert-type scale, with higher scores indicating a stronger manifestation of the respective trait (except for the non-judgmental subscale, where negative values indicate an inverse relationship).

The reliability of the instrument in this study was adequate, with Cronbach's α values ranging from 0.79 to 0.90.

3.3. Procedures and Ethics

The study was conducted in accordance with the ethical principles for research in social sciences, with approval from the institutional ethics committee. Participants were informed about the purpose of the study, its voluntary nature, anonymity, and their right to withdraw from the study at any time. Informed consent was obtained before filling in the questionnaire.

The questionnaires were administered in two ways: electronically and using the paper-and-pencil method. Participants were given detailed instructions on how to complete and submit questionnaires. To ensure accessibility, participants with visual or motor impairments could receive technical assistance from a trusted person chosen from their own environment (e.g., to read questions aloud or mark answers). The content and structure of the questionnaire remained the same for all participants. Therefore, this adaptation likely did not affect the reliability of the research results. All participants completed the part of the questionnaire, which collected socio-demographic data. It included questions about age, gender, type of disability, sports status (professional or amateur), sports branch, and meditation experience.

The completion took about 30–40 min, and all data were processed in accordance with the requirements of the General Data Protection Regulation, anonymized and analysed only in aggregate form. The data were processed employing descriptive statistical methods, correlations were calculated, regression models and mediations were developed.

3.4. Data Analysis

The collected data were analysed using descriptive statistical methods in order to determine the main characteristics of the sample. To assess the relationships between variables, Pearson correlation coefficients were calculated. The strength of the relationship was described by applying the estimates proposed by Cohen (1988) [38], where a weak relationship is $r \approx 0.10$, a moderate relationship is $r \approx 0.30$, and a strong relationship is $r \geq 0.50$. Multiple regression models were created to determine the directions and strength of the effect, and mediation analysis procedures were employed to test the possible mediation effect, using the bootstrapping method to estimate confidence intervals.

4. Results

Of 95 respondents, 68.4% were men and 31.6 percent were women. The participants' ages ranged from 18 to 65 years, and more than half of them (57.9 percent) were professional athletes. More than half of respondents (52.6 percent) had mobility disabilities, and the rest had sensory disabilities. Of note, 25.8 percent held a university degree, 29 percent held a vocational degree, and the rest studied at school, colleges, and universities. Approximately one in three athletes has been doing sports for more than twenty-five years, which indicates their significant experience and involvement in sports. Such diversity reflects different sociodemographic groups and experiences as well as allows for a comprehensive examination of links between mindfulness, emotional intelligence, and psychological self-feeling (stress, anxiety, and depression) in the context of sport for people with disabilities.

Relationships Between Emotional Intelligence, Mindfulness, and Psychological Self-Feeling

First, a correlation analysis of emotional intelligence and mindfulness (including overall scores) was performed; its results are presented in Table 1.

Table 1. Relationships of emotional intelligence with mindfulness variables.

	Appraisal of Others' Emotions	Appraisal of Own Emotions	Regulation	Social Skills	Utilization of Emotions	Emotional Intelligence (Overall)
Awareness	0.461 **	0.572 **	0.601 **	0.381 **	0.354 **	0.596 **
Non-judgmental	−0.304 **	−0.261 *	−0.346 **	−0.175 (ns)	−0.120 (ns)	−0.302 **
Refocusing	0.371 **	0.498 **	0.513 **	0.361 **	0.564 **	0.600 **
Mindfulness (overall)	0.311 **	0.477 **	0.452 **	0.333 **	0.457 **	0.522 **

Notes: $p < 0.05$ (*); $p < 0.01$ (**); ns—non-significant ($p > 0.05$).

Thus, the results show that mindfulness is positively correlated with most components of emotional intelligence, especially with the regulation of emotions (r = 0.452, $p < 0.01$) and the overall estimate (r = 0.522, $p < 0.01$). Meanwhile, the non-judgmental component showed weak negative relationships with several aspects of emotional intelligence, and the relationship with social skills was statistically insignificant (r = −0.18, $p = 0.09$). As non-judgmental scores are increasing, the estimates of emotional intelligence components are significantly decreasing, including estimates of appraisal of other people's emotions, regulation of emotions, and overall emotional intelligence (r = −0.30, $p < 0.01$). This suggests that a higher level of non-judgmental self-acceptance is related to lower indicators of the ability to recognize, regulate, and purposefully utilize emotions.

When examining the relationships between emotional intelligence and psychological self-feeling (stress, anxiety, and depression), it was found that only appraisal of others' emotions was statistically significantly correlated with all indicators reflecting negative psychological self-feeling. The strongest relationship was found with the overall estimate of self-feeling (r = 0.293, $p = 0.004$) and stress (r = 0.304, $p = 0.003$). Meanwhile, a weaker but significant correlation was identified with anxiety (r = 0.228, $p = 0.026$) and signs of depression symptoms (r = 0.243, $p = 0.018$). However, only two of the mindfulness components (non-judgmental and overall scale estimate) showed statistically significant negative relationships with psychological self-feeling (Table 2).

Table 2. Relationships of mindfulness components with negative self-feeling in athletes.

	Stress	Anxiety	Depression	Overall
Awareness	0.055	0.128	−0.060	0.042
Non-judgmental	−0.466 **	−0.384 **	−0.336 **	−0.447 **
Refocusing	−0.009	−0.172	−0.132	−0.117
Overall	−0.258 *	−0.245 *	−0.318 **	−0.312 **

Notes: $p < 0.05$ (*); $p < 0.01$ (**).

The non-judgmental component was strongly and consistently correlated with all four indicators of negative psychological self-feeling (r fluctuated from −0.336 to −0.466, $p < 0.001$), indicating that the better the athletes were able to accept their experiences without judgment, the lower the levels of their experienced stress, anxiety, and depression. Links of awareness and refocusing components with self-feeling of athletes with disabilities were not significant.

Factors predicting the level of mindfulness among athletes with disabilities were revealed by the results of regression analysis. Independent variables included sociodemographic indicators (age, gender, and education), peculiarities of doing sports (duration, level, and sports group), experience in practicing meditation, the type of disability, and the indicator showing psychological self-feeling (composed of the sum of stress, anxiety, and depression estimates).

The results show that the regression model is statistically significant ($F(10, 76) = 3.01$, $p = 0.003$) and explains 24.9% ($R^2 = 0.249$) of the variance in the mindfulness estimate (Table 3).

Table 3. Prognostic model of mindfulness. $R^2 = 0.249$.

Model		Coefficients [a]				
		Unstandardized Coefficients		Standardized Coefficients	t	Sig.
		B	Std. Error	Beta		
1	(Constant)	57.211	5.525		10.355	<0.001
	Stress, anxiety, and depression	−0.246	0.061	−0.423	−4.040	<0.001
	Practice meditation	−1.704	1.422	−0.110	−1.198	0.234
	Type of disability	−0.167	1.276	−0.016	−0.131	0.896
	Years of doing sports	0.013	0.347	0.004	0.036	0.971
	Does sports as a professional or as an amateur	4.662	1.785	0.318	2.611	0.011
	Sports group	1.742	0.732	0.235	2.378	0.020
	Gender	−1.076	1.504	−0.069	−0.715	0.477
	Age group	0.071	0.870	0.010	0.082	0.935
	Education	−1.163	0.472	−0.256	−2.463	0.016

[a] Dependent Variable: Mindfulness.

Psychological self-feeling (stress, anxiety, and depression) was the most significant predictor of mindfulness ($\beta = -0.423$, $p < 0.001$), meaning that the higher the levels of anxiety, depression, and stress, the lower the level of mindfulness. The level of doing sports (professional vs. amateur) was significantly associated with a higher estimate of mindfulness (β = 0.318, p = 0.011). That is, professional athletes distinguish themselves by a higher level of mindfulness than amateurs. Meanwhile, education had a negative effect on mindfulness (β = −0.256, p = 0.016). This suggests that mindfulness may be weaker in athletes who have disabilities and higher education. Gender, age, duration of exercising, meditation experience, and the type of disability were not statistically significant predictors ($p > 0.05$).

In order to determine which factors predict mindfulness estimates, including psychological self-feeling components (stress, anxiety, and depression) as separate predictors, the second regression model was built (Table 4).

Table 4. Prognostic model of mindfulness by detailing psychological self-feeling. $R^2 = 0.241$.

Coefficients [a]						
Model		Unstandardized Coefficients		Standardized Coefficients	t	Sig.
		B	Std. Error	Beta		
1	(Constant)	56.771	5.569		10.193	<0.001
	Practice meditation	−1.618	1.443	−0.105	−1.122	0.265
	Type of disability	−0.007	1.290	−0.001	−0.005	0.996
	Years of doing sports	0.004	0.350	0.001	0.010	0.992
	Does sports as a professional or as an amateur	4.907	1.808	0.335	2.714	0.008
	Sports group	1.539	0.760	0.208	2.026	0.046
	Gender	−1.372	1.543	−0.088	−0.889	0.376
	Age group	0.002	0.899	0.000	0.002	0.998
	Education	−1.215	0.480	−0.268	−2.529	0.013
	Stress	−0.009	0.230	−0.006	−0.040	0.968
	Anxiety	−0.347	0.236	−0.210	−1.472	0.145
	Depression	−0.392	0.207	−0.270	−1.887	0.063

[a] Dependent Variable: Mindfulness.

The results of regression analysis show that the depression signs indicator has a tendency to approach a statistically significant effect on mindfulness (β = −0.270, p = 0.063). The anxiety and stress estimates also did not have a statistically significant effect ($p > 0.1$), and their standardized coefficients were insignificant.

To examine which factors predict the overall emotional intelligence indicator among athletes who have disabilities, a regression model was constructed with independent variables, which encompassed demographic indicators, athletic factors, and psychological self-feeling components (stress, anxiety, and depression). The model was statistically significant ($F(10, 94) = 3.692$, $p < 0.001$) and explained 28.2% ($R^2 = 0.282$) of the overall variance in emotional intelligence (Table 5).

Emotional intelligence was statistically significantly predicted by stress level (β = 0.463, p = 0.004) and education (β = −0.303, p = 0.007), indicating that a higher level of education was associated with lower emotional intelligence scores. A statistically significant negative effect of meditation on emotional intelligence estimates was also found (β = −0.199, p = 0.043). The impact of other factors (anxiety, depression, duration of exercising, gender, age group, type of sports, sports group, and type of disability) was not statistically significant ($p > 0.05$).

Table 5. Prognostic model of emotional intelligence.

Coefficients [a]						
Model		Unstandardized Coefficients		Standardized Coefficients	t	Sig.
		B	Std. Error	Beta		
1	(Constant)	79.256	10.642		7.447	<0.001
	Practice meditation	−5.670	2.757	−0.199	−2.056	0.043
	Type of disability	2.223	2.465	0.119	0.902	0.370
	Years of doing sports	−0.288	0.670	−0.055	−0.431	0.668
	Does sports as a professional or as an amateur	3.121	3.455	0.115	0.903	0.369
	Sports group	1.418	1.452	0.104	0.977	0.332
	Gender	−3.650	2.947	−0.127	−1.238	0.219
	Age group	0.095	1.717	0.008	0.056	0.956
	Education	−2.537	0.918	−0.303	−2.763	0.007
	Stress	1.313	0.440	0.463	2.986	0.004
	Anxiety	−0.546	0.451	−0.179	−1.212	0.229
	Depression	−0.711	0.396	−0.266	−1.793	0.077

[a] Dependent variable: Emotional intelligence.

To answer Q3, mediation analysis was performed. It was found that emotional intelligence acted as a partial, statistically significant mediator, explaining the effect of mindfulness on negative psychological self-feeling (stress, anxiety, depression). Figure 1 presents a model of mediation pathways. A more detailed review of the statistical results is provided in Table 6.

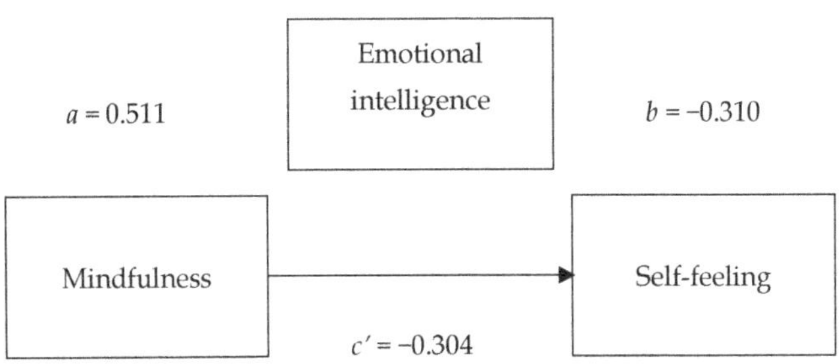

Figure 1. The mediation model.

Table 6. Results of mediation analysis.

Path	B (Unstandardized Coefficient)	SE	t	p-Value	95% PI (Bootstrap)
a: mindfulness → emotional intelligence	0.511	0.074	6.89	<0.001	[0.365, 0.655]
b: emotional intelligence → self-feeling (stress, anxiety, depression)	−0.310	0.094	−3.30	0.001	[−0.495, −0.124]
c: mindfulness → self-feeling (overall impact)	−0.462	0.095	−4.87	<0.001	[−0.648, −0.276]
c′: mindfulness → self-feeling (direct effect)	−0.304	0.098	−3.10	0.003	[−0.496, −0.112]
indirect effect (a × b)	−0.158	–	–	–	[−0.273, −0.065]

The results show that mindfulness significantly predicted emotional intelligence indicators (path a, B = 0.511, $p < 0.001$), while emotional intelligence significantly affected the negative self-feeling estimate (path b, B = −0.310, p = 0.001). There was also a statistically significant and direct effect of mindfulness on the overall self-feeling indicator (path c′, B = −0.304, p = 0.003), but it was weaker than the overall effect (path c, B = −0.462, $p < 0.001$). The indirect effect through emotional intelligence was statistically significant, and the 95% confidence interval did not include zero (indirect effect B = −0.158, 95% CI [−0.273, −0.065]).

5. Discussion

This study aimed to investigate links of mindfulness with stress, anxiety, and depression in the context of athletes who had disabilities and to reveal mechanisms through which mindfulness practices and emotional intelligence contribute to athletes' psychological well-being. Since the interrelationships between these constructs in the population of people who have disabilities have been poorly studied to date, questions were consistently raised that helped reveal not only direct but also indirect links between mindfulness and indicators of psychological self-feeling. The answers to these questions create prerequisites for a deeper understanding of the theoretical interrelationships between these phenomena and provide the basis for practical interventions aimed at strengthening the psychological well-being of athletes who have disabilities.

The first research question (Q1) aimed to find out how mindfulness was related to emotional intelligence, since it is namely this connection that creates conditions for further analysis and allows us to understand how mindfulness abilities can be linked to appraisal, regulation, and utilization of emotions in the context of sport for people with disabilities. It was found that mindfulness was significantly correlated with most components of emotional intelligence (except social skills). Social skills require the ability to recognize and understand the emotions of others, while Nadler et al. (2020) [39] found that mindfulness intervention participants had reported improvements in all components of emotional intelligence except empathy. Considering that social skills are closely related to the ability of empathy, no increase in this component might have determined a weaker relationship between mindfulness and social skills. This is consistent with previous observations that mindfulness is more likely to enhance intrapersonal emotional intelligence (self-knowledge and regulation of emotions) than interpersonal emotional intelligence (empathy, social communication) [39,40]. In addition, according to the results of a meta-analysis performed by Li et al. (2023) [41], mindfulness was associated with an increase in intrinsic motivation and with meeting basic psychological needs, such as autonomy, competence, and relatedness. This interaction suggests that mindfulness practices primarily promote intrinsic regulation and self-acceptance that is focused on the person's internal experience rather than on the demonstration of external social skills. This may explain why mindfulness was not correlated with the "social skills" scale in this study.

Notably, a higher level of non-judgmental self-acceptance was associated with lower scores of the ability to recognize, regulate, and use emotions appropriately. This result may seem contradictory, but it is consistent with the mechanism identified by Josefsson et al. (2017) [42], according to which a higher level of mindfulness (non-judgmental attitude) can reduce the tendency to rumination and enhance the ability of "reperceiving" emotional experiences. This allows athletes to "cool down" intense emotions more quickly, limit their duration, and reduce the need to actively apply conscious emotion recognition or regulation strategies. As a result, emotional intelligence indicators measured by the questionnaire may be lower, not due to poorer skills but due to a lower need to apply them.

On the other hand, the non-judgmental component was found to be strongly and consistently correlated with stress, anxiety, and depression, indicating that the better athletes are able to accept their experiences without judgment, the lower their level of psychological self-feeling. This result coincides with previous research showing that the non-judgmental acceptance approach can mitigate stressors experienced by athletes and support their psychological well-being [7,43]. According to Gu et al. (2015) [44], the said component helps reduce the automatic appraisal of negative thoughts, leading to reduced affective arousal and maintenance of better emotional balance, which can explain strong and consistent correlations with all three psychological state indicators.

Examining the role of mindfulness and emotional intelligence in predicting psychological self-feeling (Q2), it turned out that psychological self-feeling (levels of stress, anxiety, and depression) was the strongest predictor of mindfulness, revealing a negative association: higher indicators were related to lower levels of mindfulness. In addition, it was found that the level of doing sports (professional vs. amateur) significantly predicted mindfulness. Professional athletes distinguished themselves by higher mindfulness than amateurs. This can be related to higher requirements for psychological preparation and skill development, including concentration of attention and regulation of emotions. It should be emphasized that education had a negative effect on mindfulness, which could indicate that athletes with higher education may rely more on cognitive rather than mindfulness-based decision-making processes. For example, Scharfen and Memmert (2019) [45] argue that professional athletes are more characterized by developed cognitive abilities that are of great importance for decision-making. Furthermore, Waterworth et al. (2020) [46] highlight that higher education may promote a more analytical, fact-based, and logical decision-making style. This may indicate that athletes with disabilities and higher education tend to evaluate situations primarily cognitively.

These interpretations are indirectly supported by the findings of a study conducted by Noone and Hogan (2017) [47]. The results show that individuals with stronger cognitive approaches, such as a high need to seek knowledge or active open-minded thinking, benefited less from mindfulness interventions. Although their study did not directly examine the role of education, the observed interaction between cognitive style and mindfulness may help explain the negative link found in this study. It is possible that individuals with higher education are more actively engaged in cognitive processes that are less compatible with experiential, non-judgmental aspects of mindfulness. Liu and Nesbit (2024) [48] revealed in their meta-analysis that a higher need for cognition was associated with higher academic achievement, since such individuals were more inclined to deep analysis of information, reflection, and coping with cognitively complex tasks. All this suggests that the abundance of cognitive resources or the tendency towards cognitive analysis, which are usually characteristic of persons with higher-level education, may reduce their sensitivity to mindfulness practices that emphasize non-analytical, open, and non-judgmental attentiveness.

Meanwhile, demographic characteristics, meditation experience, and the type of disability did not have a significant effect, suggesting that these factors were not essential predictors of mindfulness in this context.

Emotional intelligence was significantly predicted by stress ($\beta = 0.463$, $p = 0.004$), education ($\beta = -0.303$, $p = 0.007$), and meditation practice ($\beta = -0.199$, $p = 0.043$). Fiorilli et al. (2021) [49] found that when experiencing stress, athletes who had disabilities actively used various coping mechanisms related to emotional reactions. That is, having encountered stressful situations, athletes can better mobilize and improve their ability to recognize and regulate emotions in order to effectively overcome challenges. The negative effect of education might have been related to cognitive orientation and less attention to emotional aspects [46], while the impact of meditation confirms previous research demonstrating that meditation does not always have a positive effect on emotional intelligence. For example, the study of Valim et al. (2019) [50] showed that when applying mindfulness meditation, no positive effect on the regulation of emotions was observed. Furthermore, decreasing emotional arousal may result in weakening of empathy [39,44], which is important for perceiving other people's emotions and social skills. The role of meditation intention, which is oriented to athletic achievements, cannot be ruled out either.

Being related to the person's ability to perceive and regulate emotions, emotional intelligence also plays an important role in moral decision-making. As pointed out by Vveinhardt and Deikus (2025) [51], moral decision-making is considerably affected by emotions and intuition, and synderesis allows one to correct mistakes made in this area. This indicates a broader impact of emotional intelligence, which, in addition to reducing stress and anxiety, can also promote more conscious and ethical behaviour.

Finally, the results of mediation analysis (Q3) showed that in the sample of athletes with disabilities, emotional intelligence acted as a partial mediator between mindfulness and negative psychological self-feeling (stress, anxiety, and depression). Higher level of mindfulness was associated with a better ability to perceive, regulate, and purposefully use emotions, and this ability was related to lower indicators of psychological self-feeling. The direct effect of mindfulness on self-feeling remained significant even after inclusion of emotional intelligence in the model, although its strength reduced compared with the overall effect. This shows that emotional intelligence conveys some, but not all, of the effects of mindfulness on psychological well-being. A previous study in an adolescent population demonstrated a mediating role of emotional intelligence between mindfulness and both anxiety and depression [29]. In another study of the adult population, Iau et al. (2025) [52] concluded that the ability to understand and use one's emotions might be one of the possible mechanisms through which mindfulness reduced anxiety, depression, and contributed to well-being.

The results of this study can be useful in developing the theoretical discussion on mindfulness, emotional intelligence, depression, anxiety, and stress in sports psychology, especially in the context of athletes who have disabilities. Previous studies have mainly focused on the examples of healthy athletes or the general population, while the findings of this study reveal that emotional intelligence partially explains the impact of mindfulness on psychological self-feeling among athletes who have disabilities too. Furthermore, the unusual relationship between the non-judgmental component and emotional intelligence indicators, identified in this study, provides a basis for further developing the discussion about the effects of different dimensions of mindfulness on individual components of emotional intelligence.

In practice, the findings can be valuable to sports psychologists, coaches, and rehabilitation specialists, who assist athletes with disabilities. Mindfulness and emotional intelligence practices integrated into training programs can not only directly reduce stress and anxiety but also indirectly improve self-feeling through emotion recognition and regulation abilities. Such a dual mechanism of impact can be particularly important for the long-term well-being of athletes who have disabilities. In this context, it is recommended that specialists take into account certain individual differences that determine the outcome of practices.

Considering the results of this study, it is recommended that sports psychologists and coaches working with athletes who have disabilities should incorporate structured emotional intelligence and mindfulness development programs. One such framework was presented by Laborde et al. (2022) [53], who proposed practical interventions aimed at the development of five emotional competencies: identification, expression, understanding, regulation, and use of emotions. These aspects can be developed through activities adapted to sport, such as 'discussion of emotions', 'memory of emotions', and 'sports awareness', which are based on the tripartite model of emotional intelligence (of knowledge, abilities, and traits). This framework can be combined with the MAC (Mindfulness–Acceptance–

Commitment) protocol (Gardner & Moore, 2007) [54], which integrates present-moment awareness, acceptance of internal experiences, and value-based actions. Such preliminarily proposed protocols could be further adapted to the sports environment, taking into account the specific needs and context of athletes who have disabilities.

The study has several limitations. First, the cross-sectional design does not allow to make firm conclusions about causal relationships; therefore, a longitudinal study would be needed in the future. Second, although the sample size is sufficient for statistical analysis, it is still limited, and the participants were from a single country, which limits the possibilities of making broader generalizations. Third, we were unable to find other studies that simultaneously examined the same concepts (mindfulness, emotional intelligence, depression, anxiety, and stress) in the context of sport for people with disabilities. For this reason, it was not possible to directly compare the obtained results with previous studies. Fourth, self-assessment questionnaires can be affected by social desirability and subjective perception. However, in order to mitigate these risks, several methodological solutions were applied: validated and reliable scales (DASS, MIS, and EIS) were used, and the data were collected by selecting both electronic and paper-and-pencil questionnaires adapted for participants with different types of disabilities.

Finally, the study was conducted in Lithuania, whose sociocultural context might have influenced the interpretation and application of findings in other cultures. In Lithuania, there is a lower tendency to openly express emotions, compared with, for example, the English-speaking culture (Šeškauskienė, 2020) [55], and mindfulness practices are not yet widespread; therefore, the experiences of research participants in these areas may be limited. Social stigma associated with disability (Grigaitė et al., 2025) [56] may also have influenced the openness of responses. To manage this limitation, the participants' anonymity and the possibility of choosing a response method that was acceptable to them were ensured. Although due to cultural peculiarities, the results of the study may not be fully transferable to other contexts, the applied ethical and methodological measures helped to reduce the risk of cultural influence.

6. Conclusions

This is probably one of the first studies that systematically examines links between mindfulness, emotional intelligence, and psychological self-feeling components (stress, anxiety, and depression) in the context of sport for people with disabilities. The findings have confirmed the partial mediating effect of emotional intelligence, indicating that the abilities to appraise, regulate, and utilize emotions can be one of the important mechanisms through which mindfulness practices influence the psychological well-being of people who have disabilities. This not only expands theoretical knowledge about the interaction between psychological constructs in sport for people with disabilities but also provides new insights that can contribute to the development of intervention mechanisms to improve psychological self-feeling. In this context, it is important to note that in assessing psychological self-feeling, generalized indicators of stress, anxiety, and depression are more useful than individual symptoms. The obtained results suggest the potential for applying complex interventions that would include both mindfulness and emotional intelligence enhancement methods.

Considering the limitations of this study, it is recommended that future research should use a longitudinal or intervention-based design that would allow for assessment of causal relationships between mindfulness, emotional intelligence, and psychological self-feeling indicators. Longitudinal studies would provide a better understanding of how consistent mindfulness practice affects emotional management skills over time, while interventional studies would allow us to evaluate the effectiveness of specific programs (e.g., mindfulness training sessions adapted for sports) in a group of athletes who have disabilities. It would also be appropriate to investigate the impact of different mindfulness components (e.g., attentiveness, non-judgment, and reorientation) on individual dimensions of emotional intelligence. Given the observed role of education, future research could examine in more detail the interaction between cognitive styles and the effectiveness of mindfulness practices. Finally, larger and more culturally diverse samples could help evaluate the extent to which the research findings are universal and applicable to other cultural settings.

Author Contributions: Conceptualization, D.R. and J.V.; methodology, J.V.; software, J.V.; validation, D.R. and J.V.; formal analysis, D.R.; investigation, D.R.; resources, D.R.; data curation, J.V.; writing—original draft preparation, J.V.; writing—review and editing, D.R.; visualization, J.V.; supervision, D.R.; project administration, J.V.; funding acquisition, D.R. and J.V. All authors have read and agreed to the published version of the manuscript.

Funding: This research received no external funding.

Institutional Review Board Statement: The study was conducted in accordance with the Declaration of Helsinki and approved by the Ethics Committee of Lithuanian Sports University (protocol code SMTEK-229 and 8 January 2024).

Informed Consent Statement: Informed consent was obtained from all subjects involved in the study.

Data Availability Statement: The raw data supporting the conclusions of this article will be made available by the authors upon request.

Conflicts of Interest: The authors declare no conflicts of interest.

References

1. Rees, L.; Robinson, P.; Shields, N. Media portrayal of elite athletes with disability—A systematic review. *Disabil. Rehabil.* **2017**, *41*, 374–381. [CrossRef]
2. Silva, C.F.; Howe, P.D. Dis/ability Sport for "All". In *Reflexivity and Change in Adaptive Physical Activity*; Routledge: London, UK, 2022.
3. Fagher, K.; Dahlström, Ö.; Lexell, J. Mental health, sleep, and pain in elite para athletes and the association with injury and illness—A prospective study. *Phys. Med. Rehabil. J.* **2023**, *15*, 1130–1139. [CrossRef]
4. Olive, L.S.; Rice, S.; Butterworth, M.; Clements, M.; Purcell, R. Do rates of mental health symptoms in currently competing elite athletes in paralympic sports differ from non-para-athletes? *Sports Med. Open* **2021**, *7*, 62. [CrossRef]
5. Denerel, N.; Lima, Y. Competing against COVID-19: What about the mental health problems of athletes with disabilities? *Physician Sportsmed.* **2022**, *50*, 546–552. [CrossRef] [PubMed]
6. Marconcin, P.; Silva, A.L.; Flôres, F.; Nunes, A.; Lourenço, J.F.; Peralta, M.; Minghelli, B. Association between Musculoskeletal Injuries and Depressive Symptoms among Athletes: A Systematic Review. *Int. J. Environ. Res. Public Health* **2023**, *20*, 6130. [CrossRef] [PubMed]
7. Bentzen, M.; Kenttä, G.; Derman, W.; Wik, E.H.; Havela, J.; Karls, T.; Stenman, A.; Fagher, K. Mental distress is associated with injury and illness in elite Para athletes: A 44-week prospective study over 13 860 athlete days. *BMJ Open Sport Exerc. Med.* **2025**, *11*, e002267. [CrossRef] [PubMed]
8. Augusto-Landa, J.M.; García-Martínez, I.; León, S.P. Analysis of the Effect of Emotional Intelligence and Coping Strategies on the Anxiety, Stress and Depression Levels of University Students. *Psychol. Rep.* **2022**, *127*, 1751–1770. [CrossRef]
9. Chie, H.V.; Yan-Li, S.; Nor, A.M. A systematic review of mindfulness-based stress reduction in the management of anxiety disorders among adolescents and young adults aged 13–26. *Asian J. Psychiatry* **2025**, *108*, 104497. [CrossRef]
10. Zhang, H.; Zhang, X.; Jiang, X.; Dai, R.; Zhao, N.; Pan, W.; Guo, J.; Fan, J.; Bao, S. Mindfulness-based intervention for hypertension patients with depression and/or anxiety in the community: A randomized controlled trial. *Trials* **2024**, *25*, 299. [CrossRef]
11. Jiménez-Picón, N.; Romero-Martín, M.; Ponce-Blandón, J.A.; Ramirez-Baena, L.; Palomo-Lara, J.C.; Gómez-Salgado, J. The relationship between mindfulness and emotional intelligence as a protective factor for healthcare professionals: Systematic review. *Int. J. Environ. Res. Public Health* **2021**, *18*, 5491. [CrossRef]
12. Guo, Q.; Li, S.; Liang, J.; Yu, X.; Lv, Y. Mindfulness may be associated with less prosocial engagement among high intelligence individuals. *Sci. Rep.* **2023**, *13*, 4208. [CrossRef]
13. Sukmana, M.E.; Kristiyanto, A.; Liskustyawati, H. The relationship between emotional intelligence and hardiness on stress resistance in athletes with disabilities in Indonesian national Paralympic committee. *Int. J. Health Med. Sci.* **2021**, *4*, 23–37. [CrossRef]

14. Schindler, S.; Pfattheicher, S.; Reinhard, M.A. Potential negative consequences of mindfulness in the moral domain. *Eur. J. Soc. Psychol.* **2019**, *49*, 1055–1069. [CrossRef]
15. Lambert, D.; Van Den Berg, N.H.; Mendrek, A. Adverse effects of meditation: A review of observational, experimental and case studies. *Curr. Psychol.* **2023**, *42*, 1112–1125. [CrossRef]
16. Tingaz, E.O.; Solmaz, S.; Ekiz, M.A.; Atasoy, M. The relationship between mindfulness and self-rated performance in student-athletes: The mediating role of depression, anxiety and stress. *Sport Sci. Health* **2023**, *19*, 657–663. [CrossRef]
17. Kanaujia, S.; Saraswati, P.; Singh, N.; Singh, S.; Kataria, N.; Yadav, P. Effect of yoga and mindfulness on psychological correlates in young athletes: A meta-analysis. *J. Ayurveda Integr. Med.* **2023**, *14*, 100725. [CrossRef] [PubMed]
18. de Jesus, M.S.; de Oliveira Filho, C.W.; Gebara, L.; Cases, S.S.; Santos, S.M.C.B.; Sarubbi, V., Jr.; da Silva, M.O.; Demarzo, M. Acceptability, Feasibility, and Effects of a Mindfulness-Based Intervention on the Quality of Life and Performance of the Brazilian Paralympic Boccia Team: Mixed Methods Case Study. *Qeios* **2025**, *7*, 1–18. [CrossRef]
19. Macdougall, H.; O'Halloran, P.; Sherry, E.; Shields, N. A Pilot Randomised Controlled Trial to Enhance Well-Being and Performance of Athletes in Para Sports. *Eur. J. Adapt. Phys. Act.* **2019**, *12*, 1–19. [CrossRef]
20. Gu, J.; Strauss, C.; Crane, C.; Barnhofer, T.; Karl, A.; Cavanagh, K.; Kuyken, W. Examining the factor structure of the 39-item and 15-item versions of the Five Facet Mindfulness Questionnaire before and after mindfulness-based cognitive therapy for people with recurrent depression. *Psychol Assess.* **2016**, *28*, 791–802. [CrossRef]
21. Wang, Y.; Lei, S.M.; Fan, J. Effects of Mindfulness-Based Interventions on Promoting Athletic Performance and Related Factors among Athletes: A Systematic Review and Meta-Analysis of Randomized Controlled Trial. *Int. J. Environ. Res. Public Health* **2023**, *20*, 2038. [CrossRef]
22. Salovey, P.; Mayer, J.D. Emotional Intelligence. *Imagin. Cogn. Personal.* **1990**, *9*, 185–211. [CrossRef]
23. Mayer, J.D.; Caruso, D.R.; Salovey, P. The Ability Model of Emotional Intelligence: Principles and Updates. *Emot. Rev.* **2016**, *8*, 290–300. [CrossRef]
24. Olderbak, S.; Semmler, M.; Doebler, P. Four-branch model of ability emotional intelligence with fluid and crystallized intelligence: A meta-analysis of relations. *Emot. Rev.* **2018**, *11*, 166–183. [CrossRef]
25. Mayer, J.D.; Salovey, P. What is emotional intelligence? In *Emotional Development and Emotional Intelligence: Implications for Educators*; Salovey, P., Sluyter, D., Eds.; Basic Books: New York, NY, USA, 1997; pp. 3–31.
26. Fuochi, G.; Voci, A. How mindfulness, decentering, nonattachment and rumination interact with the temporal associations between emotions and thoughts: An experience sampling study. *Int. J. Psychol.* **2024**, *59*, 1111–1120. [CrossRef]
27. Jones, D.R.; Graham-Engeland, J.E.; Smyth, J.M.; Lehman, B.J. Clarifying the associations between mindfulness meditation and emotion: Daily high-and low-arousal emotions and emotional variability. *Appl. Psychol. Health Well-Being* **2018**, *10*, 504–523. [CrossRef]
28. Preacher, K.J.; Hayes, A.F. Asymptotic and resampling strategies for assessing and comparing indirect effects in multiple mediator models. *Behav. Res. Methods* **2008**, *40*, 879–891. [CrossRef]
29. Foster, B.; Lomas, J.; Downey, L.; Stough, C. Does emotional intelligence mediate the relation between mindfulness and anxiety and depression in adolescents? *Front. Psychol.* **2018**, *9*, 2463. [CrossRef]
30. Pozeriene, J.; Reklaitiene, D. Disability Sport in Lithuania. In *The Palgrave Handbook of Disability Sport in Europe*; Van Lindert, C., Scheerder, J., Brittain, I., Eds.; Palgrave Macmillan: Cham, Switzerland, 2023. [CrossRef]
31. Lithuanian Sport Federation for the Disabled Lietuvos Neįgaliųjų Sporto Federacijos 2025–2028 Strateginis Planas. 2025. Available online: https://www.lnsf.lt/wp-content/uploads/2024/12/LIETUVOS-NEIGALIUJU-SPORTO-FEDERACIJOS-2025-2028-STRATEGINIS-PLANAS-1.pdf (accessed on 20 August 2025).
32. Pensgaard, A.M.; Sørensen, M. Empowerment through the sport context: A model to guide research for individuals with disability. *Adapt. Phys. Act. Q.* **2022**, *19*, 48–67. [CrossRef]
33. Martin, J.J. Multidimensional self-efficacy and affect in wheelchair basketball players. *Adapt. Phys. Act. Q.* **2008**, *25*, 275–288. [CrossRef]
34. Cohen, J. A power primer. *Psychol. Bull.* **1992**, *112*, 155–159. [CrossRef]
35. Lovibond, S.H.; Lovibond, P.F. *Manual for the Depression Anxiety Stress Scales*, 2nd ed.; Psychology Foundation: Sydney, Australia, 1995.
36. Thienot, E.; Jackson, B.; Dimmock, J.; Grove, R.; Bernier, M.; Fournier, J.F. Development and preliminary validation of the mindfulness inventory for sport. *Psychol. Sport Exerc.* **2014**, *15*, 72–80. [CrossRef]
37. Lane, A.M.; Meyer, B.B.; Devonport, T.J.; Davies, K.A.; Thelwell, R.; Gill, G.S.; Diehl, C.D.P.; Wilson, M.; Weston, N. Validity of the emotional intelligence scale for use in sport. *J. Sports Sci. Med.* **2009**, *8*, 289–295.
38. Cohen, J. *Statistical Power Analysis for the Behavioral Sciences*, 2nd ed.; Lawrence Erlbaum Associates: Hillsdale, NJ, USA, 1988.
39. Nadler, R.; Carswell, J.; Minda, J. Online mindfulness training increases well-being, trait emotional intelligence, and workplace competency ratings: A randomized waitlist-controlled trial. *Front. Psychol.* **2020**, *11*, 255. [CrossRef] [PubMed]

40. Geurtzen, N.; Scholte, R.H.J.; Engels, R.C.M.E.; Tak, Y.R.; van Zundert, R.M.P. Association between mindful parenting and adolescents' internalizing problems: Non-judgmental acceptance of parenting as core element. *J. Child Fam. Stud.* **2014**, *24*, 1117–1128. [CrossRef]
41. Li, L.Y.; Meng, X.; Hu, W.T.; Geng, J.S.; Cheng, T.H.; Luo, J.C.; Hu, M.Y.; Li, H.Y.; Wang, Y.; Wang, Y.Y. A meta-analysis of the association between mindfulness and motivation. *Front. Public Health* **2023**, *11*, 1159902. [CrossRef] [PubMed]
42. Josefsson, T.; Ivarsson, A.; Lindwall, M.; Gustafsson, H.; Stenling, A.; Böröy, J.; Mattsson, E.; Carnebratt, J.; Sevholt, S.; Falkevik, E. Mindfulness mechanisms in sports: Mediating effects of rumination and emotion regulation on sport-specific coping. *Mindfulness* **2017**, *8*, 1354–1363. [CrossRef]
43. Lundqvist, C.; Stahl, L.; Kentta, G.; Thulin, U. Evaluation of a mindfulness intervention for Paralympic leaders prior to the Paralympic Games. *Int. J. Sports Sci. Coach.* **2018**, *13*, 62–71. [CrossRef]
44. Gu, J.; Strauss, C.; Bond, R.; Cavanagh, K. How do mindfulness-based cognitive therapy and mindfulness-based stress reduction improve mental health and wellbeing? A systematic review and meta-analysis of mediation studies. *Clin. Psychol. Rev.* **2015**, *37*, 1–12. [CrossRef]
45. Scharfen, H.; Memmert, D. Measurement of cognitive functions in experts and elite athletes: A meta-analytic review. *Appl. Cogn. Psychol.* **2019**, *33*, 843–860. [CrossRef]
46. Waterworth, V.; Procyk, A.; Canetti, E.; Hing, W.; Gough, S. The influence of education in decision making concerning athlete's return to sport following a concussion injury: A systematic review. *J. Concussion* **2020**, *4*, 205970022094198. [CrossRef]
47. Noone, C.; Hogan, M.J. Improvements in critical thinking performance following mindfulness meditation depend on thinking dispositions. *Mindfulness* **2018**, *9*, 461–473. [CrossRef]
48. Liu, Q.; Nesbit, J.C. The relation between need for cognition and academic achievement: A meta-analysis. *Rev. Educ. Res.* **2024**, *94*, 155–192. [CrossRef]
49. Fiorilli, G.; Buonsenso, A.; Davola, N.; Martino, G.D.; Baralla, F.; Boutious, S.; Centorbi, M.; Calcagno, G.; Cagno, A.d. Stress impact of covid-19 sports restrictions on disabled athletes. *Int. J. Environ. Res. Public Health* **2021**, *18*, 12040. [CrossRef] [PubMed]
50. Valim, C.P.R.A.T.; Marques, L.M.; Boggio, P.S. A positive emotional-based meditation but not mindfulness-based meditation improves emotion regulation. *Front. Psychol.* **2019**, *10*, 647. [CrossRef]
51. Vveinhardt, J.; Deikus, M. Synderesis vs. Consequentialism and Utilitarianism in Workplace Bullying Prevention. *Soc. Incl.* **2025**, *13*, 8406. [CrossRef]
52. Iau, E.A.; Verhaeghen, P. A well-regulated mind: Emotional intelligence as a mediator between mindfulness and mental health and wellbeing. *Curr. Psychol.* **2025**, *44*, 3548–3563. [CrossRef]
53. Laborde, S.; Mosley, E.; Ackermann, S.; Mrsic, A.; Dosseville, F. Emotional intelligence in sports and physical activity: An intervention focus. In *Emotional Intelligence in Education: Integrating Research with Practice*; Springer International Publishing: Cham, Switzerland, 2018; pp. 289–320.
54. Gardner, F.L.; Moore, Z.E. *The Psychology of Enhancing Human Performance: The Mindfulness-Acceptance-Commitment (MAC) Approach: A Practitioner's Guide*; Springer: New York, NY, USA, 2007.
55. Šeškauskienė, I. Emotion or Reason? Heart as a Container in English and Lithuanian. *Kalbotyra* **2020**, *73*, 132–149. [CrossRef]
56. Grigaitė, U.; Aginskaitė, S.; Pedrosa, B.; Aluh, D.O.; Santos-Dias, M.; Silva, M.; Cardoso, G.; Caldas-de-Almeida, J.M. Experiences of women with disabilities in Lithuania when their gender, disability, domestic violence, and mental health services intertwine. *Disabil. Health J.* **2025**, *18*, 101837. [CrossRef]

sports MDPI

Article

Exploration of Commonly Used Tests to Assess Physical Qualities in Male, Adolescent Rugby League Players: Discriminative Validity Analyses and Correlations with Match Performance Metrics

Michael A. Carron [1,2,*], Aaron T. Scanlan [1] and Thomas M. Doering [1]

1 School of Health, Medical and Applied Sciences, Central Queensland University, Rockhampton, QLD 4702, Australia; a.scanlan@cqu.edu.au (A.T.S.); t.doering@cqu.edu.au (T.M.D.)
2 Health, Education, Lifestyle, and Performance (HELP) Laboratory, St Brendan's College, Yeppoon, QLD 4703, Australia
* Correspondence: m.carron@cqu.edu.au

Abstract

Tests assessing physical qualities are regularly used in youth rugby league teams for various functions. However, the utility of such tests is under-explored in this population. In this way, tests are commonly examined in terms of how well they can differentiate performances between groups that are expected to differ and how they relate to outcomes in actual competitive contexts. Therefore, the purpose of this exploratory study was to investigate the discriminative validity and relationships to match performance metrics of frequently used tests to assess physical qualities in male, adolescent rugby league players. Anthropometric (standing height and body mass) and fitness-related (20 m linear sprint, 505-Agility Test, L-run Test, medicine ball throw, countermovement jump, one-repetition maximum back squat, bench press, and prone row tests, and Multistage Fitness Test) physical qualities were measured using common tests in 42 players (16.1 ± 1.3 years). Test outcomes were compared between players in different age and positional groups for discriminative validity analyses. Relationships between test outcomes and match performance metrics gathered via global positioning system and video analysis were also determined. Compared to younger players (14–15 years), older players (16–18 years) had significantly better fitness-related physical qualities ($p < 0.05$, $d = -1.78$–1.66), but similar anthropometric qualities ($p > 0.05$, $d = -0.45$–0.20). Significant, *moderate* correlations ($p < 0.05$, $r = 0.56$–0.70) were found between (1) one-repetition maximum (1-RM) back squat and relative (per min) high-speed running distance and maximum velocity in matches; (2) 20-m sprint time and relative total distance; (3) 505-Agility Test time and relative line breaks; and (4) height and relative unsuccessful tackles. Consequently, commonly used fitness-related tests demonstrate discriminative validity in detecting differences between age groups, with standing height and the 1-RM back squat showing promising utility given their associations with key match metrics in adolescent rugby league players.

Keywords: development; paediatric; performance; GPS; video analysis; physical activity

1. Introduction

Team success during rugby league match-play is predicated on scoring more points via tries, conversions, and field goals than the opposing team. To achieve success in matches, rugby league players repeatedly engage in various physical acts during both offensive and defensive scenarios, including high-intensity runs, precise directional changes, and collisions [1]. In turn, performing these demanding tasks is heavily dependent on possessing well-developed anthropometric and fitness-related physical qualities, such as body mass, linear speed, change-of-direction (COD) speed, muscular power, muscular strength, and aerobic capacity [2]. Indeed, the importance placed on effectively developing these physical qualities has been previously documented among coaches working with adolescent rugby league players [3]. Accordingly, coaching staff of adolescent players in various settings, including schools, utilise periodic anthropometric and fitness testing to assess key physical qualities for various practical functions. For example, coaching staff may implement testing strategies to differentiate physical qualities between players for selection and/or other grouping purposes (i.e., discriminative validity) [4]. Moreover, coaching staff likely want to identify which physical qualities translate most strongly to match performance to assess player potential and readiness for competition [5].

Ensuring a test possesses adequate discriminative validity is essential before it is applied in practice for the purpose of differentiating between players. Specifically, discriminative validity refers to whether test outcomes that are unrelated between separate groups of players are actually not related [5]. Discriminative validity is typically assessed via determining differences in test outcomes between groups of players who are theorised to have varying physical qualities—for instance, differences between players competing at different playing levels or occupying different playing positions [5,6]. Accordingly, within school settings, players competing in different age-based divisions may be expected to possess different physical qualities given older players have likely accrued a higher training age with increased exposure to coaching [7] and may have undergone greater physical development via maturation during adolescence [7–9]. In this regard, differentiating between players of different age groups enables end-users to employ age-specific strategies, and identify underperforming players according to their level for appropriate intervention [10]. Importantly, limited research has been conducted on this topic involving adolescent rugby league players, with existing findings suggesting tests assessing physical qualities may hold strong discriminative validity when discerning performances between adult and adolescent age groups, but that this validity may weaken when discriminating between age groups specifically within adolescent players [6,10]. Likewise, players from different positional groups may possess different physical qualities given the varied competitive demands experienced by backs and forwards documented among male, adolescent rugby league players [10], with limited evidence on this topic strictly within this population. Consequently, current evidence on the discriminative validity of tests assessing physical qualities is limited among adolescent rugby league players, with more data needed for a definitive understanding to be established, particularly in schoolboy populations. Furthermore, existing research examining the validity of tests among adolescent players has not accounted for the most frequently adopted tests in the scientific literature, or key physical qualities, such as muscular strength, which has been shown to be important for match performance in male, senior rugby league players [11,12].

Regarding the application of tests assessing physical qualities, it is important to understand how well they relate to real sporting contexts and match performance [5] via correlation analyses between test outcomes and key match performance metrics [13]. In rugby league, global positioning system (GPS) technology and video-based analyses are predominantly used to quantify match performance [14]. However, existing correlation data between test outcomes and match performance are limited to male, senior rugby league players [11,15]. In this previous research, significant ($p < 0.05$) associations were documented between CMJ height and the number of times beating an opposing player

($r = 0.44$) [15], and between 3-RM bench press and back squat loads and tackling-related metrics ($r = 0.70$–0.77) [11]. However, no evidence exists regarding the relationship between commonly used tests to assess physical qualities and match performance metrics among adolescent rugby league players. Such population-specific data is crucial to elucidate, given that the physical qualities [6] and match demands [1] in adolescent rugby league players differ from senior players.

Therefore, the purpose of this exploratory study was to investigate the discriminative validity and relationships with match performance metrics of the most common tests and testing protocols used to measure physical qualities in male, adolescent rugby league players identified in the literature [8]. More precisely, this study sought to determine whether test outcomes: (1) demonstrate discriminative validity between players from different age (14–15 years vs. 16–18 years) and positional groups (backs vs. forwards); and (2) correlate with match performance metrics gathered using GPS and video-based technologies.

2. Methods

2.1. Subjects

Schoolboy, adolescent rugby league players ($n = 42$, 16.1 ± 1.3 years) were recruited from one secondary school in Australia to participate in this study. Players were eligible to participate if they were free from injury and illness and had completed at least six months of rugby league training (including field training and strength and conditioning) prior to testing. For discriminative validity analyses between age groups, players were eligible to participate if they had competed in the first-grade competition in either the 14–15 years age group ($n = 19$, 14.8 ± 0.4 years) or the 16–18 years age group ($n = 23$, 17.2 ± 0.7 years) across the 2023 schoolboy season. For comparisons between playing positions and correlation analyses, players were eligible to participate if they had competed in the first-grade 16–18 years competition (total sample, $n = 16$, 17.2 ± 0.7 years; backs, $n = 8$, 17.3 ± 0.9 years; forwards, $n = 8$, 17.2 ± 0.6 years) across the 2023 schoolboy season. Written informed consent was obtained from all players and their legal guardians before study commencement. Ethical approval for this study was obtained from the Human Research Ethics Committee (#23570).

2.2. Procedures

2.2.1. Study Overview

An observational, exploratory design was adopted to assess the discriminative validity and correlations to match performance metrics of the most common tests and testing protocols used to measure physical qualities in male, adolescent rugby league players identified in the literature [8].

2.2.2. Tests Assessing Physical Qualities

Table 1 outlines all tests and testing protocols used to assess physical qualities in the present study. Players completed three trials of the 20-m linear sprint, 505-Agility Test, L-run Test, MBT, and CMJ, and were permitted 60 s of passive standing rest between each trial, and between each test. For 1-RM tests, players were permitted 180 s of seated rest between each of five attempts. The best outcome from each trial/attempt was recorded for analyses in each test. The MSFT was completed only once. Tests were implemented by the lead researcher, who has demonstrated strong retest reliability in administering these tests in a similar cohort (intraclass correlation coefficient = 0.733–0.999; coefficient of variation = 0.05–4.02%) [16].

2.2.3. Discriminative Validity Assessment

To assess discriminative validity, test outcomes were compared between age groups (14–15 years vs. 16–18 years), and between positional groups (backs vs. forwards) strictly in the 16–18 years age group. The final sample size for each test within each group differed due to varied player availabilities across testing sessions (14–15 years: $n = 19$; 16–18 years: $n = 19$–23; backs: $n = 7$–8; forwards: $n = 6$–8). All tests were administered across two sessions separated by 48 h at the end of a 10-week periodised pre-season phase. Players were instructed to refrain from vigorous activity, consume their typical diet, and undertake their normal daily schedules (i.e., sleep, hydration, nutrition, and school participation) for 48 h prior to each testing session [17]. The first testing session consisted of standing height, body mass, Σ4 skinfold thickness, MBT, CMJ, and 1-RM bench press, back squat, and prone row tests, completed within an air-conditioned (~22 °C), indoor gym facility. The second testing session consisted of the 20-m linear sprint test, 505-Agility Test, L-run Test, and MSFT, completed on an outdoor, regulation (100 m in length and 68 m in width) rugby league field.

Table 1. The most common tests and testing protocols identified in the literature [8] and used in this study to assess physical qualities in male, adolescent rugby league players.

Test	Protocol
Standing height	A stadiometer (SECA 213, SECA Corp; Hamburg, Germany) was used; players stood upright with their head positioned in the Frankfurt plane and in bare feet. Standing height was measured to the nearest 0.1 cm.
Body mass	Electronic scales (SECA 813, SECA Corp; Hamburg, Germany) were used; players wore standard rugby league training attire in bare feet. Body mass was measured to the nearest 0.01 kg.
Σ4 skinfold thickness	Measurements taken at biceps, triceps, subscapular, and supra-illiac sites. Harpenden callipers (John Bull, British Indicators Ltd.; London, England) were used to assess skinfold thickness in accordance with The International Society for the Advancement of Kinanthropometry guidelines.
20 m linear sprint	Players stood in a split stance with toes on the leading foot aligned with marking tape 50 cm behind the first timing gate. Single-beam electronic timing gates (SmartSpeed Pro, Fusion Sport; Brisbane, Australia) were used to record 20 m sprint time to the nearest 0.001 s with gates set at 0 and 20 m.
505-Agility Test	Players stood in a split stance with toes on the leading foot aligned with marking tape at 0 m. Players sprinted 15 m forwards before contacting a marked line with their preferred foot and turning 180° back towards the start for a further 5 m. A single-beam electronic timing gate was positioned 10 m from the start to record performance time to the nearest 0.001 s across the 5 m directly before and after the turn.
L-run Test	Players stood in a split stance with toes on the leading foot aligned with marking tape 50 cm behind the timing gate. Players sprinted to a dome marker positioned 5 m in front, before turning 90° in the designated direction and sprinting to another dome marker positioned 5 m away and returning on that same course back to the starting point, while always moving in a forward direction and around the outside of the dome markers. Players completed the first turn at 90°, second turn at 180°, and final turn at 90°. A single-beam electronic timing gate was positioned at 0 m to record performance time to the nearest 0.001 s.
Multistage Fitness Test	The last successful shuttle completed in the MSFT was used to estimate maximal oxygen uptake ($mL \cdot kg^{-1} \cdot min^{-1}$) via a valid equation [18]. Players partook in repeated 20 m shuttle runs that progressively increased in pace as indicated by audio cues. Testing concluded when players failed to complete two successive shuttles successfully or stopped voluntarily.

Table 1. *Cont.*

Test	Protocol
Medicine ball throw	Players threw a 2 kg medicine ball (Celsius; Sydney, Australia) horizontally to achieve the maximum distance (m) possible. Players were seated on a flat bench with their back in contact with a wall, knees flexed to 90°, and feet contacting the floor. A measuring tape was fastened to the floor at the wall below the player when sitting on the bench with distance measured to the nearest 0.1 cm in a direct line to the initial floor marking made by the ball, which was covered in chalk.
Countermovement jump	Players jumped as high as possible with a countermovement phase to displace the highest vane possible on a yardstick device (Swift; Lismore, Australia). A self-selected squat depth and arm swing were permitted during the countermovement with jump height measured to the nearest 1 cm.
One-repetition maximum	One-repetition maximum tests for bench press, back squat, and prone row exercises were conducted, in this order, in accordance with procedures specified by the National Strength and Conditioning Association. All tests were conducted using a 2.13 m Olympic bar (20 kg). The bench press was performed maintaining a supine position on a flat bench with hands pronated using a hook grip. The back squat was performed using a high position and a pronated hook grip, with a self-selected footing, where players were required to squat until their thighs were parallel to the floor. The prone row was performed laying in a prone position on a flat bench, where players pulled the bar towards their body until making contact with the underside of the bench (12 cm thickness) using a pronated hook grip.

2.2.4. Correlations Between Test Outcomes and Match Performance Metrics

For correlation analyses, players completed the same tests across two separate sessions during the in-season phase immediately following a series of competitive matches. More precisely, players completed three consecutive weekly matches in weeks 12–15 of the 16-week in-season. Players then completed testing one week later in the same manner as described for discriminative validity analyses. The final sample size for each test differed due to varied player availabilities across testing sessions (n = 11–16). Various metrics were measured via GPS and video-based techniques during each match as performance indicators.

2.2.5. Global Positioning System Procedures and Metrics

Prior to each match, a microsensor device with GPS technology (Catapult S5, OptimEyeTM S5, firmware version 7.22, dimensions: 96 mm × 52 mm × 14 mm; mass: 67 g; Catapult Sports, Melbourne, Australia [which remained firmware version 7.22 for the duration of the study]) was placed securely inside a manufacturer-supplied vest (Catapult Sports; Melbourne, Australia) worn by each player throughout match-play. The same device was worn across all matches by the same player to avoid inter-device variability in outcomes [19]. Each device was turned on at least 20 min before the warm-up prior to matches, which were held on outdoor grassed fields with no obstructions to adequately synchronise with satellites. GPS technology was used to quantify peak velocity ($m \cdot s^{-1}$), total distance covered (m), and total distance covered performing high-speed running (HSR) > 5 $m \cdot s^{-1}$ (m). The cut-point of >5 $m \cdot s^{-1}$ chosen to detect HSR has been previously established across the literature in rugby league players [20]. Both total distance and total HSR distance were determined relative (per min) to the total individualised time each player was on the field accumulated across all matches. Total time on the field excluded half-time breaks and interchanged periods when not actively participating in matches, which were manually recorded by the lead researcher. Across the three matches combined, players had an average total time of 136.7 ± 41.5 min (range: 59.8–188.5 min) on the field.

2.2.6. Video-Based Procedures and Metrics

Video analyses were used to measure various match performance metrics adapted from an established rugby league video analysis framework [21]. Specifically, modifications to the original framework included development of attacking metrics that mirrored the descriptors provided for defensive metrics. For instance, descriptors provided in the original framework for a dominant tackle position on defence were modified for application to line contacts on offence. In this way, players undergoing line contacts were scored based on the position (e.g., positive) they occupied following line contact when in possession of the ball. While several metrics were provided in the original framework, the limited counts observed for some performance metrics (e.g., fends) precluded their inclusion, so only metrics that were performed at least once in a match by all players were included for analysis. Consequently, six performance metrics (Table 2) derived from video footage were included in this study. Video footage was recorded for each match by a professional videographer using a Sony HDC-4300 camcorder (60 frames per second at 1/120th shutter). Video footage was analysed and coded by the lead researcher using Hudl (Agile Sports Technologies Inc., Lincoln, NE, USA). Video-based performance metrics were recorded as frequency counts tabulated across all matches and made relative (per min) to total individualised time on the field for each player. All video-based performance metrics were analysed by the lead researcher, with 101 video clips (21 min and 53 s of footage) randomly analysed on a separate occasion to determine the intra-rater reliability across metrics (r = 0.823, Cohen's Kappa = 0.905).

Table 2. Video-based match performance metrics used in this study that were taken, or adapted, from an established rugby league video analysis framework [21].

Metric	Description
Defensive	
Accelerates into line for tackles	The tackler deliberately speeds up towards the line before making contact.
Unsuccessful tackles	The ball carrier was not held by the tackler; the ball or a ball-carrier's hand did not make contact with the ground or was not stopped from making further progress towards the try line.
Dominant tackles	The ball carrier was held by the tackler, and advanced backwards (negative progress) towards their own try line.
Offensive	
Dominant line contact	The ball carrier had gained territory towards the opposing try line during the contact phase.
Accelerates into line contact	The ball carrier deliberately speeds up towards the line before making contact.
Line break	The ball carrier passes what is determined as the defensive line and advances toward the opposition try line.

2.3. Statistical Analysis

Normality and homogeneity of variance for each test outcome variable were confirmed using the Shapiro–Wilk and Levene's tests. Accordingly, all data are reported descriptively as mean ± standard deviation (SD). For discriminative validity analyses, separate independent t-tests were used to detect significant differences in test outcomes between age groups and between positional groups. Magnitudes of differences for pairwise comparisons were determined as mean differences (with 95% confidence intervals [CI]) and Cohen's d effect size calculated using a published spreadsheet [22] (with 95% CI) with effect magnitudes interpreted as *trivial*, <0.20; *small*, 0.20–0.49; *medium*, 0.50–0.79; or *large*, $\geq$ 0.80 [23]. Pearson correlations (r) were also determined between test outcomes and match performance metrics. Correlation magnitudes were interpreted as *trivial* = <0.20, *small* = 0.20–0.49, *moderate* = 0.50–0.79, or *large* = $\geq$0.80 [23]. Statistical significance was accepted where alpha was <0.05. All analyses were conducted using IBM SPSS software (version 24 IBM Corp.; Armonk, NY, USA) or Microsoft Excel (version 15, Microsoft Corp.; Redmond, WA, USA).

3. Results

3.1. Discriminative Validity Analyses

Table 3 shows the descriptive data for test outcomes alongside discriminative validity analyses between age groups. The 16–18 years group performed significantly better in all fitness-related tests ($p \leq 0.05$, d = −1.78–1.66, *medium–large*), but not in anthropometric tests ($p > 0.05$, d = −0.45–0.20, *trivial–small*). Table 4 shows the descriptive data for test outcomes with discriminative validity analyses between positional groups. No significant differences ($p > 0.05$, d = −0.40–0.73, *trivial–large*) were evident for any test outcome between positional groups.

Table 3. Descriptive data and discriminative validity analyses of common tests used to assess physical qualities in male, adolescent rugby league players via comparisons between age groups.

Test	Age Group		p	Mean Difference (95% CI)	Cohen's d (95% CI)
	14–15 Years	16–18 Years			
Standing height (cm)	178.5 ± 4.9	179.4 ± 4.3	0.566	−0.85 (−3.80, 2.11)	0.20 (−0.43, 0.82)
Body mass (kg)	79.2 ± 10.5	78.2 ± 9.1	0.738	1.06 (−5.32, 7.45)	−0.10 (−0.73, 0.53)
Σ4 skinfolds (mm)	52.77 ± 9.46	48.47 ± 9.85	0.174	4.31 (−1.99, 10.60)	−0.45 (−1.08, 0.19)
20 m linear sprint (s)	3.125 ± 0.138	2.991 ± 0.137	0.003 *	0.13 (0.05, 0.22)	−0.98 (−1.62, −0.33)
505-Agility Test (s)	2.232 ± 0.152	2.331 ± 0.089	0.013 *	−0.10 (−0.18, −0.02)	0.81 (0.17, 1.45)
L-run test (s)	5.995 ± 0.268	5.585 ± 0.191	<0.001 *	0.41 (0.27, 0.56)	−1.78 (−2.51, −1.06)
MSFT (mL·kg^{-1}·min^{-1})	41.1 ± 5.3	45.3 ± 3.9	0.006 *	−4.21 (−7.14, −1.29)	0.91 (0.27, 1.56)
CMJ (cm)	53.06 ± 8.9	63.2 ± 5.7	<0.001 *	−10.12 (−14.74, −5.49)	1.38 (0.70, 2.06)
MBT (m)	6.79 ± 0.60	7.14 ± 0.54	0.049 *	−0.36 (−0.72, 0.00)	0.62 (−0.01, 1.24)
1-RM bench press (kg)	82.1 ± 13.9	100.5 ± 19.1	0.001 *	−18.33 (−28.94, −7.72)	1.09 (0.44, 1.75)
1-RM back squat (kg)	94.2 ± 17.1	125.7 ± 20.3	<0.001 *	−31.44 (−43.30, −19.58)	1.66 (0.96, 2.30)
1-RM prone pow (kg)	63.2 ± 12.2	82.2 ± 13.3	<0.001 *	−19.02 (−27.04, −11.00)	1.48 (0.80, 2.17)

Notes: Sample size for each test ranged between 39 and 42; data are presented as mean ± standard deviation; * denotes significant difference between groups. Abbreviations: CI, confidence intervals; MSFT, Multistage Fitness Test; MBT, medicine ball throw; CMJ, countermovement jump; 1-RM, one-repetition maximum.

Table 4. Descriptive data and discriminative validity analyses of common tests used to assess physical qualities in male, adolescent rugby league players via comparisons between positional groups.

Test	Positional Group		p	Mean Difference (95% CI)	Cohen's d (95% CI)
	Backs	Forwards			
Standing height (cm)	182.9 ± 3.0	183.4 ± 9.0	0.901	−0.43 (−7.78, 6.92)	0.08 (−0.97, 1.12)
Body mass (kg)	77.6 ± 7.3	85.3 ± 19.0	0.310	−7.692(−23.52, 8.13)	0.54 (−0.53, 1.60)
Σ4 skinfolds (mm)	46.82 ± 9.69	57.68 ± 17.86	0.168	−10.86 (−26.98, 5.26)	0.70 (−0.33, 1.84)
20 m linear sprint (s)	3.107 ± 0.237	3.080 ± 0.175	0.821	0.03 (−0.23, 0.29)	−0.13 (−1.22, 0.96)
505-Agility Test (s)	2.268 ± 0.159	2.227 ± 0.179	0.688	0.04 (−0.18, 0.26)	−0.24 (−1.38, 0.89)
L-run test (s)	5.691 ± 0.239	5.766 ± 0.337	0.658	−0.08 (−0.44, 0.29)	0.26 (−0.88, 1.39)
MSFT (mL·kg^{-1}·min^{-1})	47.9 ± 2.7	47.2 ± 2.9	0.698	0.67 (−3.12, 4.46)	−0.25 (−1.44, 0.94)
CMJ (cm)	63.88 ± 5.72	60.88 ± 9.09	0.443	3.00 (−5.15, 11.15)	−0.40 (−1.39, 0.59)
MBT (m)	6.53 ± 0.59	6.33 ± 0.99	0.640	0.20 (−0.70, 1.09)	−0.24 (−1.26, 0.78)
1-RM bench press (kg)	85.6 ± 4.2	94.3 ± 17.4	0.194	−8.66 (−22.33, 5.01)	0.67 (−0.38, 1.71)
1-RM back squat (kg)	118.8 ± 10.9	130.0 ± 20.0	0.200	−11.25 (−29.34, 6.84)	0.70 (−0.31, 1.71)
1-RM prone row (kg)	75.0 ± 9.3	83.8 ± 14.3	0.169	−8.75 (−21.69, 4.19)	0.73 (−0.28, 1.74)

Notes: Sample size for each test ranged between 11 and 16; data are presented as mean ± standard deviation. Abbreviations: CI, confidence intervals; MSFT, Multistage Fitness Test; MBT, medicine ball throw; CMJ, countermovement jump; 1-RM, one-repetition maximum.

3.2. Correlation Analyses

Table 5 shows the correlation coefficients between anthropometric qualities and match performance metrics. A significant, *moderate* correlation was found between standing height and unsuccessful tackles ($p < 0.05$, $r = 0.57$).

Table 5. Pearson correlations (with 95% confidence intervals) between common tests used to assess anthropometric qualities and match performance metrics in male, adolescent rugby league players.

Test	Match Performance Metric								
	Distance	HSR Distance	Peak Velocity	Accelerates into Tackles	Unsuccessful Tackles	Dominant Tackles	Dominant Line Contacts	Accelerations into Line	Line Breaks
Standing height	0.32 (−0.25, 0.73)	0.15 (−0.41, 0.63)	0.09 (−0.46, 0.60)	−0.01 (−0.54, 0.53)	0.57 (0.05, 0.84) *	−0.14 (−0.63, 0.42)	0.19 (−0.38, 0.65)	0.06 (−0.49, 0.57)	−0.02 (−0.54, 0.52)
Body mass	0.24 (−0.31, 0.67)	−0.07 (−0.56, 0.46)	0.00 (−0.51, 0.51)	0.21 (−0.34, 0.66)	0.32 (−0.23, 0.72)	−0.01 (−0.61, 0.49)	0.24 (−0.32, 0.67)	0.22 (−0.33, 0.66)	0.13 (−0.41, 0.60)
Σ4 skinfolds	−0.00 (−0.55, 0.55)	−0.54 (−0.84, 0.01)	−0.24 (−0.70, 0.36)	0.09 (−0.49, 0.61)	0.08 (−0.49, 0.61)	0.29 (−0.31, 0.73)	−0.19 (−0.67, 0.41)	−0.19 (−0.67, 0.41)	−0.06 (−0.59, 0.51)

Notes: * denotes significant correlation ($p < 0.05$). Unshaded cells indicate *trivial* relationships (r = <0.20), lightly shaded cells indicate *small* relationships (r = 0.20–0.49), and darker shaded cells indicate *moderate* relationships (r = 0.50–0.79). All performance metrics were determined relative to on-field time, except for peak velocity. Abbreviations: HSR, high-speed running.

Table 6 shows the correlation coefficients between fitness-related physical qualities and match performance metrics. Significant, moderate correlations were found between 1-RM back squat performance and relative HSR distance as well as peak velocity during matches ($p < 0.05$, r = 0.56–0.70). In addition, significant, moderate correlations were apparent between 20-m linear sprint time and relative total distance (r = 0.61), between 505-Agility Test time and relative number of line breaks (r = 0.60), and between standing height and relative number of times accelerating into tackles (r = 0.57).

Table 6. Pearson correlations (with 95% confidence intervals) between common tests used to assess fitness-related physical qualities and match performance metrics in male, adolescent rugby league players.

Test	Match Performance Metric								
	Distance	HSR Distance	Peak Velocity	Accelerates into Tackles	Unsuccessful tackles	Dominant Tackles	Dominant Line Contacts	Accelerations into Line	Line Breaks
20 m sprint	0.61 (0.09, 0.87) *	−0.30 (−0.73, 0.31)	−0.23 (−0.69, 0.37)	−0.12 (−0.63, 0.47)	0.36 (−0.24, 0.76)	−0.15 (−0.65, 0.43)	0.04 (−0.52, 0.58)	−0.13 (−0.64, 0.45)	0.20 (−0.40, 0.68)
505-Agility Test	0.32 (−0.32, 0.75)	0.38 (−0.25, 0.78)	0.27 (−0.36, 0.73)	−0.27 (−0.73, 0.36)	0.14 (−0.48, 0.66)	−0.22 (−0.71, 0.41)	0.49 (−0.11, 0.83)	0.51 (−0.10, 0.84)	0.60 (0.04, 0.87) *
L-run test	0.14 (−0.47, 0.66)	0.11 (−0.49, 0.65)	0.15 (−0.47, 0.67)	0.03 (−0.55, 0.60)	0.17 (−0.45, 0.68)	−0.22 (−0.71, 0.40)	0.44 (−0.18, 0.81)	0.45 (−0.17, 0.81)	−0.09 (−0.63, 0.51)
MSFT	−0.30 (−0.76, 0.37)	0.14 (−0.50, 0.68)	0.02 (−0.58, 0.62)	0.48 (−0.17, 0.84)	0.01 (−0.60, 0.61)	0.07 (−0.56, 0.64)	−0.13 (−0.68, 0.51)	−0.15 (−0.69, 0.49)	−0.21 (−0.72, 0.45)
CMJ	−0.09 (−0.55, 0.42)	0.24 (−0.29, 0.66)	−0.01 (−0.50, 0.49)	−0.39 (−0.74, 0.13)	−0.03 (−0.52, 0.47)	−0.48 (−0.79, 0.02)	−0.10 (−0.57, 0.42)	−0.08 (−0.55, 0.44)	−0.06 (−0.54, 0.45)
MBT	−0.02 (−0.53, 0.50)	0.30 (−0.26, 0.70)	0.30 (−0.25, 0.70)	−0.09 (−0.57, 0.45)	−0.13 (−0.60, 0.41)	−0.32 (−0.72, 0.23)	0.38 (−0.17, 0.75)	0.40 (−0.14, 0.76)	0.30 (−0.25, 0.70)
1-RM bench press	0.38 (−0.16, 0.75)	0.01 (−0.46, 0.57)	0.07 (−0.46, 0.57)	0.26 (−0.29, 0.68)	0.30 (−0.25, 0.70)	−0.21 (−0.65, 0.34)	0.33 (−0.22, 0.72)	0.26 (−0.29, 0.68)	0.06 (−0.47, 0.56)
1-RM back squat	0.06 (−0.49, 0.57)	0.56 (0.04, 0.84) *	0.70 (−0.27, 0.90) *	−0.10 (−0.60, 0.45)	0.11 (−0.44, 0.61)	−0.30 (−0.72, 0.28)	0.09 (−0.46, 0.59)	0.10 (−0.46, 0.60)	−0.11 (−0.60, 0.45)
1-RM prone row	0.03 (−0.48, 0.51)	−0.12 (−0.62, 0.35)	0.23 (−0.30, 0.65)	0.18 (−0.35, 0.62)	−0.02 (−0.51, 0.48)	−0.09 (−0.56, 0.43)	0.33 (−0.20, 0.71)	0.31 (−0.22, 0.70)	0.36 (−0.17, 0.72)

Notes: * denotes significant correlation (p <0.05). Unshaded cells indicate *trivial* relationships (r = <0.20), lightly shaded cells indicate *small* relationships (r = 0.20 –0.49), and darker shaded cells indicate *moderate* relationships (r = 0.50–0.79). All performance metrics were determined relative to on-field time, except for peak velocity. Abbreviations: HSR, high-speed running; MSFT, Multistage Fitness Test; CMJ, countermovement jump; MBT, medicine ball throw; 1-RM, one-repetition maximum.

4. Discussion

This exploratory study is the first to assess the discriminative validity of the most common tests and testing protocols used to measure physical qualities in male, adolescent rugby league players. Moreover, it is the first study to examine the correlations between physical qualities and match performance metrics derived from both GPS and video-based technologies in wider rugby league research. The main findings from this study are as follows: (1) fitness-related but not anthropometric tests differentiate physical qualities between 14–15 years and 16–18 years first-grade schoolboy, adolescent players; (2) similar physical qualities were apparent between backs and forwards in 16–18-year-old players using these tests; and (3) outcomes from standing height, 20-m sprint, 505-Agility Test, and 1-RM back squat assessments were significantly correlated with match performance metrics among schoolboy, adolescent rugby league players.

Findings from this study suggest that the most common tests and testing protocols used to measure fitness-related physical qualities in male, adolescent rugby league players identified in the literature [8] can be used to differentiate between age groups within a first-grade school context. In this way, most tests may hold suitable discriminative validity to apply for player selection purposes perhaps when factoring in various sources of evidence to decide on team line-ups or identifying potential players with suitable qualities. Moreover, given that these tests can differentiate between age groups within the school context, they may be used to assign players to appropriate playing levels. In this way, participating within an appropriate competition relative to their physical ability may increase player enjoyment, improve long-term retention in sports participation, and ultimately strengthen health outcomes in this population. Importantly, results from this study partially agree with those reported previously by Dobbin et al. [6], who found that the CMJ, MBT, and prone Yo-YoIRT differentiated (d = 0.23–1.00) between male youth (15.1 ± 0.8 years) and academy (17.5 ± 2.0 years) adolescent rugby league players, with superior results among the older age group. However, these authors [6] reported that 20-m linear sprint (d = −0.06) and COD speed (d = 0.10) tests did not differentiate between youth and academy players, but height and body mass were greater among academy players. Indeed, these contrasting results reported by Dobbin et al. [6] may be interrelated given that they speculated that the heavier mass among academy players may require greater relative force generation to overcome body inertia during the accelerative phases of the 20-m sprint and COD tests. Stemming from this supposition, variations in findings between studies may relate to the nature of the samples investigated, whereby players in the older age group in the study by Dobbin et al. [6] were heavier than the players in the present study of a similar age (87.5 ± 11.7 kg vs. 78.2 ± 9.1 kg), potentially explaining the discrepancies reported between age groups for linear and COD speed. Additionally, the present findings regarding better linear and COD speed among older players may be explained by the introduction of specialised resistance training among this group and not younger players in the school training environment examined. While the training regimes of the different age groups were not specified in previous research by Dobbin et al. [6], the introduction of specialised resistance training among older players in the present study likely enhanced their ability to rapidly generate force and overcome body inertia while improving technical capacities in linear sprinting and COD manoeuvres [24]. Importantly, differences in performance outcomes in the present study may stem from the older group (16–18 years) having undergone greater maturation than the younger group (14–15 years). Indeed, previous research has shown that adolescent rugby league players (in under-13, -14, and -15-year categories) with greater maturity demonstrate superior physical qualities than their less matured counterparts [7]. However, the present study is limited in this way, given maturation status was not assessed due to precluding factors prohibiting its measurement. Nonetheless, the findings from the present study are broadly consistent with the current body of evidence concerning expected differences in anthropometric and physical qualities among adolescents [6,25].

The findings from the current study show non-significant differences in test outcomes between positional groups within first-grade, 16–18 years players. However, it is worth noting that body mass, Σ4 skinfolds, and 1-RM bench press, back squat, and prone row performances were *moderately* ($d = 0.54$–0.73) greater in forwards compared to backs. Moreover, non-significant differences may be a reflection of the small sample in this analysis. As such, contrary to findings from the present study, Gabbett [10] found that male, adolescent rugby league players (16–18 years) in the prop position had significantly greater ($p < 0.05$) height, body mass, and Σ4 skinfold thickness, and significantly worse ($p < 0.05$) 10- and 20-m linear sprint times, COD performance time, and aerobic capacity than all other positions (i.e., hookers, halves, backrowers, and outside backs). However, Gabbett [10] examined sub-elite rugby league players who likely occupy certain positions more consistently throughout a season compared to players in school settings who may rotate between positions due to more generalised roles. As such, the similarities in physical qualities observed between backs and forwards in the present study may be explained by homogenous training strategies in school contexts which focus on general physical development across positional groups due to resource and time constraints among student-athletes [26]. Moreover, playing positions were categorised more broadly as backs and forwards in the present study compared to the more precise positional groups adopted by Gabbett [10], given that this approach has been used elsewhere [27] and maximises the sample size for each positional group due to the restricted recruitment within a single school in this study. In this way, broader positional grouping may diminish the extent of potential position-related differences in physical qualities.

This is the first study to examine correlations between tests assessing physical qualities and match performance metrics among schoolboy, adolescent rugby league players. Although most correlations were non-significant and *trivial*-to-*small* in magnitude, some notable relationships were observed. Specifically, correlation analyses revealed that players with greater maximal lower-body muscular strength, assessed via the 1-RM back squat test, tended to cover greater relative HSR distance and achieve greater peak velocities during matches. Although no studies have examined correlations between performance in the 1-RM back squat test and match performance metrics among schoolboy, adolescent rugby league players, Johnston et al. [28] showed that male, sub-elite rugby league players (19.2 ± 0.7 years) categorised as having a high 3-RM back squat performance covered greater HSR distances (>5.1 $m{\cdot}s^{-1}$) during matches than those categorised as having a low 3-RM back squat performance ($d = 1.00$, $p = 0.01$). Consequently, the collective findings across previous research [28] and from this study indicate that maximal lower-body muscular strength may be a critical correlate of intense running outputs in rugby league match-play among adolescent players. These findings might be reflective of the various adaptive mechanisms associated with resistance training to develop strength-related qualities such as enhanced musculotendinous stiffness, motor unit recruitment, and rate of force development [24]. Moreover, a significant, positive correlation was found between standing height and unsuccessful tackles. In this regard, the players investigated in the current study were likely undergoing varied rates of physical growth as commonly seen in the adolescent developmental phase [29]. Given that heightened rates of physical growth are associated with motor incoordination [29], players who were taller may have exhibited poorer movement execution and subsequently been more likely to miss tackles.

Regarding other notable relationships, a significant, positive correlation was found between 20-m sprint time and relative total distance, indicating that slower players cover greater distances per minute of play. Indeed, this finding suggests that the ability to maintain movement consistently across matches (i.e., high average speed) is not predicated on the ability to simply sprint quickly in a single bout, with previous research in male, professional rugby league players also suggesting other physical attributes (repeated-sprint ability, repeated-high-intensity running capacity, and aerobic capacity) have limited association with relative total distance in matches [30]. Consequently, a combination of physical qualities alongside other factors (e.g., technical and tactical elements) likely contributes to the relative total distance covered in rugby league match-play, which warrants further exploration. Similar to this finding, a significant, positive correlation was also found between 505-Agility Test time and relative line breaks, indicating that players with slower COD speed penetrate the defensive line more often. Indeed, this correlation indicates that executing line breaks may not overly depend on COD speed, which is partially supported by data reported during rugby union match-play demonstrating that most line breaks involve no change in running angle [31]. Alternatively, this result might relate to the design of the 505-Agility Test, whereby players are required to perform a pre-planned 180° turn that more resembles gaining position within the defensive line between tackles during matches. In contrast, a test involving a COD while maintaining movement in a forward direction (e.g., side-step manoeuvre) [32] and involving a reactive component (e.g., simulated opponent) [33] may better translate to player potential in breaking the defensive line during matches via responding to and evading opponents. As further reasoning, the correlations between 20-m sprint time and relative total distance, and between 505-Agility Test time and relative line breaks may have been impacted by the narrow dispersion in performance times observed in these tests (e.g., 20 m linear sprint: 3.094 ± 0.203 s, n = 42; 505-Agility Test: 2.282 ± 0.070 s, n = 41). This tight range in performance times across the sample in this study may have been due to similarly developed accelerative abilities among players in this population [34] and in turn could have influenced the correlations observed [35].

This study is not without limitations, which should be acknowledged when interpreting the findings. First, the correlation analysis involved a single schoolboy team with some players not able to complete all tests, limiting the final sample sizes. Small samples increase the likelihood of encountering statistical testing errors in correlation analyses, [36] which may have also contributed to the counterintuitive relationships observed between some variables. Moreover, many physical (and non-physical) aspects likely underpin the complex multifaceted nature of competitive performance in team sports [35,37], with their associations not necessarily being linear in shape. However, the small sample limited the number of datapoints that could have been used to uncover more complex relationships via multivariate and non-linear analyses in this study. Therefore, future work is encouraged to expand on the analyses conducted in this work by recruiting larger samples from multiple schools. Ultimately, interpretations of the correlational findings from this exploratory study should be carried out with caution—especially those that are counterintuitive—given that they are population-specific and limited to the small sample able to be recruited. Second, the sample comprised two different age groups both competing at a first-grade level, as opposed to different levels or grades within the same age group. However, given that players compete within their respective chronological age group in school settings, this approach was logical for the current study. Third, a selection of tests and testing protocols identified as the most commonly used to measure physical qualities in male, adolescent rugby league players in the literature [8] was utilised in this study. Consequently, contemporary tests gaining increased popularity in recent years such as the isometric midthigh pull [38], and tests implemented by industry bodies in practice but not the literature, were not included in this study. Future research should examine other tests in male, adolescent rugby league players as they become more widely adopted in research and practice.

Lastly, the video analysis was limited to six performance metrics due to the infrequent occurrence of the wider set of metrics during matches across the players investigated. This approach restricted the scope of performance analysis able to be performed from the original video analysis framework [21], and may have limited our ability to elucidate meaningful relationships between physical qualities and match performance.

Practical Applications

The present findings show that common tests used to measure fitness-related physical qualities in male, adolescent rugby league players appear to adequately differentiate between first-grade age groups (i.e., 14–15 and 16–18 years) in an Australian schoolboy context, meaning they may be useful for player assignment to appropriate playing levels, which, in turn, may enhance long-term retention and health outcomes in this population. The lack of differences in physical qualities between positional groups may be due to player development strategies within school settings being generic in nature rather than specific to playing position due to time and resource constraints. Consequently, it is probable that physical qualities may be rather homogenous across positional groups when players are categorised broadly as backs and forwards in a schoolboy, adolescent cohort. Furthermore, while findings from the present study show that most physical qualities did not significantly correlate with match performance metrics, some notable relationships were observed. In this way, the significant associations between 1-RM back squat performance and relative HSR distance as well as peak velocity during matches indicates that this test may provide outcomes that inform player potential to execute intense running demands in match-play. In turn, the significant correlation between standing height and unsuccessful tackles might inform player selection strategies for specific positions (e.g., those that require extensive tackling requirements) or encourage suitable technical intervention to circumnavigate this issue in taller players.

5. Conclusions

The most common tests and testing protocols used to measure fitness-related, but not anthropometric qualities, in male, adolescent rugby league players significantly differentiated between age groups in first-grade schoolboy players. Moreover, there were no significant differences in physical qualities between playing positions when generalised as backs and forwards, likely due to homogenous development strategies being applied across positional groups in school settings. In turn, while most correlations between physical qualities and match performance metrics were non-significant and *trivial*-to-*small* in magnitude, the 1-RM back squat test and standing height may hold some translation to match-play given their significant, *moderate* associations with performance metrics. Future studies involving larger samples of adolescent rugby league players across diverse school settings are encouraged to build upon these findings, contributing to a broader and more robust evidence base on this topic. Given the exploratory nature of the present study, the findings may help guide the generation of hypotheses in future confirmatory research with adequate error control [39]. In this regard, based on the present findings, future studies may hypothesise that commonly used tests assessing fitness-related physical qualities effectively discriminate between high-level (e.g., first-grade), adolescent, schoolboy rugby league players participating in different competitions predicated on chronological age (e.g., 14–15 years vs. 16–18 years). Moreover, it may be hypothesised that lower tackling proficiency is related with a taller standing height and that stronger 1-RM back squat performance is related with greater high-intensity running outputs in matches among players.

Author Contributions: All authors contributed equally to the current study. All authors contributed to the study's conception and design. Material preparation, data collection, and analysis were performed by the lead author. The first draft of the manuscript was written by the lead author. All authors reviewed and edited the manuscript, before approving the final manuscript. All authors have read and agreed to the published version of the manuscript.

Funding: The lead author is the recipient of a Scholarship and the recipient of an International Excellence Award administered by the host institution. This scholarship and award is titled the St Brendan's College and Central Queensland University Elevate Scholarship and International Excellence Award (100% tuition).

Institutional Review Board Statement: The study was conducted in accordance with the Declaration of Helsinki and approved by the Central Queensland University Human Research Ethics Committee (code: #23570; date: 19 May 2022).

Informed Consent Statement: Informed consent was obtained prior to conducting this original investigation.

Data Availability Statement: The original contributions presented in this study are included in the article. Further inquiries can be directed to the corresponding author.

Conflicts of Interest: The authors declare no conflicts of interest.

References

1. Gabbett, T.J.; Jenkins, D.G.; Abernethy, B. Relationships between physiological, anthropometric, and skill qualities and playing performance in professional rugby league players. *J. Sports Sci.* **2011**, *29*, 1655–1664. [CrossRef] [PubMed]
2. Gabbett, T.J.; Jenkins, D.G.; Abernethy, B. Correlates of tackling ability in high-performance rugby league players. *J. Strength. Cond. Res.* **2011**, *25*, 72–79. [CrossRef] [PubMed]
3. McCormack, S.; Jones, B.; Till, K. Training practices of academy rugby league and their alignment to physical qualities deemed important for current and future performance. *Int. J. Sports Sci. Coach.* **2020**, *15*, 512–525. [CrossRef]
4. Gabbett, T.; Kelly, J.; Ralph, S.; Driscoll, D. Physiological and anthropometric characteristics of junior elite and sub-elite rugby league players, with special reference to starters and non-starters. *J. Sci. Med. Sport.* **2009**, *12*, 215–222. [CrossRef]
5. Weakley, J.; Black, G.; McLaren, S.; Scantlebury, S.; Suchomel, T.J.; McMahon, E.; Watts, D.; Read, D.B. Testing and profiling athletes: Recommendations for test selection, implementation, and maximizing information. *Strength Cond. J.* **2024**, *46*, 159–179. [CrossRef]
6. Dobbin, N.; Highton, J.; Moss, S.L.; Twist, C. The discriminant validity of a standardized testing battery and its ability to differentiate anthropometric and physical characteristics between youth, academy, and senior professional rugby league players. *Int. J. Sports Physiol. Perform.* **2019**, *14*, 1110–1116. [CrossRef]
7. Till, K.; Cobley, S.; O'Hara, J.; Cooke, C.; Chapman, C. Considering maturation status and relative age in the longitudinal evaluation of junior rugby league players. *Scand. J. Med. Sci. Sports* **2014**, *24*, 569–576. [CrossRef]
8. Carron, M.A.; Scanlan, A.T.; Power, C.J.; Doering, T.M. What tests are used to assess the physical qualities of male, adolescent rugby league players? A systematic review of testing protocols and reported data across adolescent age groups. *Sports Med. Open* **2023**, *9*, 106. [CrossRef]
9. Malina, R.M.; Rogol, A.D.; Cumming, S.P.; Coelho e Silva, M.J.; Figueiredo, A.J. Biological maturation of youth athletes: Assessment and implications. *Br. J. Sports Med.* **2015**, *49*, 852–859. [CrossRef]
10. Gabbett, T.J. A comparison of physiological and anthropometric characteristics among playing positions in junior rugby league players. *Br. J. Sports Med.* **2005**, *39*, 675–680. [CrossRef]
11. Sparanza, M.J.; Gabbett, T.J.; Johnston, R.D.; Sheppart, J.M. Muscular strength and power correlates of tackling ability in semiprofessional rugby league players. *J. Strength. Cond. Res.* **2015**, *29*, 2071–2078. [CrossRef] [PubMed]
12. Gabbett, T.J.; Seibold, A.J. Relationship between tests of physical qualities, team selection, and physical match performance in semiprofessional rugby league players. *J. Strength. Cond. Res.* **2013**, *27*, 3259–3265. [CrossRef] [PubMed]
13. Andrade, C. Internal, external, and ecological validity in research design, conduct, and evaluation. *Ind. J. Psychol. Med.* **2018**, *40*, 498–499. [CrossRef] [PubMed]
14. Hausler, J.; Halaki, M.; Orr, R. Application of global positioning system and microsensor technology in competitive rugby league match-play: A systematic review. *Sports Med.* **2016**, *46*, 559–588. [CrossRef]
15. Gabbett, T.; Kelly, J.; Pezet, T. Relationship between physical fitness and playing ability in rugby league players. *J. Strength. Cond. Res.* **2007**, *21*, 1126–1133.

16. Carron, M.A.; Scanlan, A.T.; Doering, T.M. The restest reliability of common tests to assess physical qualities in adolescent rugby league players. *Pediatr. Exerc. Sci.* **2024**, *6*, 1–8. [CrossRef]
17. Gabbett, T.; Kelly, J.; Sheppard, J. Speed, change of direction speed, and reactive agility of rugby league players. *Strength Cond. J.* **2008**, *22*, 174–181. [CrossRef]
18. Ramsbottom, R.; Brewer, J.; Williams, C. A progressive shuttle run test to estimate maximal oxygen uptake. *Br. J. Sports Med.* **1988**, *22*, 141–144. [CrossRef]
19. Jennings, D.; Cormack, S.; Coutts, A.J.; Boyd, L.J.; Aughey, R.J. Variability of GPS units for measuring distance in team sport movements. *Int. J. Sports Physiol. Perform.* **2010**, *5*, 565–569. [CrossRef]
20. Glassbrook, D.; Doyle, T.; Alderson, J.; Fuller, J. The demands of professional rugby league match-play: A meta-analysis. *Sports Med. Open* **2019**, *5*, 24. [CrossRef]
21. Hopkinson, M.; Bissas, A.; Nicholson, G.; Beggs, C.; Scantlebury, S.; Hendricks, S.; Jones, B. A video analysis framework for the rugby league tackle. *Sci. Med. Footb.* **2022**, *6*, 15–28. [CrossRef] [PubMed]
22. Lakens, D. Calculating and reporting effect sizes to facilitate cumulative science: A practical primer for t-tests and ANOVAs. *Front. Psychol.* **2013**, *4*, 863. [CrossRef] [PubMed]
23. Cohen, J. *Statistical Power Analysis for the Behavioral Sciences*, 2nd ed.; Routledge: London, UK, 1988.
24. Swinton, P.A.; Lloyd, R.; Keogh, J.W.; Agouris, I.; Stewart, A.D. Regression models of sprint, vertical jump, and change of direction performance. *J. Strength. Cond. Res.* **2014**, *28*, 1839–1848. [CrossRef]
25. Dobbin, N. Sprint mechanical properties of professional rugby league players according to playing standard, age and position, and the association with key physical characteristics. *J. Sports Med. Phys. Fit.* **2022**, *62*, 467–475. [CrossRef] [PubMed]
26. Usher, W. National Rugby League's Junior Performance and Participation Initiatives: Evaluating Stratergies. 2019. Available online: https://research-repository.griffith.edu.au/server/api/core/bitstreams/86046b66-43c8-4064-a9bb-035de58d69b3/content (accessed on 1 May 2025).
27. Till, K.; Tester, E.; Jones, B.; Emmonds, S.; Fahey, J.; Cooke, C. Anthropometric and physical characteristics of English academy rugby league players. *J. Strength. Cond. Res.* **2014**, *28*, 319–327. [CrossRef]
28. Johnston, R.D.; Gabbett, T.J.; Jenkins, D.G.; Hulin, B.T. Influence of physical qualities on post-match fatigue in rugby league players. *J. Sci. Med. Sport* **2015**, *18*, 209–213. [CrossRef]
29. Brown, K.A.; Patel, D.R.; Darmawan, D. Participation in sports in relation to adolescent growth and development. *Transl. Pediatr.* **2017**, *6*, 150–159. [CrossRef]
30. Gabbett, T.J.; Stein, J.G.; Kemp, J.G.; Lorenzen, C. Relationship between tests of physical qualities and physical match performance in elite rugby league players. *J. Strength. Cond. Res.* **2013**, *27*, 1539–1545. [CrossRef]
31. den Hollander, S.; Brown, J.; Lambert, M.; Treu, P.; Hendricks, S. Skills associated with line breaks in elite rugby union. *J. Sports Sci. Med.* **2016**, *15*, 501–508.
32. Wheeler, K.W.; Askew, C.D.; Sayers, M.G. Effective attacking strategies in rugby union. *Eur. J. Sport Sci.* **2010**, *10*, 237–242. [CrossRef]
33. Sheppard, J.M.; Young, W.B. Agility literature review: Classifications, training and testing. *J. Sports Sci.* **2006**, *24*, 919–932. [CrossRef] [PubMed]
34. Dobbin, N.; Hunwicks, R.; Highton, J.; Twist, C. A reliable testing battery for assessing physical qualities of elite academy rugby league players. *J. Strength. Cond. Res.* **2018**, *32*, 3232–3238. [CrossRef] [PubMed]
35. Janse, R.J.; Hoekstra, T.; Jager, K.J.; Zoccali, C.; Tripepi, G.; Dekker, F.W.; van Diepen, M. Conducting correlation analysis: Important limitations and pitfalls. *Clin. Kidney J.* **2021**, *14*, 2332–2337. [CrossRef] [PubMed]
36. Mujika, I.; Halson, S.; Burke, L.M.; Balgue, G.; Farrow, D. An intergrated, multifactorial approach to periodization for optimal performance in individual and team sprots. *Int. J. Sports Physiol. Perform.* **2018**, *13*, 538–561. [CrossRef]
37. Aggarwal, R.; Ranganthan, P. Common pitfalls in statistical analysis: The use of correlation techniques. *Perspect. Clin. Res.* **2016**, *7*, 187–190.
38. Martin, E.A.; Beckham, G.K. Isometric mid-thigh pull performance in rugby players: A systematic literature review. *J. Funct. Morphol. Kinesiol.* **2020**, *5*, 91. [CrossRef]
39. Ditroilo, M.; Mesquida, C.; Abt, G.; Lakens, D. Exploratory research in sport and exercise science: Perceptions, challenges, and reccomendations. *J. Sports Sci.* **2025**, *43*, 12. [CrossRef]

sports

MDPI

Article

Understanding External Peak Demands in Elite vs. Non-Elite Male Basketball Players

Yoel Antoranz [1], Enrique Alonso-Pérez-Chao [2,3], Carlos Mª Tejero-González [1], Hugo Salazar [4,5], Juan del Campo-Vecino [1] and Sergio L. Jiménez-Sáiz [6,*]

1 Department of Physical Education, Sport and Human Movement, Universidad Autónoma de Madrid, 28049 Madrid, Spain; yoel.antoranz@estudiante.uam.es (Y.A.); carlos.tejero@uam.es (C.M.T.-G.); juan.delcampo@uam.es (J.d.C.-V.)
2 Department of Physical Activity and Sports Science, University Alfonso X el Sabio, 28691 Villanueva de la Cañada, Spain; ealonsoperezchao@gmail.com
3 Department of Real Madrid Graduate School, Faculty of Medicine, Health and Sports, Universidad Europea de Madrid, 28670 Madrid, Spain
4 Department of Physical Activity and Sports Sciences, Faculty of Health Sciences, Euneiz University, 01013 Vitoria-Gasteiz, Spain; hsalazar002@gmail.com
5 Faculty of Education and Sport, University of Basque Country (UPV/EHU), 48940 Vitoria-Gasteiz, Spain
6 Sport Sciences Research Centre, Faculty of Education & Sport Sciences and Interdisciplinary Studies, Universidad Rey Juan Carlos, 28942 Fuenlabrada, Spain
* Correspondence: sergio.jimenez.saiz@urjc.es

Abstract: Background: Understanding the physical demands of basketball at different competitive levels is essential for optimizing training and performance. While elite players are often assumed to experience the highest physical loads, evidence comparing peak external demands (PDs) between elite and non-elite athletes using time-window analysis is limited. Therefore, the aim of this study was to examine how player level (Elite vs. Non-Elite) influences the external PDs experienced by male basketball players. Methods: This study examined PlayerLoad™ (PL) PDs in elite (n = 10) and non-elite (n = 11) male basketball players during the 2023–2024 season. Players were monitored using inertial measurement units (IMUs) during official and friendly matches (elite = 8 games; non-elite = 29 games). Peak PL values were computed using rolling averages across 30-s, 1-min, and 3-min time windows. Linear mixed-effects models were employed to examine differences between groups, adjusting for age and match nature. A secondary analysis was carried out including only friendly matches. Results: Non-elite players exhibited significantly higher PL PDs across all the time windows ($p < 0.001$), with effect sizes ranging from small to very large in the main analysis (ES = −0.41 to −2.11) and from very large to extremely large in the secondary analysis (ES = −2.68 to −5.06). Differences were more pronounced in longer durations. These results suggest that non-elite athletes sustain higher physical loads, possibly due to less efficient movement patterns and lower tactical regulation. Conclusions: Elite players display lower peak external loads than their non-elite counterparts, likely due to superior cognitive, tactical, and perceptual abilities that enhance movement economy. Training programs should incorporate tasks that combine physical intensity with decision-making demands to foster efficiency and potentially reduce injury risk.

Keywords: most demanding scenarios; PlayerLoad; team sport; worst-case scenarios; physical demands; accelerometry; athlete health management

1. Introduction

Basketball is an intermittent sport [1,2], characterized by alternating periods of high-intensity actions and low-intensity or recovery phases [2]. The measurement and monitoring of these actions have evolved significantly over time. Initially, these were conducted through observational methods such as time–motion analysis, which required significant time and was prone to human error [1,3]. Currently, devices such as Electronic Performance Tracking Systems, which typically encompass inertial movement units (IMUs) and/or local positioning systems (LPS), are primarily used in indoor sports, as they provide valid and reliable measurements for estimating external load, particularly peak demands (PDs) or the most demanding scenarios (MDS) [3,4]. External load refers to the measurement of variables such as the number of jumps, the number and intensity of accelerations and decelerations, changes of direction, player load, distance covered at different intensities, or walking distance [4–6].

Basketball performance can be influenced by numerous technical, tactical, physical, mental, and psychological factors, as well as contextual elements such as the quality of the opponent, competition schedule, athlete recovery, diet, or sleep quality [7–12]. Therefore, competitive demands may also be affected by these variables.

The analysis of PDs is conducted using moving time windows, which help prevent underestimation of the values reached, as can happen when using average values [13,14]. The rolling average method is preferred, as it ensures no peak load is overlooked, unlike the fixed-window method [15]. Measurement windows can be either short (15, 30, 45 s, or 1 min), which helps identify peak load values, or long (2, 3, 4, or 5 min), allowing for comparisons with average values or training tasks [4].

An intriguing avenue for future PD analysis could be to explore whether it is influenced by the type of competition or the athlete's level. Athlete-level classification can vary depending on criteria or population distribution, with current classifications including world-class, elite (international level), highly trained (national level), trained (local level), or recreational (active) [16]. Elite athletes are those who compete at the international level, representing approximately 0.0025% of the global population [16]. Other authors argue that athlete classification does not conform to fixed categories but rather represents a continuum in which various variables must be considered [17]. For the purpose of this study, the classification system described first will be used.

Despite its relevance, few studies in the literature have examined differences in external load—particularly PDs and MDS—between elite and non-elite basketball players. From a traditional standpoint, studies using time–motion analysis typically employ average values to compare elite and non-elite athletes. The work by Scanlan et al., which compared Australian basketball players, concluded that elite athletes experience higher external load demands during a game, although load peaks or "bursts" are greater in sub-elite athletes, with longer recovery times [18]. A similar study conducted with rugby players showed that average values are similar for both elite and semi-elite athletes, although elite players exhibit higher load demands during the first half [19]. Finally, a study conducted with basketball players compared fast break actions (successful transition from defense to offense) found no significant differences in the actions or their effectiveness between elite and sub-elite players [20].

In contrast, two studies have gone beyond time–motion analysis [21,22]. The first, which employed LPS for measurement, compared basketball players in different positions (guard, forward, and center) from an elite-level team and a semi-elite team. However, they did not use measurement windows but instead relied on average values. The results showed that sub-elite athletes performed more accelerations and decelerations than elite athletes, although, for forward players, the maximum accelerations and decelerations were of greater intensity at the elite level [21].

The second study compared two elite-level teams: one competing in the Euroleague (the top-tier European competition) and the other in the EuroCup (the second-tier European competition). Using IMU devices and measurement windows of 30 s, 60 s, and 180 s, the study found that the EuroCup team (a lower elite level) reached higher peak values in accelerations, decelerations, changes of direction, and jumps, with effect sizes ranging from 0.34 to 1.15 [22].

Moreover, understanding these physical demands has crucial implications for athlete health management. Higher external peak demands have been linked to increased injury risk [23], highlighting the importance of tailoring training to match competition demands and reduce the potential for overuse injuries and long-term physical deterioration.

As noted, there is a scarcity of research examining PDs in elite versus non-elite basketball players. Therefore, the aim of this study was to examine how player level (elite vs. non-elite) influences the external PDs experienced by male basketball players across three specific time frames (30-s, 1min, and 3-min). Based on the reviewed literature [18,20–22], we hypothesize that elite athletes will exhibit lower PD values compared to non-elite athletes.

2. Methods

2.1. Participants

The study sample consisted of two distinct teams, each representing differing levels of athletic proficiency. A convenience sampling method was employed, recruiting participants based on accessibility from both teams. One team comprised elite players engaged in competitive matches within the EuroLeague and Spain's First Basketball Division. The elite players (n = 10, mean ± standard deviation: age: 25.9 ± 3.2 years, height: 197.5 ± 8.1 cm, body mass: 91.8 ± 4.3 kg) were closely monitored throughout 8 friendly games during the 2023–2024 season. In contrast, the non-elite team consisted of players competing in the Spanish 4th Division. These non-elite players (n = 11, mean ± standard deviation: age: 20.72 ± 4.2 years, height: 196.2 ± 9.9 cm, body mass: 88.8 ± 14.3 kg) were monitored during 26 official and 3 friendly games in the same season, 2023–2024. All participants signed a written informed consent form prior to participation, and the study was approved by the local ethics committee (CEI-137-2955), in accordance with the Declaration of Helsinki.

For inclusion in the final analysis, game samples required players to have completed at least 5 min of device-recorded playing time in each game. In this way, playing time included all stoppages, such as free throws, fouls, and out-of-bounds, but excluded break periods between quarters, time-outs, or moments when players were substituted [24]. Consequently, five game samples were excluded for failing to meet this criterion. Furthermore, players were only considered eligible for inclusion in the study if they had participated in at least 50% of the games (elite team = 4/8 games and non-elite team = 15/29 games). Moreover, data from any game were excluded from the analysis if a player withdrew due to injury or if the device battery was depleted during play. Overall, 300 game samples (elite = 56 samples; non-elite = 244 samples) across the 21 male players (elite = 10 players; non-elite = 11 players) were included in the analyses.

2.2. Design

This observational comparative study analyzed and compared PlayerLoad™ (PL) between elite and non-elite male basketball players during official and friendly matches over the 2023–2024 season. Throughout the games, each player utilized a monitoring device (S7, Catapult Sports, Melbourne, Australia) discretely integrated into a tailored neoprene vest beneath standard playing attire and positioned accurately over the upper thoracic spine, between the scapulae [25]. Each device was equipped with microsensor technology, including an accelerometer (±16 g, 100 Hz), a magnetometer (±4900 µT, 100 Hz), and a gyroscope (up to 2000 deg/s, 100 Hz). To ensure consistency and minimize potential output discrepancies, each player continued to use the same device throughout the entire study period [26].

2.3. Physical Variables

PDs for PL were computed in absolute terms and were extracted individually for each player across various time windows (30-s, 1-min, and 3-min). PL is a variable that represents, in arbitrary units, the sum of movement occurring in each of the planes of motion during physical activity, taking into account the squared rates of change in acceleration for each of those planes [27]. These PDs were directly derived from the Catapult software (version 3.11.0). Peak values were identified using rolling averages, which offer a more accurate approach for measuring peak demands compared to fixed time interval methods [15] and have been previously applied in basketball research [4]. Subsequently, the extracted PDs were inputted into customized Microsoft Excel spreadsheets (version 16.0, Microsoft Corporation, Redmond, WA, USA) for further analysis.

2.4. Statistical Analysis

All data analyzed were presented as mean values, along with their standard deviation and coefficient of variation. To assess differences in PL PDs between groups, linear mixed models were employed, followed by Bonferroni post hoc analysis. A separate linear mixed model was conducted for each time window (30-s, 1-min, 3-min), incorporating player level (elite or non-elite) as a fixed factor, the athlete as a random factor, and the interaction between player level and athlete also as a random factor. Age was included as a covariate in all models to control for its effect, added both as a fixed-effects factor and as a random-effects factor in its interaction with player level and the athlete. To account for the effect of match nature, it was introduced as an adjustment variable, treated as a dummy variable, with a value of 0 for friendly matches and 1 for official matches. This variable was included as a fixed-effects factor and as a random-effects factor in the interaction. In all models, PL was considered the independent variable. Given the nature of linear mixed models, normality was assessed post hoc through the examination of residuals [28]. This assumption was verified using the Shapiro–Wilk and Kolmogorov–Smirnov tests.

To quantify the difference between groups for each time window, effect size (ES) was calculated using Cohen's d. Descriptive statistics, linear mixed-effects models, and Bonferroni post hoc comparisons were performed using the SPSS software (Version 28, IBM Corp., Armonk, NY, USA), with statistical significance set at 95% ($p < 0.05$). Effect sizes and their corresponding 95% confidence intervals (CIs) were computed using a custom-configured Excel spreadsheet (Version 16.0, Microsoft Corp., Redmond, WA, USA). ES values were interpreted as trivial (≤0.20), small (0.21–0.60), moderate (0.61–1.20), large (1.21–2.00), very large (2.01–4.00), and extremely large (>4.00) [29] and were analyzed in conjunction with their 95% CIs to assess the precision and potential triviality of the estimates. If the 95% CI overlapped zero, the ES was interpreted as trivial, regardless of the point estimate.

Although the variable match nature was used as an adjustment variable to control for its effect, given that official matches for the elite team were unavailable, a second complementary analysis was conducted. In this second analysis, only friendly matches were considered: 8 matches from the elite team and 3 from the non-elite team. Similarly, player level was introduced as a fixed effect, the athlete as a random-effects factor, and age as a covariate or adjustment variable, following the steps previously described.

3. Results

The findings of the primary analysis are displayed through tables and figures. The mean, standard deviation, and coefficient of variation are shown for each group and measurement window in the PL variable (see Table 1 and Figure 1). Additionally, the differences found in the comparisons for each measurement window are presented, along with the effect size and CIs for each (See Table 2 and Figure 2).

Table 1. Descriptive statistics for each group and their corresponding time windows.

Descriptive											
30-s Time Window				1-min Time Window				3-min Time Window			
Variable	Group	Mean ± SD	%CV	Variable	Group	Mean ± SD	%CV	Variable	Group	Mean ± SD	%CV
Player Load (PL)	Elite	13.59 ± 1.15	9.2%	Player Load (PL)	Elite	22.38 ± 2.02	10.0%	Player Load (PL)	Elite	43.54 ± 6.41	15.7%
	Non-elite	19.39 ± 2.95	14.9%		Non-elite	42.71 ± 6.27	14.5%		Non-elite	62.80 ± 9.65	15.1%

Note: Age adjusted to 21.48 years. Match nature adjusted as dummy variable to 0.73 (0 = non-official; 1 = official).

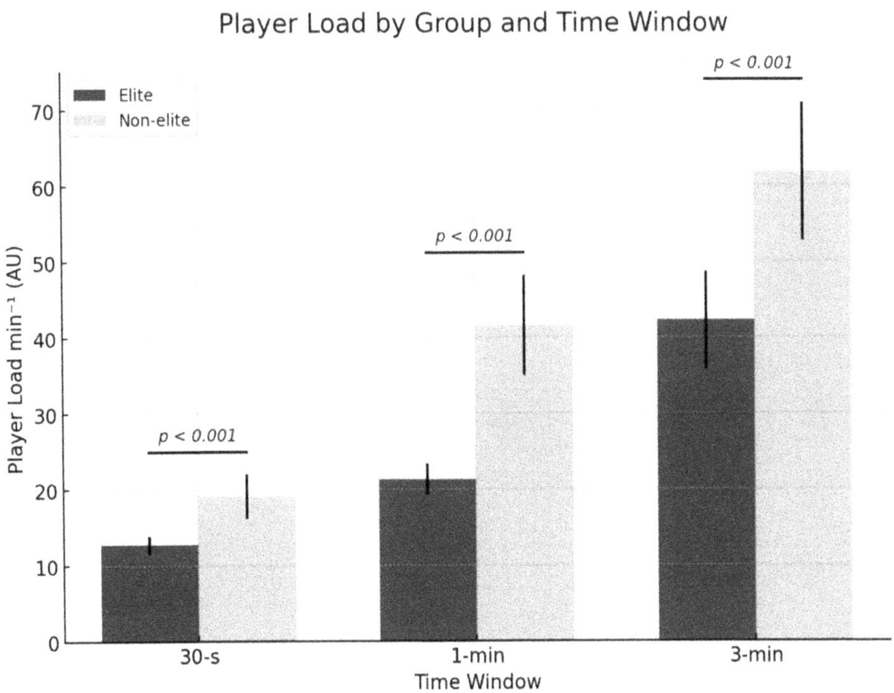

Figure 1. Player load values for each group across the time windows. The p-values for between-group differences are shown for each time window, derived from linear mixed models adjusted for age and match nature.

Significant differences were found ($p < 0.001$) for all analyses conducted, with ES ranging from −0.41 to −2.11 (small—very large) and 95% CIs ranging from −0.70 to −0.12 (30-s), −1.78 to −1.16 (1-min), and −2.44 to −1.77 (3-min). All ESs were accompanied by 95% CIs, and none of them overlapped zero, indicating meaningful group differences.

The results of the secondary analysis are presented in the form of tables. For the PL variable, the mean, standard deviation, and coefficient of variation are reported for each group and measurement window (see Table 3). Furthermore, the results of the pairwise comparisons across the different measurement windows are displayed, including the effect sizes and corresponding CIs (see Table 4).

Table 2. Comparison of the differences and effect size between groups for each of the time windows.

Mean Differences and Effect Sizes			
Sample Duration	**Effect Size**	**95%CI**	***p***
30-s time window, elite vs. non-elite	−0.41	−0.70, −0.12	<0.001
1-min time window, elite vs. non-elite	−1.47	−1.78, −1.16	<0.001
3-min time window, elite vs. non-elite	−2.11	−2.44, −1.77	<0.001

Note: Age adjusted to 21.48 years. Match nature adjusted as dummy variable to 0.73 (0 = non-official; 1 = official).

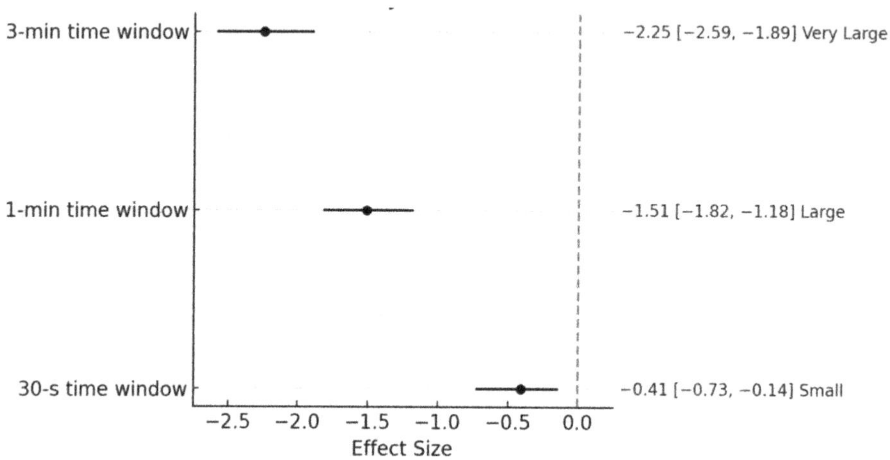

Figure 2. Effect size and CIs for each of the time windows.

Table 3. Descriptive statistics for each group and their corresponding measurement windows in the non-official match sample.

Descriptive (Non-Official Matches)											
30-s Time Window				1-min Time Window				3-min Time Window			
Variable	**Group**	**Mean ± SD**	**%CV**	**Variable**	**Group**	**Mean ± SD**	**%CV**	**Variable**	**Group**	**Mean ± SD**	**%CV**
Player Load (PL)	Elite	12.73 ± 1.15	9.2%	Player Load (PL)	Elite	21.28 ± 2.02	10.0%	Player Load (PL)	Elite	42.18 ± 6.41	15.7%
	Non-elite	19.05 ± 2.93	14.9%		Non-elite	41.51 ± 6.58	15.1%		Non-elite	61.76 ± 9.06	15.1%

Note: Age adjusted to 24.09 years.

All analyses revealed statistically significant differences ($p < 0.001$), with effect sizes ranging from −2.68 to −5.06, indicating large to extremely large effects and 95% CIs ranging from −3.27 to −2.03 (30-s), −5.91 to −4.11 (1-min), and −4.03 to −2.64 (3-min).

Table 4. Comparison of the differences and effect sizes between groups for each of the measurement windows in the friendly match sample.

Mean Differences and Effect Sizes (Non-Official Matches)			
Sample Duration	**Effect Size**	**95%CI**	***p***
30-s time window, elite vs. non-elite	−2.68	−3.27, −2.03	<0.001
1-min time window, elite vs. non-elite	−5.06	−5.91, −4.11	<0.001
3-min time window, elite vs. non-elite	−3.36	−4.03, −2.64	<0.001

Note: Age adjusted to 24.09 years.

4. Discussion

This study aimed to investigate the influence of player level (elite vs. non-elite) on the external PDs encountered by male basketball players over three distinct time windows (30-s, 1-min, and 3-min). Statistically significant differences were observed between the groups for the PL variable across all three time windows. Given the significant age difference between the elite (25.9 $\pm$ 3.2) and non-elite groups (20.72 $\pm$ 4.2; $p < 0.05$), age was included as a covariate to control for its potential effect on the findings. Furthermore, match nature was statistically adjusted as a dummy variable.

As previously noted, significant differences were found regarding the differences between groups. Across all measurement windows, the peak PL values attained by the non-elite athletes were higher than those of the elite players. In the longer windows, the differences were meaningfully greater, as indicated by the magnitude of the ES and 95% CIs not overlapping zero. The ES for the 30-s time window was qualitatively considered small (ES = −0.41; 95% CI = −0.70 to −0.12, $p < 0.001$). For the 1 min window, the ES was considered large (ES = −1.47; 95% CI = −1.78 to −1.16, $p < 0.001$). Finally, for the 3-min window, the ES obtained was the highest in qualitative terms, rated as very large (ES = −2.11; 95% CI = −2.44 to −1.77, $p < 0.001$). These findings have been related to those obtained in the study by Trapero et al. [21], in which it was observed that non-elite athletes performed a higher number of accelerations and decelerations compared to the elite group [21]. However, as mentioned in the introduction, that study did not use time windows but rather average values.

The only study we found that used time windows was the one comparing two elite teams, in this case, one from the Euroleague and the other from the Eurocup, with the latter being of a lower competitive level. In this study, despite both teams being elite-level, the Eurocup team achieved higher PDs in various peak and average physical performance variables compared to the Euroleague team [22], which aligns with the data obtained in the present study.

Regarding the other studies previously mentioned, which were analyzed using time–motion analysis, comparisons are somewhat more challenging due to the different measurement methodologies employed and the absence of time windows. In contrast to the findings of Scanlan et al. [18], where elite athletes exhibited higher external load values, our results showed lower PDs among elite players. However, although the comparison is neither precise nor reliable, it appears that the external load peaks, or "bursts", as referred to by the authors, were higher in the sub-elite group [18], which seems to correlate with the higher PDs recorded by the mobile windows system used in the present study, which does not rely on average values in order to avoid underestimating external load. Finally, the results obtained by Sirotic et al. and Conte et al., in this case, with rugby players, could not be confirmed, as no significant differences were found between the elite and semi-elite groups in the variables analyzed [19,20].

Considering only the results from the second analysis, which involved friendly matches, the results follow the same trend. Across all three time windows, non-elite athletes reached significantly higher PL values ($p < 0.001$) compared to the elite group, with effect sizes greater than those observed in the main analysis. The values were considered very large for the 30-s (ES = −2.68; 95% CI = −3.27 to −2.03, $p < 0.001$) and 3-min (ES = −3.36; 95% CI = −4.03 to −2.64, $p < 0.001$) windows and extremely large for the 1-min window (ES = −5.06; 95% CI = −5.91 to −4.11, $p < 0.001$). These results may seem surprising, as it is often assumed that higher-level athletes will demonstrate superior physical performance. Firstly, it is important to consider that the complexity of a sport or activity does not depend solely on physical and/or coordinative factors [30]. Marteniuk's model suggests that sports skill depends on perceptual ability, decision-making, and execution [30–32]. Therefore, physical factors would only address one part of these three critical elements. As mentioned in a previous study, higher-level competitive athletes did not exhibit higher PDs compared to those of lower levels or those with less significance within their team [33]. In relation to Marteniuk's model, authors such as Sampaio et al. [34] have suggested that physical performance is influenced by cognitive factors. Higher-level athletes, in this case, NBA All-Star players, performed slower or less intense actions, but ones that were more effective, allowing them to better manage their physical resources by making better decisions during the game [34]. Decision-making and cognitive factors are fundamental to agility in team sports [35] and, more specifically, in basketball [36]. A study conducted with Australian state-level players concluded that decision-making time and response speed were critical determinants of athletes' agility and that training methods aimed at improving decision-making should be integrated into training programs [37].

Elite male basketball players exhibit superior psychological skills, such as selective attention, memory retention, and environmental analysis, compared to lower-level athletes [38]. A study that conducted an electroencephalographic analysis comparing elite and non-elite basketball players concluded that cortical activity was greater in the elite group [39]. However, this study was performed under highly controlled conditions, analyzing only free-throw shooting, a closed skill. Thus, its findings cannot be directly extrapolated to our research context.

Various studies conducted on other sports also reveal cognitive differences between elite and non-elite athletes. Two trials involving young football players found that elite-level athletes exhibit better inhibitory control, greater cognitive flexibility, and enhanced metacognition, as well as superior self-regulation, which enables them to be more effective in their environment by being aware of their skills and weaknesses [40,41]. Finally, a study on hockey players indicated that the primary difference between elite and non-elite athletes was related to procedural knowledge, specifically in terms of decision-making and positioning [42].

Therefore, one possible hypothesis for the difference between elite and non-elite players in the present study is related to cognitive and decision-making factors. These factors can be developed and enhanced through tasks such as small-sided games—by modifying rules, playing spaces, or the number of players—or through more analytical drills, such as change-of-direction (COD) exercises involving responses to visual or auditory stimuli [43].

While physical and conditional factors are relevant, achieving higher PDs does not appear to be the sole determinant of high sports performance. In this study, the data show that ES is greater in longer windows. That is, as the measurement duration increases, the difference in PL becomes more pronounced. This finding aligns with previous observations.

In shorter time windows, if a high or very high-intensity action is required, leading to increased demands, the difference between teams of different levels may not be as evident. However, this is not necessary throughout the entire game, as basketball is an intermittent sport [1,2]. Consequently, in periods of longer duration, greater differences may emerge, given that elite players might more effectively select the moments when such intensity should be applied, as opposed to other instances where it may not be necessary, thereby optimizing their movement efficiency [34]. Considering all the aforementioned aspects, it is crucial to acknowledge that basketball performance is multifactorial. It may depend on physical, technical, tactical, and contextual factors—such as the opponent's characteristics or the game situation—as well as mental and psychological components [12]. Therefore, analyses that consider only limited factors should be interpreted with caution.

From an injury prevention standpoint, optimizing physical and cognitive efficiency could lower the cumulative mechanical load on musculoskeletal structures, thereby reducing the incidence of acute and overuse injuries [23,44]. Training approaches that combine high-intensity demands with decision-making tasks not only enhance performance but may also serve as a protective strategy for athlete longevity and well-being. Structured load management, individualized intensity monitoring, and task-specific perceptual–cognitive training should be emphasized as part of comprehensive athlete health programs.

From a health perspective, improving efficiency in high-intensity actions could help reduce cumulative fatigue and lower injury risk, especially in congested competition periods. Emphasizing cognitive–perceptual training alongside physical development may foster more intelligent effort distribution, preserving athletes' well-being while sustaining high performance levels.

Two important limitations should be considered. First, the number of monitored games differed substantially between the groups: the non-elite team participated in 29 matches, while the elite team played only 8. Second, all games for the elite group were friendly matches, while the non-elite group played a mix of official and friendly matches. Although statistical adjustments were made for match nature, these differences could still contribute to the observed effects and should be taken into account when interpreting the results. Despite this, a previous study conducted on a non-elite sample found no significant differences in PL PDs between official and non-official matches [33]. However, there is limited scientific evidence analyzing this phenomenon from the perspective of MDS. Consequently, a second analysis was conducted exclusively with friendly matches from both teams to validate the proposed hypothesis. Another limitation of the present study is the mean age difference between the two samples. To address this, the possible effect of age on PL was considered by including it as an adjustment variable in the statistical analysis. Finally, an additional limitation is the lack of access to positional data (such as distances covered or running speeds), as well as the absence of analysis of other inertial parameters, including jumping actions. Such data would provide greater insight into the demands of external load and offer a more comprehensive comparison of the results.

These findings highlight the importance of tailoring training programs not merely to maximize physical output but to optimize it within the context of game situations. Coaches and strength and conditioning professionals should integrate high-intensity tasks with decision-making challenges—such as small-sided games or agility drills with perceptual stimuli—to better replicate the demands experienced during competition. Since elite players appear to regulate their efforts more efficiently across longer durations, promoting movement economy and tactical awareness may be more beneficial than simply increasing training volume or intensity.

From a future research perspective, it would be interesting to conduct this type of analysis by including other related variables, such as accelerations, decelerations, jumps, and running at different intensities. This could provide greater depth and richness to both the data and the understanding of this area of research. Furthermore, it would be advisable to monitor several different teams, both elite and non-elite, over more than one season, including both friendly and official matches.

5. Conclusions

The peak demands of PL experienced by non-elite players are significantly higher compared to elite players. While physical factors play a crucial role, they are not the most decisive in athletic performance. Higher-level athletes, in this case, elite players, appear to be more efficient or economical in executing high-intensity actions, making better decisions. This effect was more pronounced in longer windows. In the primary analysis, the 1-min window showed a large effect (ES = −1.47; 95% CI = −1.78 to −1.16, $p < 0.001$), and the 3-min window a very large effect (ES = −2.11; 95% CI = −2.44 to −1.77, $p < 0.001$), compared to the shortest window (30-s, ES = −0.41; 95% CI = −0.70 to −0.12, $p < 0.001$). In the secondary analysis (friendly matches only), effect sizes were even greater: ES = −5.06 for the 1-min window (95% CI = −5.91 to −4.11), ES = −3.36 for the 3-min window (95% CI = −4.03 to −2.64), and ES = −2.68 for the 30-s window (95% CI = −3.27 to −2.03), all with $p < 0.001$.

The primary practical application of this study lies in the value of understanding these data. Performance improvement does not stem solely from increasing the workload imposed on athletes. Training tasks should incorporate exercises that combine high intensity with decision-making and perceptual abilities in real-game situations. This approach enables athletes to optimize their movement efficiency, reducing physical exertion while achieving better results. Incorporating these strategies into athlete development programs may not only boost performance but also contribute to injury prevention and long-term health maintenance, ultimately supporting sustainable elite careers.

Author Contributions: Y.A., E.A.-P.-C., C.M.T.-G., H.S., J.d.C.-V. and S.L.J.-S.; methodology, Y.A., E.A.-P.-C. and S.L.J.-S.; formal analysis, Y.A., C.M.T.-G., H.S. and E.A.-P.-C.; investigation, Y.A., E.A.-P.-C., C.M.T.-G., H.S., J.d.C.-V. and S.L.J.-S.; writing—original draft preparation, Y.A., E.A.-P.-C. and S.L.J.-S.; writing—review and editing, E.A.-P.-C., C.M.T.-G., H.S., J.d.C.-V. and S.L.J.-S.; supervision, E.A.-P.-C. and S.L.J.-S. All authors have read and agreed to the published version of the manuscript.

Funding: This research received no external funding.

Institutional Review Board Statement: This study was conducted in accordance with the Declaration of Helsinki and approved by the Research Ethics Committee of the Autonomous University of Madrid (CEI-137-2955), the approval date is 18 April 2024.

Informed Consent Statement: All participants provided written informed consent prior to inclusion in this study.

Data Availability Statement: The original contributions presented in this study are included in the article; further inquiries can be directed to the authors.

Conflicts of Interest: The authors declare no conflicts of interest.

References

1. Taylor, J.B.; Wright, A.A.; Dischiavi, S.L.; Townsend, M.A.; Marmon, A.R. Activity Demands During Multi-Directional Team Sports: A Systematic Review. *Sports Med.* **2017**, *47*, 2533–2551. [CrossRef]
2. Sosa, C.; Lorenzo, A.; Trapero, J.; Ribas, C.; Alonso, E.; Jimenez, S.L. Specific Absolute Velocity Thresholds during Male Basketball Games Using Local Positional System; Differences between Age Categories. *Appl. Sci.* **2021**, *11*, 4390. [CrossRef]
3. Fox, J.L.; Scanlan, A.T.; Stanton, R. A Review of Player Monitoring Approaches in Basketball: Current Trends and Future Directions. *J. Strength Cond. Res.* **2017**, *31*, 2021–2029. [CrossRef]

4. Alonso Pérez-Chao, E.; Portes, R.; Gómez, M.Á.; Parmar, N.; Lorenzo, A.; Jiménez-Sáiz, S.L. A Narrative Review of the Most Demanding Scenarios in Basketball: Current Trends and Future Directions. *J. Hum. Kinet.* **2023**, *89*, 231–245. [CrossRef]
5. Halson, S.L. Monitoring Training Load to Understand Fatigue in Athletes. *Sports Med.* **2014**, *44*, 139. [CrossRef]
6. Gonçalves, G.; Neta, P.; Ribeiro, J.; Guimaraes, E. Internal and External Loads during Formal Training and Competition, Physical Capacities, and Technical Skills in Youth Basketball: A Comparison between Starters and Rotation Players. *J. Hum. Kinet.* **2025**, *96*, 53–67. [CrossRef]
7. Williams, C.; Rollo, I. Carbohydrate Nutrition and Team Sport Performance. *Sports Med.* **2015**, *45*, 13–22. [CrossRef]
8. Calleja-González, J.; Terrados, N.; Mielgo-Ayuso, J.; Delextrat, A.; Jukic, I.; Vaquera, A.; Torres, L.; Schelling, X.; Stojanovic, M.; Ostojic, S.M. Evidence-Based Post-Exercise Recovery Strategies in Basketball. *Physician Sportsmed.* **2016**, *44*, 74–78. [CrossRef]
9. Ochoa-Lácar, J.; Singh, M.; Bird, S.P.; Charest, J.; Huyghe, T.; Calleja-González, J. How Sleep Affects Recovery and Performance in Basketball: A Systematic Review. *Brain Sci.* **2022**, *12*, 1570. [CrossRef]
10. França, C.; Gomes, B.B.; Gouveia, É.R.; Ihle, A.; Coelho-E-silva, M.J. The Jump Shot Performance in Youth Basketball: A Systematic Review. *Int. J. Environ. Res. Public Health* **2021**, *18*, 1–12. [CrossRef]
11. Esteves, P.T.; Mikolajec, K.; Schelling, X.; Sampaio, J. Basketball Performance Is Affected by the Schedule Congestion: NBA Back-to-Backs under the Microscope. *Eur. J. Sport. Sci.* **2021**, *21*, 26–35. [CrossRef]
12. Cao, S.; Geok, S.K.; Roslan, S.; Sun, H.; Lam, S.K.; Qian, S. Mental Fatigue and Basketball Performance: A Systematic Review. *Front. Psychol.* **2022**, *12*, 819081. [CrossRef]
13. Fox, J.L.; Conte, D.; Stanton, R.; McLean, B.; Scanlan, A.T. The Application of Accelerometer-Derived Moving Averages to Quantify Peak Demands in Basketball: A Comparison of Sample Duration, Playing Role, and Session Type. *J. Strength Cond. Res.* **2021**, *35*, S58–S63. [CrossRef]
14. Alonso, E.; Miranda, N.; Zhang, S.; Sosa, C.; Trapero, J.; Lorenzo, J.; Lorenzo, A. Peak Match Demands in Young Basketball Players: Approach and Applications. *Int. J. Environ. Res. Public Health* **2020**, *17*, 2256. [CrossRef]
15. Cunningham, D.J.; Shearer, D.A.; Carter, N.; Drawer, S.; Pollard, B.; Bennett, M.; Eager, R.; Cook, C.J.; Farrell, J.; Russell, M.; et al. Assessing Worst Case Scenarios in Movement Demands Derived from Global Positioning Systems during International Rugby Union Matches: Rolling Averages versus Fixed Length Epochs. *PLoS ONE* **2018**, *13*, e0195197. [CrossRef]
16. McKay, A.K.A.; Stellingwerff, T.; Smith, E.S.; Martin, D.T.; Mujika, I.; Goosey-Tolfrey, V.L.; Sheppard, J.; Burke, L.M. Defining Training and Performance Caliber: A Participant Classification Framework. *Int. J. Sports Physiol. Perform.* **2022**, *17*, 317–331. [CrossRef]
17. Swann, C.; Moran, A.; Piggott, D. Defining Elite Athletes: Issues in the Study of Expert Performance in Sport Psychology. *Psychol. Sport. Exerc.* **2015**, *16*, 3–14. [CrossRef]
18. Scanlan, A.; Dascombe, B.; Reaburn, P. A Comparison of the Activity Demands of Elite and Sub-Elite Australian Men's Basketball Competition. *J. Sports Sci.* **2011**, *29*, 1153–1160. [CrossRef]
19. Sirotic, A.C.; Coutts, A.J.; Knowles, H.; Catterick, C. A Comparison of Match Demands between Elite and Semi-Elite Rugby League Competition. *J. Sports Sci.* **2009**, *27*, 203–211. [CrossRef]
20. Conte, D.; Favero, T.G.; Niederhausen, M.; Capranica, L.; Tessitore, A. Determinants of the Effectiveness of Fast Break Actions in Elite and Sub-Elite Italian Men's Basketball Games. *Biol. Sport.* **2017**, *34*, 177–183. [CrossRef]
21. Trapero, J.; Trapero, J.; Sosa, C.; Zhang, S.; Portes, R.; Gómez-Ruano, M.Á.; Bonal, J.; Jiménez, S.L.; Lorenzo, A. Comparison of the Movement Characteristics Based on Position-Specific Between Semi-Elite and Elite Basketball Players. *Rev. de Psicol. Del Deporte* **2019**, *28*, 140–145.
22. Ujaković, F.; Salazar, H.; Pleša, J.; Svilar, L. Elite Basketball Game External Load Varies Between Different Teams and Competition. *Kinesiology* **2024**, *56*, 145–152. [CrossRef]
23. Gabbett, T.J. The Training-Injury Prevention Paradox: Should Athletes Be Training Smarter and Harder? *Br. J. Sports Med.* **2016**, *50*, 273–280. [CrossRef] [PubMed]
24. Alonso Pérez-Chao, E.; Lorenzo, A.; Scanlan, A.; Lisboa, P.; Sosa, C.; Gómez, M.Á. Higher Playing Times Accumulated Across Entire Games and Prior to Intense Passages Reduce the Peak Demands Reached by Elite, Junior, Male Basketball Players. *Am. J. Mens. Health* **2021**, *15*. [CrossRef]
25. Hodder, R.W.; Ball, K.A.; Serpiello, F.R. Criterion Validity of Catapult ClearSky T6 Local Positioning System for Measuring Inter-Unit Distance. *Sensors* **2020**, *20*, 3693. [CrossRef]
26. Castellano, J.; Casamichana, D.; Calleja-González, J.; Román, J.S.; Ostojic, S.M. Reliability and Accuracy of 10 Hz GPS Devices for Short-Distance Exercise. *J. Sports Sci. Med.* **2011**, *10*, 233.
27. Bredt, S.D.G.T.; Chagas, M.H.; Peixoto, G.H.; Menzel, H.J.; Andrade, A.G.P.D. Understanding Player Load: Meanings and Limitations. *J. Hum. Kinet.* **2020**, *71*, 5. [CrossRef]
28. Barr, D.J.; Levy, R.; Scheepers, C.; Tily, H.J. Random Effects Structure for Confirmatory Hypothesis Testing: Keep It Maximal. *J. Mem. Lang.* **2013**, *68*, 255–278. [CrossRef]

29. Hopkins, W.G.; Marshall, S.W.; Batterham, A.M.; Hanin, J. Progressive Statistics for Studies in Sports Medicine and Exercise Science. *Med. Sci. Sports Exerc.* **2009**, *41*, 3–12. [CrossRef]
30. Broadbent, D.P.; Causer, J.; Williams, A.M.; Ford, P.R. Perceptual-Cognitive Skill Training and Its Transfer to Expert Performance in the Field: Future Research Directions. *Eur. J. Sport. Sci.* **2015**, *15*, 322–331. [CrossRef]
31. Marteniuk, R.G. Cognitive Information Processes in Motor Short-Term Memory and Movement Production. In *Motor Control*; Elsevier: Amsterdam, The Netherlands, 1976; pp. 175–186. [CrossRef]
32. Hayes, K.C.; Marteniuk, R.G. Dimensions of Motor Task Complexity. In *Motor Control*; Elsevier: Amsterdam, The Netherlands, 1976; pp. 201–228. [CrossRef]
33. Antoranz, Y.; Alonso-Pérez-Chao, E.; Tejero-González, C.M.; Salazar, H.; Del Campo-Vecino, J.; Jiménez-Sáiz, S.L. Exploring External Peak Demands: The Influence of Contextual Factors on Male Basketball Players. *Appl. Sci.* **2024**, *14*, 10542. [CrossRef]
34. Sampaio, J.; McGarry, T.; Calleja-González, J.; Jiménez Sáiz, S.; Schelling I Del Alcázar, X.; Balciunas, M. Exploring Game Performance in the National Basketball Association Using Player Tracking Data. *PLoS ONE* **2015**, *10*, e0132894. [CrossRef] [PubMed]
35. Paul, D.J.; Gabbett, T.J.; Nassis, G.P. Agility in Team Sports: Testing, Training and Factors Affecting Performance. *Sports Med.* **2016**, *46*, 421–442. [CrossRef] [PubMed]
36. Morrison, M.; Martin, D.T.; Talpey, S.; Scanlan, A.T.; Delaney, J.; Halson, S.L.; Weakley, J. A Systematic Review on Fitness Testing in Adult Male Basketball Players: Tests Adopted, Characteristics Reported and Recommendations for Practice. *Sports Med.* **2022**, *52*, 1491. [CrossRef]
37. Scanlan, A.; Humphries, B.; Tucker, P.S.; Dalbo, V. The Influence of Physical and Cognitive Factors on Reactive Agility Performance in Men Basketball Players. *J. Sports Sci.* **2014**, *32*, 367–374. [CrossRef]
38. Kioumourtzoglou, E.; Derri, V.; Tzetzis, G.; Theodorakis, Y. Cognitive, Perceptual, and Motor Abilities in Skilled Basketball Performance. *Percept. Mot. Ski.* **1998**, *86*, 771–786. [CrossRef]
39. Keshvari, F.; Farsi, A.; Abdoli, B. Investigating the EEG Profile of Elite and Non-Elite Players in the Basketball Free Throw Task. *J. Mot. Behav.* **2024**, *56*, 91–102. [CrossRef]
40. Huijgen, B.C.H.; Leemhuis, S.; Kok, N.M.; Verburgh, L.; Oosterlaan, J.; Elferink-Gemser, M.T.; Visscher, C. Cognitive Functions in Elite and Sub-Elite Youth Soccer Players Aged 13 to 17 Years. *PLoS ONE* **2015**, *10*, e0144580. [CrossRef]
41. Toering, T.T.; Elferink-Gemser, M.T.; Jordet, G.; Visscher, C. Self-Regulation and Performance Level of Elite and Non-Elite Youth Soccer Players. *J. Sports Sci.* **2009**, *27*, 1509–1517. [CrossRef]
42. Elferink-Gemser, M.T.; Kannekens, R.; Lyons, J.; Tromp, Y.; Visscher, C. Knowing What to Do and Doing It: Differences in Self-Assessed Tactical Skills of Regional, Sub-Elite, and Elite Youth Field Hockey Players. *J. Sports Sci.* **2010**, *28*, 521–528. [CrossRef]
43. Serpell, B.G.; Young, W.B.; Ford, M. Are the Perceptual and Decision-Making Components of Agility Trainable? A Preliminary Investigation. *J. Strength Cond. Res.* **2011**, *25*, 1240–1248. [CrossRef]
44. Soligard, T.; Schwellnus, M.; Alonso, J.M.; Bahr, R.; Clarsen, B.; Dijkstra, H.P.; Gabbett, T.; Gleeson, M.; Hägglund, M.; Hutchinson, M.R.; et al. How Much Is Too Much? (Part 1) International Olympic Committee Consensus Statement on Load in Sport and Risk of Injury. *Br. J. Sports Med.* **2016**, *50*, 1030–1041. [CrossRef]

sports

MDPI

Article

Mental Fatigue Impairs Temporal Perceptual Prediction: A Study on Boxing Performance Across Skill Levels

Chang-Hong Wu [1,*], Yi Yang [2], Xia Xu [3], Ning Wang [1], Qiao Li [1], Lu Geng [1] and Shan-Jun Bao [4,*]

[1] School of Sports Medicine, Wuhan Sports University, Wuhan 430079, China; 2022410170@whsu.edu.cn (N.W.); 2022410168@whsu.edu.cn (Q.L.); 2021420010@whsu.edu.cn (L.G.)
[2] Sports Drug Rehabilitation Center of Physical Education, Southwest University, Chongqing 400715, China; yangyi99@email.swu.edu.cn
[3] Key Lab of Exercise Training and Monitoring, Wuhan Sports University, Wuhan 430079, China; xuxia@whsu.edu.cn
[4] School of Sports Training, Wuhan Sports University, Wuhan 430079, China
* Correspondence: 2021420013@whsu.edu.cn (C.-H.W.); 2004075@whsu.edu.cn (S.-J.B.)

Abstract: Objective: This study investigated the impact of mental fatigue on the temporal perceptual prediction of action recognition among boxers of different skill levels. Methods: A mixed experimental design of two (groups: Mental Fatigue Expert Group and Mental Fatigue Novice Group) × two (technique types: attack and defense) × three (time shields: −80 ms, −40 ms, and action start) was implemented. Twenty expert and novice boxers participated in this study. Mental fatigue was induced using a 45-min Stroop paradigm, and the effects were assessed using the VAS, Brog-20, BRUMS-F, and BRUMS-V. The experimental procedure for time perception was developed using E-prime 3.0, incorporating 36 videos depicting various attack and defense techniques, and reaction time and accuracy were recorded. Results: (1) A significant main effect on reaction time (RT) was observed ($F(1,38) = 5.97$, $p < 0.05$, $\eta^2 = 0.14$) but not on accuracy (ACC), suggesting a pronounced influence of mental fatigue on novice boxers' temporal perceptual prediction in action recognition; (2) significant main effects of skill types were noted in both RT ($F(1,38) = 9.03$, $p < 0.05$, $\eta^2 = 0.19$) and ACC ($F(1,38) = 18.496$, $p < 0.05$, $\eta^2 = 0.327$), indicating disparities in the recognition of offensive and defensive skills under mental fatigue; (3) temporal shielding significantly influenced both RT ($F(2,76) = 31.42$, $p < 0.05$, $\eta^2 = 0.45$) and ACC ($F(2,76) = 125.727$, $p < 0.05$, $\eta^2 = 0.768$), with −80 ms showing a lower RT and ACC compared to −40 ms and action initiation; (4) second-order interaction effects were present in both RT ($F(2,76) = 9.85$, $p < 0.05$, $\eta^2 = 0.21$) and ACC ($F(2,76) = 8.773$, $p < 0.05$, $\eta^2 = 0.188$), with the RT interaction suggesting a negative impact on perceptual prediction at −80 ms and a faster offensive RT than defensive RT. The ACC interaction indicated that under mental fatigue, −40 ms approached and exceeded −80 ms in both offensive and defensive actions, with higher ACC in offense than defense; and (5) a third-order interaction effect among group, technique type, and time shielding on RT ($F(2,76) = 3.92$, $p < 0.05$, $\eta^2 = 0.09$) suggests that mental fatigue more significantly affects novice defensive technique RT than offensive technique. Conclusions: (1) The 45-min Stroop task effectively induced mental fatigue. (2) Mental fatigue negatively impacts both expert and novice boxers, with a more pronounced effect on experts' defensive skills. (3) The −40 ms time perception is crucial for predicting action recognition as it approaches action initiation.

Keywords: mental fatigue; boxing performance; time perceptual prediction; motion recognition

 https://doi.org/10.3390/sports13050154

1. Introduction

Boxing demands high temporal and spatial perception from athletes, as they are required to make swift judgments and decisions in the field to capitalize on the best attack opportunities [1]. This process involves the perception, identification, and analysis of relevant environmental information, followed by the selection of appropriate responses by athletes [2]. Perception prediction, which utilizes partial or prior information to anticipate unknown events and facilitate information processing, plays a crucial role in this process and is vital for athletes in open sports [3]. Therefore, perceptual prediction in sports can be understood as the process where expert athletes selectively attend to more relevant cues to limit the amount of information processed, thereby generating a perceptual representation. This is essentially a process of making predictions based on limited cues [4]. These include action recognition, visual searches, and predictive processes [5]. Time and spatial perception predictions are specialized perceptions in boxing, in which athletes must coordinate their movements in both dimensions to optimize their athletic performance [6]. In boxing, it is not only crucial to emphasize strength and skill but also to possess accurate movement recognition to quickly identify an opponent's technical moves and tactical intentions during a match. Action recognition is closely related to perceptual prediction. Action recognition can provide important informational support for perceptual prediction, helping athletes more accurately predict their opponents' movements and the outcomes of competitions, thereby enhancing their performance [7]. Both offensive and defensive decisions are critical in boxing; effective offensive techniques, such as straight punches, swing punches, or hook punches, can score points or even knock down an opponent, while effective defensive techniques, such as dodging, blocking, or sliding, can help athletes avoid the opponent's scoring and provide opportunities for effective counterattacks [8].

Mental fatigue is a psychobiological state resulting from prolonged high-intensity cognitive activity [9]. This state is characterized by exhaustion and discomfort due to mental stress and emotional strain [10]. According to the resource depletion theory, mental fatigue arises from the exhaustion of available cognitive resources due to the continuous allocation of attention [11]. It not only induces subjective feelings of fatigue and lack of energy but also adversely affects an individual's physical and mental health, including emotional, cognitive, motivational, and physiological aspects [10]. In sports, mental fatigue can impair cognitive performance [12], such as perceptual prediction abilities, thereby negatively impacting athletic performance [13]. Specifically, studies have shown that mental fatigue can lead to significant declines in perceptual prediction, which is crucial for high-performance athletes [11]. Particularly after high-intensity training and competition, athletes undergo significant psychological preparation and adjustment, increasing the burden on their mental resources [14]. Consequently, mental fatigue may affect an individual's neurobiological state, thereby influencing perceptual prediction abilities, including temporal and spatial perception prediction abilities. Time perception prediction, defined in conjunction with previous research [15], involves the use of incomplete sensory information to infer and predict the duration and sequence of objective events in sports. Time masking can be used to predict time perception [16]. This technique involves blocking video materials at different time points to form an observation period and obtain a progressive series, revealing perceptual prediction information during key time periods. The selection of temporal shielding points (−80 ms, −40 ms, and action initiation) was based on empirical evidence from perceptual prediction studies in combat sports. Specifically, −80 ms represents the early preparatory phase of an opponent's action, allowing for the assessment of anticipatory skills, while −40 ms captures the critical window for rapid decision-making just prior to movement execution [4]. These time points align with the temporal dynamics of boxing, where split-second adjustments are required to predict and counter offensive and defensive maneuvers. According to a previous study [17], in terms of time shielding, −80 ms and −40 ms can demonstrate differences between expert athletes and novices. In the context of boxing, previous research has highlighted the importance of accurate movement recognition for effective offensive and defensive actions [1]. However, the specific impact of mental fatigue on the temporal perceptual prediction of action recognition in boxing remains less explored.

Despite these findings, several gaps remain in the literature. First, most existing studies have focused on the effects of mental fatigue on general cognitive performance, with limited research specifically addressing its impact on time perception prediction in sports like boxing [18,19]. Second, the differences in the effects of mental fatigue on offensive and defensive techniques have not been fully investigated [20–22]. Third, the critical time points for action recognition under mental fatigue conditions have not been clearly identified [23]. Finally, the interaction between skill level and mental fatigue in the context of temporal perceptual prediction has not been adequately explored [24].

To address these gaps, the present study aims to examine the impact of mental fatigue on the temporal perceptual prediction of action recognition among boxers of different skill levels. Specifically, we investigate whether mental fatigue differentially affects the recognition of offensive and defensive techniques and identify the critical time points for action recognition under mental fatigue conditions. Based on the literature and the nature of boxing performance, we hypothesize that (1) mental fatigue will significantly impair temporal perceptual prediction, primarily by increasing reaction time (RT) rather than reducing accuracy (ACC); (2) novice boxers will exhibit greater vulnerability to mental fatigue compared to experts, especially in defensive techniques; (3) offensive techniques will maintain relatively stable temporal perceptual prediction under mental fatigue, whereas defensive techniques will be more affected; and (4) the −40 ms time shield point will be critical for action recognition, as it provides sufficient information for accurate prediction, unlike the −80 ms point. This study will provide valuable insights into how mental fatigue influences boxing performance and inform future training and competition strategies.

2. Subjects and Methods

2.1. Subjects

Participants were recruited from among 20 individuals (16 males and 4 females) from a sports training major at a renowned sports university, all of whom were national first-class elite boxers.

The participants' characteristics included the average age (20.30 ± 1.66 years), average height (1.76 ± 6.47 m), average body weight (72.43 ± 9.91 kg), and average training duration (6.58 ± 2.71 years). Additionally, a novice group comprising 20 male boxing beginners was recruited with an average age of (21.45 ± 1.99 years), average height of (1.75 ± 6.52 m), and an average weight of (73.89 ± 10.82 kg). Participants were recruited from among 20 individuals (16 males and 4 females) from a sports training major at a renowned sports university, all of whom were national first-class elite boxers.

All the participants exhibited normal intelligence and physical health, had no history of mental illness, and had either normal or corrected-to-normal vision. They had not previously engaged in any perceptual prediction exercise or received related guidance. Each participant voluntarily consented to participate in this study; abstained from alcohol, caffeine, and sleep deprivation within 24 h before this experiment; and received a gift upon completion. The study protocol was approved by the Ethics Committee of the School of Sports Medicine at Wuhan Sports University (approval number: 2024013).

2.2. Experiment Design

The experimental design employed a mixed-factorial approach with three factors: 2 (groups: Mental Fatigue Expert Group and Mental Fatigue Novice Group) × 2 (technique types: attack and defense) × 3 (time blocking: −80 ms, −40 ms, and action initiation). The group factor was a between-subjects factor, whereas technique type and time blocking were within-subject factors. The dependent variables were accuracy and reaction time for predicting motion decisions based on temporal perception.

2.3. Experiment Material

Mental fatigue was induced using the Stroop paradigm [19,25], which has been established to be more stable over a 45-min duration compared to a 30-min induction [26]. The Stroop task was programmed using E-prime 3.0 (Psychology Software Tools, Inc., Pittsburgh, PA, USA) software and initiated with the following instructions:

Thank you for this test. Please maintain your focus at the center of the screen throughout the test. A '+' fixation point appears, followed by a colored word. Your task is to determine whether the font color matches the meaning of the word. If they match, press the 'F' key; if they do not, press the 'J' key. Respond as quickly and accurately as possible with feedback provided after each response. Failure to respond within 1.5 s or incorrect responses were recorded as errors. The test calculates accuracy and reaction time, with the top three performers receiving additional rewards. Press any key to begin.

After instructions, a 500 ms fixation point '+' was presented, followed by a 1500 ms stimulus. Participants need to respond to the stimulus by pressing a button, and there will be 500 ms feedback after each stimulus. The Stroop paradigm consisted of three blocks, each with 300 traits lasting 15 min, for a total of 900 traits lasting 45 min.

The materials for the motion decision-making task based on time perception prediction were filmed using an iPhone 12 from the perspective of the subjects, with three boxers invited to a training center for video recording. The phone was positioned approximately 0.5 m above the ground and 2 m away from the athletes. Athletes were instructed to face the camera, assume a ready stance, and perform in-place technical movements for both attack and defense. Offensive actions included straight punches, hook punches, and swinging punches, and defensive actions included arm hugging, dodging, and blocking. Each movement was performed twice within 2 s. The videos were edited using Adobe Premier (Adobe Inc., San Jose, CA, USA), resulting in 99 videos (54 offensive and 45 defensive) based on the three blocking conditions. After evaluation by a coach and three graduate boxing students using a five-point rating scale, 77 videos were deemed suitable for experimental testing. The experimental program, developed using E-prime 3.0, included 36 formal experimental videos and 4 practice videos. Inter-rater reliability was ensured through a five-point rating scale used by the coach and three graduate boxing students to evaluate the videos, ensuring the final selection of 77 suitable videos for experimental testing.

Due to the negative impact of mental fatigue on subjective evaluations, several subjective rating scales have been validated as effective tools for assessing the state of mental fatigue. These include the Brunel Mood Scale (BRUMS-C, V, and F), the Visual Analog Scale (VAS), and the Borg-20 rating scale of perceived exertion (Borg-20) [11]. The following scales were used to assess the state of mental fatigue: The Visual Analog Scale (VAS) has demonstrated high reliability in mental fatigue research, with a test–retest reliability (ICC) of 0.69 (95% CI: 0.53–0.81) [27]. The Chinese version of the Brunel Mood Scale (BRUMS-C) has shown good reliability and validity in cross-cultural validation, with internal consistency (Cronbach's α) ranging from 0.77 (fatigue) to 0.87 (anger) across its subscales. Confirmatory factor analysis (CFA) confirmed its structural validity (CFI $\geq$ 0.90, RMSEA $\leq$ 0.06), indicating its suitability for assessing mood states in Chinese academic settings [28]. The Borg-20 scale, widely used and validated, demonstrates high validity in assessing subjective fatigue [29] Table S1.

2.4. Experiment Process

This experiment was divided into two sessions: practice and formal. The practice session consisted of 4 trials, while the formal session comprised 36 trials, with 18 offensive and 18 defensive techniques. The experimental duration was approximately 3–4 min to closely simulate the duration of an actual boxing round.

The participants were invited to the laboratory for testing. Upon arrival, they signed an informed consent form, were assigned a code, and provided their demographic information (name, sex, age, major, grade, height, weight, group, and training years). Height and weight were measured onsite. Participants completed the Chinese versions of the Brunel Mood Scale (BRUMS-C), Visual Analog Scale (VAS), and Borg-20 rating scale of perceived exertion (Borg-20) before commencing formal testing. They then completed a 45-min Stroop paradigm to induce mental fatigue. After the task, BRUMS-C, VAS, and Brog-20 measurements were taken again, followed by the perceptual prediction task for motion decision-making. Videos of the boxing techniques were played randomly on a computer screen, and the participants were required to judge the techniques based on the observed content. For 'straight punching', press 1; for 'hook punching', press 2; for 'swing punching', press 3; for 'arm hugging', press 4; for 'dodging', press 5; and for 'blocking', press 6. The participants were required to respond within a given timeframe, with failure to respond to the considered errors. A practice session consisting of four trials was conducted before the formal experiment to familiarize the participants with the process. Final measurements of the BRUMS-C, VAS, and Borg-20 were performed upon completion (Figure 1). In subsequent expressions, 1, 2, and 3, respectively, refer to the subjective evaluation scores at three different time points.

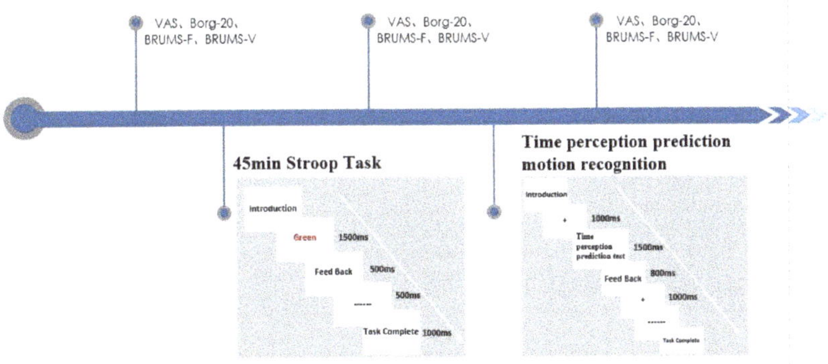

Figure 1. Experimental process of time perception prediction motion recognition.

2.5. Statics and Analysis

The experimental results mainly include descriptive statistics of RT and ACC in the Stroop paradigm, BRUMS-C scale only recording two subdimensions of BRUMS-F (fatigue) and BRUMS-V (vitality), one-way ANOVA of VAS and Borg-20, descriptive statistics of time perception prediction for action recognition and motion decision-making, and three-factor repeated measures ANOVA. SPSS 26.0 software was used for data analysis and processing, and Graphpad Prism 8 was used for plotting.

The experimental results primarily included descriptive statistics of reaction time (RT) and accuracy (ACC) in the Stroop paradigm, BRUMS-C scale recordings of the BRUMS-F (fatigue) and BRUMS-V (vitality) subdimensions, one-way ANOVA of VAS and Borg-20, descriptive statistics of time perception prediction for action recognition and motion decision making, and three-factor repeated measures ANOVA. Before conducting the repeated measures ANOVA, we tested the assumptions of normality and sphericity. Normality was assessed using the Shapiro–Wilk test, and sphericity was tested using Mauchly's test. In case of violations of sphericity, we applied the Greenhouse–Geisser correction. Additionally, homogeneity of variance was tested using Box's test. To provide a comprehensive understanding of the effect sizes reported in our study, we have included the interpretation thresholds for the partial eta-squared (η^2) values. According to commonly accepted guidelines, η^2 values can be interpreted as follows: a small effect size ($\eta^2 = 0.01$) indicates a weak relationship between variables, which may not be very significant in practical applications; a medium effect size ($\eta^2 = 0.06$) indicates a moderate relationship between variables, which is usually detectable through data analysis; and large effect size ($\eta^2 \geq 0.14$) indicates a strong relationship between variables, which is typically very evident and has practical significance [30]. Data analysis and processing were conducted using SPSS software (version 26.0), and GraphPad Prism 8 (GraphPad Software Inc., San Diego, CA, USA) was used for data visualization.

3. Results

The study findings are presented herein, encompassing data on mental fatigue induction, Visual Analog Scale (VAS), and Borg-20 scale scores, and an analysis of response times and accuracy rates in time perception prediction.

3.1. Mental Fatigue (MF)

The induction of mental fatigue was induced using the Stroop paradigm for 45 min. The mean and standard deviation of RT and ACC in the Stroop paradigm for the MF boxing expert group and MF boxing novice group are described statistically, as shown in Table 1.

Table 1. RT and ACC of MF boxing expert group and MF boxing novice group in Stroop task.

Group	Mean	SD
MF Boxing Expert (RT)	571.50	62.19
MF Boxing Novice (RT)	576.50	55.17
MF Boxing Expert (ACC)	97.02	1.61
MF Boxing Novice (ACC)	96.94	1.82

There were 20 subjects in both groups, N = 40.

3.2. VAS, Borg-20, BRUMS-F, and BRUMS-V Scale Scores

The VAS scores revealed a significant difference between the MF expert and novice groups (F (1,18) = 8.36, $p = 0.005 < 0.05$), with the novice group exhibiting higher scores than the expert group. Within the expert group, a significant increase was observed from VAS1 to VAS2 ($p < 0.05$) and from VAS1 to VAS3 ($p < 0.05$), with no significant difference between VAS2 and VAS3 ($p > 0.05$). The findings of the novice group mirrored these findings. This indicates that both groups experienced a significant increase in VAS scores after the Stroop task compared to pre-task levels.

Borg-20 scale scores showed no significant differences between the expert and novice groups (F (1,18) = 2.37, $p = 0.126 > 0.05$). However, in the expert group, a significant increase was noted from Brog-20 scale 1 to Borg-20 scale 2 ($p < 0.05$) and from Borg-20 scale 1 to Borg-20 scale 3 ($p < 0.05$), with no significant difference between Borg-20 scale 2 and Borg-20 scale 3 ($p > 0.05$). The novice group exhibits a similar trend. These results suggest that both groups had significantly elevated Borg-20 scale scores following the Stroop task compared with pre-task levels.

The VAS, Borg-20, and BRUMS-F scores collectively indicated an increase in subjective fatigue after the Stroop task. Conversely, the BRUMS-V vitality dimension scores decreased after the task, indicating reduced vitality (Figure 2).

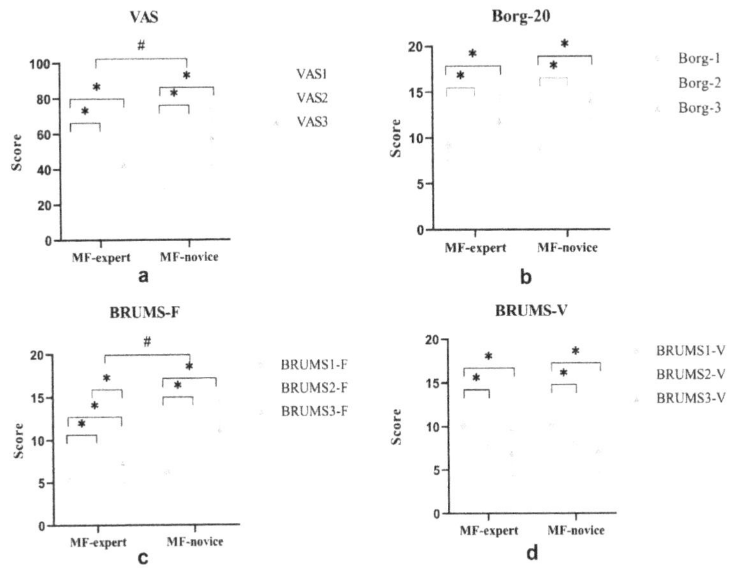

Figure 2. VAS, Borg-20, BRUMS-F, and BRUMS-V scale scores for MF expert group and MF novice group. * indicates a significance level of 0.05. "#" indicates that there is a significant difference between the MF-expert group and the MF-novice group. (**a**) VAS scores of expert and novice groups at three time points in mental fatigue; (**b**) Borg-20 scores of expert and novice groups at three time points in mental fatigue; (**c**) BRUMS-F scores of expert and novice groups at three time points in mental fatigue; and (**d**) BRUMS-V scores of expert and novice groups at three time points in mental fatigue.

3.3. Reaction Time (RT)

Descriptive statistics for RT in the time perception prediction and motion decision-making experiments are presented in Table 2. Inferential statistical analysis was conducted using repeated-measures analysis of variance (ANOVA) within subjects. Box's test for homogeneity of variance indicated variance homogeneity across groups ($p = 0.376 > 0.05$). Multivariate ANOVA revealed significant main effects of the technique type ($p = 0.005$, $p < 0.01$), whereas the interaction between the technique type and group was not significant ($p = 0.087$, $p > 0.05$). The main effect of shielding time was significant ($p = 0.000$, $p < 0.01$), as was the interaction between technique type and shielding time ($p = 0.001$, $p < 0.01$), and the three-way interaction involving group, technique type, and shielding time ($p = 0.031$, $p < 0.05$). The main effect of the group was significant ($p = 0.019$, $p < 0.05$). Sphericity assumptions were not violated by technique type, and the time-shielding effects were consistent with the sphericity assumption ($p = 0.156$, $p > 0.05$). The main effect of the group was significant, with $F(1,38) = 5.97$, $p < 0.05$, $\eta^2 = 0.14$. The main effect of technique type was significant, with $F(1,38) = 9.03$, $p < 0.05$, $\eta^2 = 0.19$. The interaction between group and technique type was not significant, with $F(1,38) = 3.10$, $p > 0.05$, $\eta^2 = 0.075$. The main effect of shielding time was significant, $F(2,76) = 31.42$, $p < 0.05$, $\eta^2 = 0.45$. The interaction between group and time shielding was not significant, with $F(2,76) = 0.18$, $\eta^2 = 0.01$; the interaction between technique type and time shielding was significant, with F (2,76) = 9.85, $p < 0.05$, $\eta^2 = 0.21$; and the three-way interaction was significant, with F (2,76) = 3.92, $p < 0.05$, $\eta^2 = 0.09$. The results of the multivariate ANOVA were consistent with those of the univariate ANOVA.

Table 2. Descriptive statistics of RT for time perception prediction motion recognition (M ± SD).

	Attack			Defense		
	−80 ms	**−40 ms**	**Start**	**−80 ms**	**−40 ms**	**Start**
BE	744.51 ± 62.02	811.16 ± 67.51	856.69 ± 71.30	855.86 ± 71.19	729.44 ± 60.08	784.64 ± 65.37
BN	833.73 ± 74.78	914.81 ± 82.05	919.79 ± 82.49	849.69 ± 76.20	932.45 ± 83.63	830.57 ± 74.55

BE is the boxing expert group, and BN is the boxing novice group.

Multiple comparisons were conducted due to the significant main effect of time shielding and its three levels. The interaction between technique type and shielding time was significant, necessitating simple effects tests. The three-way interaction involving group, technique type, and time shielding was also significant and requires further investigation.

Multiple comparison results for time shielding revealed a significant difference between level 1 (−80 ms) and level 3 (action initiation) of factor C, indicating that the RT at −80 ms was shorter than that at action initiation ($p = 0.005$, $p < 0.05$). There was also a significant difference between level 1 (−80 ms) and level 2 (−40 ms), indicating that the RT was shorter at −80 ms compared to −40 ms. No significant difference was observed between level 2 (−40 ms) and level 3 (action initiation) ($p = 0.421$, $p > 0.05$).

Simple effects tests for the interaction of technique type and time shielding (B × C) indicated no significant difference between −80 ms and −40 ms time shields under offensive conditions. However, the difference between −80 ms time shielding and action initiation was significant ($p < 0.05$), with action initiation RT being higher than −80 ms. Similarly, there was a significant difference between −40 ms and action initiation, with −40 ms shielding time being faster than action initiation. Under defensive conditions, a significant difference in time shielding was observed between −80 ms and −40 ms ($p < 0.05$), with RT being faster at −40 ms than at −80 ms. No significant difference was found between −80 ms and action initiation, while a significant difference was observed between −40 ms and action initiation ($p < 0.05$), with −40 ms being faster than action initiation.

In terms of time blocking, a significant difference in offensive and defensive techniques was observed at −80 ms ($p < 0.05$), with no significant difference at −40 ms ($p > 0.05$). Under the action initiation conditions, no significant differences in offensive and defensive techniques were found ($p > 0.05$). This suggests that there is a difference in RT between offensive and defensive techniques at −80 ms, with offensive techniques having shorter action recognition times.

The simple effects test results showed no significant difference between the MF expert and novice groups at −40 ms ($p = 0.44$, $p > 0.05$). At −80 ms, no significant difference was observed ($p = 0.08$, $p > 0.05$). At action initiation, a marginally significant difference was observed ($p = 0.06$). Under defensive conditions, a significant difference was found between the MF expert and novice groups at −40 ms ($p = 0.005$, $p < 0.05$). At −80 ms, no significant difference was observed ($p = 0.20$, $p > 0.05$). At action initiation, a marginally significant difference was observed ($p = 0.06$). The MF expert group may exhibit a shorter perceived reaction time than the MF novice group when initiating both offensive and defensive actions. Additionally, the MF expert group may recognize defensive actions earlier than the MF novice group at −40 ms.

Under the MF expert group conditions, significant differences in attack and defense technical types were observed at −40 ms ($p = 0.00$, $p < 0.05$), with no significant differences at −80 ms ($p = 0.27$, $p > 0.05$). At action initiation, significant differences in attack and defense technical types were observed ($p = 0.04$, $p < 0.05$). Under the MF novice group conditions, no significant differences in attack and defense technical types were observed at −40 ms and similarly at −80 ms ($p = 0.77$, $p > 0.05$). No significant differences were observed in action initiation ($p = 0.68$, $p > 0.05$). The MF expert group demonstrated a shorter reaction time to defensive movements and faster recognition of whether the opponent intended to attack or defend under −40 ms and action initiation conditions, whereas no such difference was observed in the MF novice group. This suggests that the MF novice group had weaker recognition of attack and defense technical types compared to the MF expert group under the three blocking conditions. Under the MF expert group conditions, no significant difference was observed in time blocking between −40 ms and −80 ms when the technical type was offensive ($p = 0.98$, $p > 0.05$), and a significant difference was found in time blocking between −40 ms and −80 ms when the technical type was defensive ($p = 0.012$, $p < 0.05$). No significant difference was observed in time blocking between −40 ms and −80 ms when the technical type was defensive, and no significant difference was observed in time blocking between −40 ms and −80 ms when the technical type was offensive. A significant difference was observed in time blocking between −40 ms and −80 ms when the technical type was offensive in the MF novice group ($p = 0.004$, $p < 0.05$). The difference between −40 ms and action initiation was not significant ($p = 0.28$, $p > 0.05$), while the difference between −80 ms and action initiation time shielding was significant ($p = 0.004$, $p < 0.05$); when the technical type was defense, there was a significant difference in time blocking between −40 ms and −80 ms ($p = 0.002$, $p < 0.05$), but there was no significant difference in time blocking between −40 ms and action initiation ($p = 0.98$, $p > 0.05$), and there was a significant difference in time blocking between −80 ms and action initiation ($p = 0.007$, $p < 0.05$). This indicates that in the MF expert group, the time perception judgment of offensive techniques is faster at −40 ms than at action initiation, while the time perception judgment of defensive techniques is faster at −40 ms than at −80 ms, and the time perception of action initiation is also faster at −80 ms. The MF novice group showed slower time perception in action initiation for offensive techniques compared to −80 ms, while defensive techniques had longer time perception reaction times for −40 ms compared to −80 ms and longer time perception reaction times for −80 ms compared to action initiation (Figure 3).

3.4. Accuracy (ACC)

Descriptive statistics for the ACC in the motion decision experiment based on time perception prediction are detailed in Table 3. Inferential statistical analyses were performed using repeated-measures measures ANOVA of variance. Box's test for homogeneity of variance indicated variance heterogeneity across groups ($p = 0.042$, $p < 0.05$), prompting the use of the Greenhouse–Geisser correction. Multivariate ANOVA revealed significant main effects of the technique type ($p = 0.000$, $p < 0.01$), whereas the interaction between the technique type and group was not significant ($p = 0.413$, $p > 0.05$). The main effect of time shielding was significant ($p = 0.000$, $p < 0.01$), as was the interaction between technique type and time shielding ($p = 0.004$, $p < 0.01$) but not the interaction between group and time shielding ($p = 0.467$, $p > 0.05$) or the three-way interaction ($p = 0.360$, $p > 0.05$). The main effect of the group was not significant ($p = 0.482$). Sphericity assumptions were not violated by technique type, and the time-shielding effects were consistent with the sphericity assumption ($p = 0.526$, $p > 0.05$). The main effect of the group was not significant, with F (1,38) = 0.898, $p < 0.05$, $\eta^2 = 0.023$. The main effect of technique type was significant, with F (1,38) = 18.496, $p < 0.05$, $\eta^2 = 0.327$. The interaction between group and technique type was not significant, with F (1,38) = 0.684, $p > 0.05$, $\eta^2 = 0.018$. The main effect of time shielding was significant, with F (2,76) = 125.727, $p < 0.05$, $\eta^2 = 0.768$. The interaction between group and time shielding was not significant, F (2,76) = 0.937, $\eta^2 = 0.024$; the interaction between technique type and time shielding was significant, F (2,76) = 8.773, $p < 0.05$, $\eta^2 = 0.188$. The three-way interaction was not significant with F (2,76) = 1.018, $p < 0.05$, $\eta^2 = 0.026$. The results of the multivariate ANOVA were consistent with those of the univariate ANOVA.

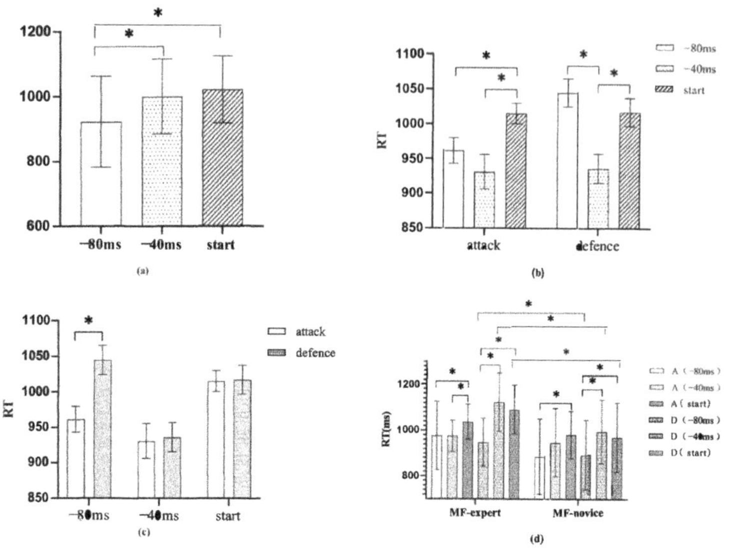

Figure 3. (**a**) is the main effect of time shielding, (**b**,**c**) is the second-order interaction effect (RT) between technology type and time shielding, and (**d**) is the third-order interaction effect (RT) between group, technology type, and time shielding. * indicates a significance level of 0.05.

Table 3. Descriptive statistics of ACC for time perception prediction motion recognition (M ± SD).

	Attack			Defense		
	−80 ms	**−40 ms**	**Start**	**−80 ms**	**−40 ms**	**Start**
BE	20.90 ± 18.58	75.25 ± 18.11	75.15 ± 11.51	20.00 ± 15.93	45.75 ± 22.89	56.80 ± 28.80
BN	23.60 ± 20.49	64.30 ± 21.01	67.45 ± 21.51	20.45 ± 18.86	47.30 ± 20.62	53.35 ± 24.19

BE is the boxing expert group, and BN is the boxing novice group.

Multiple comparisons were conducted due to the significant main effect of time shielding and its three levels. The interaction between technique type and shielding time was significant, necessitating simple effects tests.

Multiple comparison results for time shielding revealed a significant difference between level 1 (−80 ms) and level 2 (−40 ms) of factor C, with ACC at −40 ms being higher than ACC at −80 ms ($p = 0.000$, $p < 0.05$). There was also a significant difference between levels 1 (−80 ms) and 3 (action initiation), with the ACC at action initiation being higher than that at −80 ms ($p = 0.000$, $p < 0.05$). No significant difference was observed between levels 2 and 3, indicating no difference between the ACC at −80 ms and the ACC at action initiation ($p = 0.380$, $p > 0.05$).

The results of the BC simple effects test showed that in terms of technical type (B), there was a significant difference ($p > 0.05$) between the −40 ms time shield and the −80 ms time shield under the attack (B1) condition, with ACC under the attack condition being higher at −40 ms than at −80 ms. There was no significant difference between 40 ms and action initiation ($p > 0.05$). There was a significant difference ($p < 0.05$) between the 80 ms time shield and action initiation, with the ACC of action initiation under offensive conditions being higher than −80 ms. Under defensive conditions (B2), there was a significant difference ($p < 0.05$) between the −40 ms time shield and the −80 ms time shield, with the ACC of the −40 ms time shield being higher than that of the −80 ms time shield. There was no significant difference ($p > 0.05$) between the 40 ms shielding time and action initiation. The difference between 80 ms and action initiation was significant ($p < 0.05$), with ACC at action initiation being higher than that at −80 ms time masking. In terms of time shielding (C), under the condition of −40 ms (C1), there was a significant difference in the technical types of attack and defense ($p < 0.05$), with the ACC of attack being higher than that of defense. Under the condition of −80 ms (C2), there was no significant difference in the technical types of attack and defense ($p > 0.05$). However, under the condition of action initiation (C3), there was also a significant difference in the technical types of attack and defense ($p < 0.05$), with the ACC of attack being higher than that of defense (Figure 4).

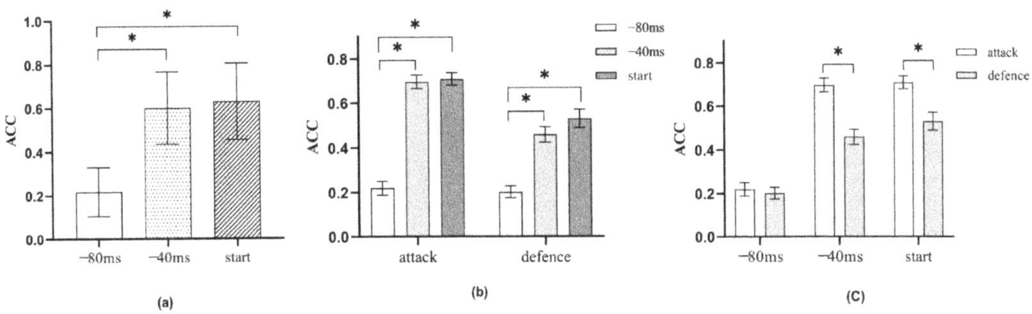

Figure 4. (**a**) is the main effect of time shielding, and (**b**,**c**) is the second-order interaction effect (ACC) between technology type and time shielding. * indicates a significance level of 0.05.

4. Discussion

This study was designed to investigate the effects of mental fatigue on the temporal perceptual prediction of action recognition among boxers with varying skill levels. Utilizing the Stroop paradigm for 45 min, we successfully induced mental fatigue and subsequently assessed the recognition of offensive and defensive technical movements by expert and novice boxers at three distinct time-blocking points [2,19,25].

Our findings indicate that the 45-min Stroop task effectively induced mental fatigue, as evidenced by significant changes in subjective fatigue and vitality indicators, such as the VAS, Brog-20, and BRUMS-F, before and after the task. This aligns with previous research suggesting that prolonged cognitive tasks can lead to mental fatigue, affecting cognitive performance, including perceptual prediction [9,12,13].

The main effect of the group on reaction time (RT) was significant, but not on accuracy (ACC), suggesting that while there was a significant difference in reaction time between expert and novice boxers, accuracy remained unaffected. This discrepancy may be attributed to the expert group's long-term specialized training, which confers an advantage in RT but not necessarily in ACC, potentially due to the impact of mental fatigue on decision-making accuracy [31,32]. The current study also revealed a dissociation between reaction time and accuracy. This dissociation is believed to be caused by mental fatigue resulting from prolonged cognitive tasks, which leads to reduced activity in brain regions associated with control [33]. Consequently, athletes adjust their strategies during the information integration phase, extending processing time to maintain basic decision-making accuracy.

Regarding technique type, both the RT and ACC exhibited main effects, highlighting the differences in the recognition of offensive and defensive techniques during mental fatigue. Our results suggest that offensive techniques are recognized more quickly and accurately than defensive techniques, which is consistent with previous research indicating that cognitive fatigue has a greater impact on offensive actions [12,22]. Compared to defense, offense may activate more primitive action patterns (such as automated processing dominated by the basal ganglia), while defense involves more complex cognitive monitoring (such as conflict detection by the dorsolateral prefrontal cortex). This suggests that mental fatigue may have a greater impact on automated processing [34].

The main effect of time shielding was also significant for both RT and ACC, with the −80 ms time point showing lower RT and ACC compared to −40 ms and action initiation. This finding suggests that as action initiation approaches, the advantage of expert boxers diminishes, potentially because of the influence of mental fatigue on information utilization [23,35].

The significant second-order interaction effects between technique type and time shielding on both RT and ACC indicate that the −40 ms time shield point provides sufficient information for participants to recognize action patterns. Furthermore, the third-order interaction effects between group, technique type, and time shielding on RT suggest that mental fatigue has a more pronounced impact on novice defensive techniques than on offensive techniques [4,21]. In line with previous studies supporting the Cognitive Resource Depletion Model [36], it is suggested that time-specific attentional focus training be adopted under mentally fatigued conditions to optimize decision-making strategies. This approach will allow for a better understanding of how athletes utilize situational information in competitions and facilitate the development of effective training programs that can be transferred from training to competition [37].

Previous studies demonstrated that mental fatigue can affect the accuracy of passing decisions in ball sports and increase reaction times during decision-making. However, the impact of mental fatigue on decision-making in different sports varies, with the current research focusing primarily on ball sports such as football and basketball [19,20,38]. Our findings contribute to the understanding of how mental fatigue affects perceptual predictions in boxing, a domain that has been less explored in the literature.

To mitigate the adverse effects of mental fatigue (MF) on temporal prediction in sports training, targeted interventions can be strategically applied: Non-invasive neuromodulation techniques, such as anodal transcranial direct current stimulation (tDCS) targeting the dorsolateral prefrontal cortex (DLPFC), have been shown to enhance cognitive control under MF, with studies in cyclists and swimmers demonstrating preserved reaction time and decision accuracy during fatigue. This approach could be synergized with sport-specific drills (e.g., video simulations of opponent actions at −80/−40 ms time points) to optimize temporal anticipation in boxing. Acute caffeine supplementation (3–6 mg/kg) antagonizes adenosine receptors, sustaining alertness and dopamine-driven motivation, which is critical for rapid defensive adjustments (e.g., blocking at −40 ms) in combat sports. Mindfulness training, such as brief breath-focused meditation sessions, reduces task-irrelevant thoughts and improves attentional focus, as evidenced by volleyball players exhibiting faster decision-making post-intervention, a strategy transferable to boxing scenarios requiring split-second predictions. Additionally, olfactory interventions using neutral pleasant odors (e.g., citrus) activate reward-related brain regions, potentially resetting cognitive load during rest intervals and enhancing temporal anticipation in subsequent training rounds. These evidence-based strategies, tailored to sport-specific demands, offer practical solutions to counteract MF-induced declines in temporal prediction, though further validation in combat sports contexts is needed to refine implementation protocols [11].

In conclusion, the current study provides evidence that mental fatigue negatively affects both expert and novice boxers, with a more significant effect on defensive skills among experts. The −40 ms time perception is identified as a critical point for action recognition, and the effects of mental fatigue are not linear across various levels of expertise, types of techniques, and time-blocking points [18,39,40].

5. Conclusions

This study provided several key findings regarding the impact of mental fatigue on temporal perceptual prediction in boxers with varying skill levels. In this section, we summarize our conclusions and implications.

First of all, the 45-min Stroop task effectively induced mental fatigue, as evidenced by significant changes in subjective fatigue and vitality indicators such as the VAS, Brog-20, and BRUMS-F scores before and after the task. In the second place, in a state of mental fatigue, the reaction time (RT) and accuracy (ACC) of the offensive techniques were higher than those of the defensive techniques. This suggests that mental fatigue may disproportionately affect the execution and recognition of defensive actions in boxing. Furthermore, the extraction of information at −40 ms was identified as a key time point for action recognition compared to −80 ms and action initiation. This indicates that the temporal window of −40 ms may be crucial for predicting action recognition in boxing. Lastly, mental fatigue can have negative effects on experts and beginners, offense and defense, and different time-blocking points; however, this effect is not linear. This finding underscores the complexity of how mental fatigue influences boxing performance and suggests that the impact may vary depending on the specific context and individual characteristics.

These conclusions contribute to the growing body of literature on the effects of mental fatigue in sports, particularly in high-intensity and high-skill sports, such as boxing. Future research should explore the nuances of mental fatigue and its interaction with various performance metrics to develop targeted interventions for athletes.

6. Limitation and Future Research Outlook

While the current study provides valuable insights into the effects of mental fatigue on boxing performance, further research is warranted to explore the intricate relationships among mental fatigue, perceptual prediction, and decision-making in sports. The sample size in the current study was determined based on the researchers' prior experience; a more rigorous approach would involve calculating an optimal sample size using G-power. Second, while the current study focused on temporal perception prediction under mental fatigue, future research could include a control group without mental fatigue to investigate differences in temporal perception prediction between states with and without mental fatigue. Another notable limitation is the gender imbalance in our participant sample, with only four female experts compared to 16 male experts and 20 male novices. This imbalance is due to the relatively low number of female participants in boxing, a sport traditionally dominated by males. Future research should aim to recruit a more balanced gender distribution to better understand the effects of mental fatigue across different genders. However, the limitation of our study is that while we reported effect sizes for the reaction time and accuracy data, we did not include effect sizes for the questionnaire data (VAS, BRUMS, and Brog-20). Future research should consider including effect sizes for all statistical analyses to provide a more comprehensive understanding of the results. While our results indicate that −40 ms is a statistically significant point for temporal perceptual prediction, the magnitude of the interaction effects suggests that this should be interpreted with caution in practical contexts.

The findings of this study have significant potential implications for practice and sports training. Coaches can design more targeted training programs based on the study results, considering the athletes' mental fatigue status and the characteristics of offensive and defensive techniques. For example, by optimizing training plans, the negative impact of fatigue on athletes' decision-making abilities can be reduced; in defensive technique training, the ability to recognize key information (such as at −40 ms) can be enhanced; and in offensive technique training, the athletes' rapid recognition of offensive cues can be utilized to improve decision-making efficiency.

Furthermore, future research on the topic of mental fatigue and perceptual prediction in athletes could benefit from the application of advanced technologies such as eye-tracking, ERPs (Event-Related Potentials), and fNIRS (functional Near-Infrared Spectroscopy). These technologies can provide deeper insights into the neural mechanisms underlying the effects of mental fatigue on athletes' performance. Additionally, this research topic is not only relevant to the field of sports but also holds potential for interdisciplinary collaboration. Collaboration with experts in psychology, physiology, and artificial intelligence could lead to more comprehensive and effective solutions for managing mental fatigue in sports.

Supplementary Materials: The following supporting information can be downloaded at: https://www.mdpi.com/article/10.3390/sports13050154/s1, Table S1:summary table listing.

Author Contributions: Conceptualization, C.-H.W. and L.G.; software, N.W.; methodology, X.X.; resources, S.-J.B.; data curation, C.-H.W., N.W., and Q.L.; writing—original draft preparation, C.-H.W.; writing—review and editing, Y.Y.; supervision, L.G.; project administration, X.X. All authors have read and agreed to the published version of the manuscript.

Funding: This research received no external funding.

Institutional Review Board Statement: This study was conducted in accordance with the Declaration of Helsinki and approved by the Ethics Committee of Medical Ethics Committee of Wuhan Sports University (protocol code:2024013, 4 March 2024).

Informed Consent Statement: Informed consent was obtained from all subjects involved in this study. Written informed consent has been obtained from the patients to publish this paper.

Data Availability Statement: The data underlying this study are not publicly available at this time, as they are part of an ongoing research effort and are currently being further analyzed and integrated into a larger research context. The data were derived from a doctoral dissertation that is in the process of finalization. We plan to make the data available upon the completion of the dissertation and after ensuring that all necessary ethical and privacy considerations have been addressed. We will update this statement with the relevant data access information once the data are ready for public release.

Acknowledgments: We would like to express our sincere gratitude to all the authors for their remarkable teamwork throughout this research project.

Conflicts of Interest: The authors declare no conflicts of interest.

References

1. Wu, R.; Yang, Q.; Cui, W.; Gao, D.; Luo, Y.; Wang, D. Relationship between visual ability assessment and punch performance in competition in male amateur boxers. *Front. Physiol.* **2024**, *15*, 1429554. [CrossRef] [PubMed]
2. Baker, J.; Cote, J.; Abernethy, B. Sport-Specific Practice and the Development of Expert Decision-Making in Team Ball Sports. *J. Appl. Sport. Psychol.* **2003**, *15*, 12–25. [CrossRef]
3. Fortes, L.S.; Nascimento-Júnior, J.R.A.; Mortatti, A.L.; Lima-Júnior, D.R.A.A.; Ferreira, M.E.C. Effect of Dehydration on Passing Decision Making in Soccer Athletes. *Res. Q. Exerc. Sport.* **2018**, *89*, 332–339. [CrossRef]
4. Causer, J.; Smeeton, N.J.; Williams, A.M. Expertise differences in anticipatory judgements during a temporally and spatially occluded task. *PLoS ONE* **2017**, *12*, e171330. [CrossRef]
5. Mann, D.T.; Williams, A.M.; Ward, P.; Janelle, C.M. Perceptual-cognitive expertise in sport: A meta-analysis. *J. Sport. Exerc. Psychol.* **2007**, *29*, 457–478. [CrossRef] [PubMed]

6. Travassos, B.; Duarte, R.; Vilar, L.; Davids, K.; Araújo, D. Practice task design in team sports: Representativeness enhanced by increasing opportunities for action. *J. Sport. Sci.* **2012**, *30*, 1447–1454. [CrossRef] [PubMed]
7. Unenaka, S.; Ikudome, S.; Mori, S.; Nakamoto, H. Concurrent Imitative Movement During Action Observation Facilitates Accuracy of Outcome Prediction in Less-Skilled Performers. *Front. Psychol.* **2018**, *9*, 1262. [CrossRef] [PubMed]
8. Fortes, L.S.; Gantois, P.; de Lima-Júnior, D.; Barbosa, B.T.; Ferreira, M.E.C.; Nakamura, F.Y.; Albuquerque, M.R.; Fonseca, F.S. Playing videogames or using social media applications on smartphones causes mental fatigue and impairs decision-making performance in amateur boxers. *Appl. Neuropsychol. Adult* **2023**, *30*, 227–238. [CrossRef]
9. Proost, M.; Habay, J.; De Wachter, J.; De Pauw, K.; Rattray, B.; Meeusen, R.; Roelands, B.; Van Cutsem, J. How to Tackle Mental Fatigue: A Systematic Review of Potential Countermeasures and Their Underlying Mechanisms. *Sports Med.* **2022**, *52*, 2129–2158. [CrossRef]
10. Congyuxin, Y.S.S.F. Mental Fatigue in Sports: Causes, Effects, and Coping Strategies—A Review Study. *Int. J. Acad. Res. Progress. Educ. Dev.* **2024**, *13*, 1103–1109.
11. Wu, C.; Zhao, Y.; Yin, F.; Yi, Y.; Geng, L.; Xu, X. Mental Fatigue and Sports Performance of Athletes: Theoretical Explanation, Influencing Factors, and Intervention Methods. *Behav. Sci.* **2024**, *14*, 1125. [CrossRef]
12. Sun, H.; Soh, K.G.; Roslan, S.; Wazir, M.R.W.N.; Soh, K.L. Does mental fatigue affect skilled performance in athletes? A systematic review. *PLoS ONE* **2021**, *16*, e258307. [CrossRef]
13. Chen, X.; Ji, Z.; Wang, Y.; Xu, J.; Wang, L.; Wang, H. Bibliometric analysis of the effects of mental fatigue on athletic performance from 2001 to 2021. *Front. Psychol.* **2023**, *13*, 1019417. [CrossRef] [PubMed]
14. Lu, C.; Xu, J. Influences of Physical, Environment, Task, Timing, Learning, Emotion, Perspective (PETTLEP) Intervention on Psychological Resilience, Psychological Skills, Anxiety and Depression of Athletes. *Iran. J. Public. Health* **2023**, *52*, 87–96. [CrossRef] [PubMed]
15. Huang, X.; Song, Q. Thinking about the Orical Model of Time Cognition. *J. Southwest China Norm. Univ.* **2004**, *30*, 25–28. [CrossRef]
16. Scharlau, I. Temporal processes in prime–mask interaction: Assessing perceptual consequences of masked information. *Adv. Cogn. Psychol.* **2007**, *3*, 241–255. [CrossRef] [PubMed]
17. Hong-peng, Z.; Zhao-yang, G. Predict Behavior and Neural Mechanism of Excellent Sanda Athletes Under Different Situations. *J. Shenyang Sport. Univ.* **2014**, *33*, 27–32.
18. Smith, M.R.; Zeuwts, L.; Lenoir, M.; Hens, N.; De Jong, L.M.; Coutts, A.J. Mental fatigue impairs soccer-specific decision-making skill. *J. Sports Sci.* **2016**, *34*, 1297–1304. [CrossRef]
19. Pageaux, B.; Lepers, R. The effects of mental fatigue on sport-related performance. *Prog. Brain Res.* **2018**, *240*, 291–315. [CrossRef]
20. Fortes, L.S.; Lima-Junior, D.; Nascimento-Júnior, J.R.A.; Costa, E.C.; Matta, M.O.; Ferreira, M.E.C. Effect of exposure time to smartphone apps on passing decision-making in male soccer athletes. *Psychol. Sport. Exerc.* **2019**, *44*, 35–41. [CrossRef]
21. Gantois, P.; Caputo, F.M.; Lima-Junior, D.; Nakamura, F.Y.; Batista, G.R.; Fonseca, F.S.; Fortes, L.S. Effects of mental fatigue on passing decision-making performance in professional soccer athletes. *Eur. J. Sport. Sci.* **2020**, *20*, 534–543. [CrossRef]
22. Le Mansec, Y.; Pageaux, B.; Nordez, A.; Dorel, S.; Jubeau, M. Mental fatigue alters the speed and the accuracy of the ball in table tennis. *J. Sports Sci.* **2018**, *36*, 2751–2759. [CrossRef]
23. Sun, W.F.; Wang, B.; Guo, D.; Zhang, D.X.; Lin, R.H. Research on Processing Superiority of Advance Cues for Elite Sanda. *Athl. J. Cap. Univ. Phys. Educ. Sports* **2021**, *33*, 268–275.
24. Martin, K.; Staiano, W.; Menaspà, P.; Hennessey, T.; Marcora, S.; Keegan, R.; Thompson, K.G.; Martin, D.; Halson, S.; Rattray, B. Superior Inhibitory Control and Resistance to Mental Fatigue in Professional Road Cyclists. *PLoS ONE* **2016**, *11*, e159907. [CrossRef]
25. Staiano, W.; Bosio, A.; Piazza, G.; Romagnoli, M.; Invernizzi, P.L. Kayaking performance is altered in mentally fatigued young elite athletes. *J. Sports Med. Phys. Fit.* **2019**, *59*, 1253–1262. [CrossRef]
26. Yang, W.; Li, J.; Zhao, S. Comparison of the effects of mental fatigue induction tasks. *Chin. J. Tissue Eng. Res.* **2024**, *28*, 3722–3728. [CrossRef]
27. Brietzke, C.; Vinícius, Í.; Franco-Alvarenga, P.E.; Canestri, R.; Goethel, M.F.; Santos, L.E.R.; Viana, B.; Santos, T.M.; Pires, F.O. Proof-of-Concept and Test-Retest Reliability Study of Psychological and Physiological Variables of the Mental Fatigue Paradigm. *Int. J. Env. Res. Pub He* **2021**, *18*, 9532. [CrossRef]
28. Hasan, M.M.; Khan, M.H.A. Bangla version of the Brunel Mood Scale (BRUMS): Validity, measurement invariance and normative data in non-clinical sample. *Heliyon* **2022**, *8*, e9666. [CrossRef]
29. Pancardo, P.; Hernández-Nolasco, J.A.; Acosta-Escalante, F. A Fuzzy Logic-Based Personalized Method to Classify Perceived Exertion in Workplaces Using a Wearable Heart Rate Sensor. *Mob. Inf. Syst.* **2018**, *2018*, 1–17. [CrossRef]
30. Fritz, C.O.; Morris, P.E.; Richler, J.J. Effect size estimates: Current use, calculations, and interpretation. *J. Exp. Psychol. Gen.* **2012**, *141*, 2–18. [CrossRef]
31. Shu-Ming, W.; Jian-chen, Z.; Xiao-jian, Y. A Research on Performance of Perceptual-motor Skill Training For Badminton Players. *J. Beijing Sport. Univ.* **2009**, *32*, 46–49. [CrossRef]

32. Smith, M.R.; Thompson, C.; Marcora, S.M.; Skorski, S.; Meyer, T.; Coutts, A.J. Mental Fatigue and Soccer: Current Knowledge and Future Directions. *Sports Med.* **2018**, *48*, 1525–1532. [CrossRef]
33. Van Cutsem, J.; Van Schuerbeek, P.; Pattyn, N.; Raeymaekers, H.; De Mey, J.; Meeusen, R.; Roelands, B. A drop in cognitive performance, whodunit? Subjective mental fatigue, brain deactivation or increased parasympathetic activity? It's complicated! *Cortex* **2022**, *155*, 30–45. [CrossRef]
34. Nakamoto, H.; Mori, S. Experts in fast-ball sports reduce anticipation timing cost by developing inhibitory control. *Brain Cogn.* **2012**, *80*, 23–32. [CrossRef]
35. Hong-peng, Z.; Cheng-lin, Z. Features and Neural Mechanism of Feature Searching of Elite Sanda Athlete. *J. Shanghai Univ. Sport.* **2010**, *34*, 74–77.
36. van der Linden, D.; Frese, M.; Meijman, T.F. Mental fatigue and the control of cognitive processes: Effects on perseveration and planning. *Acta Psychol.* **2003**, *113*, 45–65. [CrossRef]
37. Williams, A.M.; Jackson, R.C. Anticipation in sport: Fifty years on, what have we learned and what research still needs to be undertaken? *Psychol. Sport. Exerc.* **2019**, *42*, 16–24. [CrossRef]
38. Fortes, L.S.; De Lima-Junior, D.; Fiorese, L.; Nascimento-Junior, J.; Mortatti, A.L.; Ferreira, M. The effect of smartphones and playing video games on decision-making in soccer players: A crossover and randomised study. *J. Sports Sci.* **2020**, *38*, 552–558. [CrossRef]
39. Fortes, L.S.; Lima-Junior, D.; Barbosa, B.T.; Faro, H.K.C.; Ferreira, M.E.C.; Almeida, S.S. Effect of mental fatigue on decision-making skill and visual search behaviour in basketball players: An experimental and randomised study. *Int. J. Sport. Exerc. Psychol.* **2022**, *ahead-of-print*, 1–20. [CrossRef]
40. Trecroci, A.; Boccolini, G.; Duca, M.; Formenti, D.; Alberti, G. Mental fatigue impairs physical activity, technical and decision-making performance during small-sided games. *PLoS ONE* **2020**, *15*, e238461. [CrossRef]

sports

MDPI

Article

Physical Training Considerations for Futsal Players According to Strength and Conditioning Coaches: A Qualitative Study

Rafael Albalad-Aiguabella [1,2], David Navarrete-Villanueva [2,3,4], Elena Mainer-Pardos [1], Oscar Villanueva-Guerrero [1], Borja Muniz-Pardos [2,5,6,7,8,*] and Germán Vicente-Rodríguez [2,3,5,6,7,8]

1 Health Sciences Faculty, Universidad San Jorge, Autov A23 km 299, Villanueva de Gállego, 50830 Zaragoza, Spain; ralbalad@usj.es (R.A.-A.); epardos@usj.es (E.M.-P.); oscarvillanuevaguerrero@gmail.com (O.V.-G.)
2 EXER-GENUD (Growth, Exercise, NUtrition and Development) Research Group (S72_23R), FIMS Collaborating Center of Sports Medicine, University of Zaragoza, 50013 Zaragoza, Spain; dnavarrete@unizar.es (D.N.-V.); gervicen@unizar.es (G.V.-R.)
3 AgroFood Institute of Aragon (IA2), Universidad de Zaragoza, 50009 Zaragoza, Spain
4 Faculty of Health Science, University of Zaragoza, Domingo Miral, s/n, 50009 Zaragoza, Spain
5 Physiopathology of Obesity and Nutrition Networking Biomedical Research Centre (CIBERObn), Instituto de Salud Carlos III, 28029 Madrid, Spain
6 Exercise and Health Spanish Research Network, 50009 Zaragoza, Spain
7 Faculty of Health and Sport Science (FCSD), University of Zaragoza, Ronda Misericordia 5, 22001 Huesca, Spain
8 Department of Physiatry and Nursing, University of Zaragoza, 50009 Zaragoza, Spain
* Correspondence: bmuniz@unizar.es

Abstract: The professionalization of futsal requires greater physical demands on players, requiring strength and conditioning coaches to manage loads, optimize performance, and prevent injuries. This study aimed to describe the current practices of high-level strength and conditioning coaches and determine the elements needed to optimize their performance. Two video-recorded focus groups consisting of eight strength and conditioning coaches from the Spanish futsal league's first and second divisions were transcribed, translated, and analyzed using a content analysis approach with open-ended questions on physical preparation and current practices. Results showed that strength and conditioning coaches prioritized five main areas: (1) competitive demands, (2) training load control and monitoring, (3) injury risk mitigation strategies, (4) contextual factors and interpersonal relationships, and (5) training methodologies to optimize performance. However, they also claim to deal with several limitations such as lack of time, limited resources and access to facilities, insufficient staff, problems related to combining sport with other activities (e.g., work), or the difficulty to individualize, which limits the optimization of their practices. Based on these findings, practical applications include implementing neuromuscular and strength training sessions at least twice a week, using cost-effective load monitoring tools (e.g., RPE and wellness questionnaires) to manage workloads, individualizing training programs to address the specific demands and characteristics of each player, and fostering close multidisciplinary collaboration to optimize performance and reduce injury risks. These insights can guide current and aspiring strength and conditioning coaches toward optimized practices. This study can assist novice strength and conditioning coaches in identifying the key focus areas of elite physical trainers and understanding their challenges and limitations, fostering collaboration among sports professionals to create a more optimized environment.

Keywords: sport; futsal; performance; coaching; player monitoring; individualization

1. Introduction

Futsal is a team sport of cooperation and opposition and it is considered an intermittent discipline with incomplete recovery periods, where high-intensity efforts predominate and occur continuously throughout the match [1–3]. Competitive schedules are often saturated with numerous competitions, with little time for recovery and training between matches [4]. In recent years, the physical demands of futsal have increased, leading to an ever-growing demand for players' technical, tactical, physical, physiological, and psychological capabilities [5,6]. This demand has required strength and conditioning coaches (S&CCs) to optimize training methodologies to maximize athletic performance, prepare players for competition, and maintain high physical conditioning throughout the season [7,8].

The role of an S&CC is complex and heterogeneous, encompassing the development and maintenance of diverse and essential physical capacities for optimal performance [9]. S&CCs are focused on planning adequate workloads, balancing training and recovery to ensure optimal periodization while minimizing injury risk [10–13], and are also required to collaborate within multidisciplinary teams [14]. Different tools for load quantification and monitoring are frequently used in both training and competitions, providing valuable data that help in the decision-making process during training [15,16]. The training load can be understood according to two main components: internal and external loads [17]. Internal load refers to physiological and psychological responses to training [18], with commonly used markers such as heart rate [19,20], biochemical variables [21,22], subjective perception of effort (RPE), and well-being questionnaires [23,24]. External load refers to the objective and measurable demands of training [25], with the emergence of tracking technologies, such as global positioning systems (GPS), local positioning systems (LPS), or indoor accelerometers [26,27], aiding in the assessment of key variables, such as total distance covered, player load, accelerations, deceleration, or distance covered at high intensity, among others [1,7]. Strength and conditioning coaches must enhance a range of physical capacities in players, including strength, sprint performance, and change-of-direction ability. In addition to routine futsal training, several studies have demonstrated that incorporating supplemental training, such as resistance training, plyometrics, agility exercises, or combined strength–speed workouts, can significantly improve these capacities [28–31]. Evidence suggests that one to two additional training sessions per week, effective from low to moderate intensities and lasting between 15 and 45 min, depending on the type of training, are sufficient to elicit meaningful performance improvements [15,29,31].

Additionally, individualizing training loads according to individual player characteristics such as age, gender, training history, or physical fitness is also essential for S&CCs at the professional level [32–34]. Notably, optimizing the physical preparation requires accounting for other confounding variables, such as competition schedules, club environments, player characteristics, and interpersonal relationships [35,36]. For this purpose, S&CCs should have a wide perspective, so all these factors are considered.

While an increasing number of studies have analyzed the physical demands of futsal [7,8,35,37,38], little research has been conducted on the usual practices of S&CCs and their influence on the aforementioned variables involved in their practice. In other sports, previous studies have explored the methodologies used by S&CCs through closed-ended surveys and questionnaires [39–45]. To date, in futsal, only one study has been found that analyzed the practices of S&CCs [15]. However, this research employed closed-ended survey questions, which limited the depth of the insights.

Given this gap in the literature and the inherent strengths of the focus group with open questions, the present study conducted focus groups with futsal S&CCs to achieve two main objectives: (1) to identify the fundamental principles and specific practices guiding their training methodologies and (2) to determine the nonconditioning-related factors that significantly impact their professional responsibilities (e.g., related to context, inter-individual relationships). The findings of the present work contribute to both research and applied practice, providing valuable insights for futsal S&CCs.

2. Materials and Methods

2.1. Study Design

This study used a descriptive, qualitative, cross-sectional design to analyze and understand the usual practices of futsal S&CCs (first or second-division) during the competitive season to increase the physical performance of their players and prevent injuries. Two focus groups were performed in October 2023. Each group comprised four S&CCs from the first- or second-division men's and women's futsal teams of the Spanish league. Access to data was exclusively limited to the researchers. Data were encoded to ensure anonymity and were destroyed once the study was completed.

2.2. Participants

Initially, 10 professional S&CCs from the first- and second-division men's and women's futsal teams in the Spanish league were contacted to voluntarily participate in the study. Eight of the 10 S&CCs responded positively and agreed to participate in this research. Before conducting the focus group discussions, all participants signed an informed consent to participate in the research and agreed to have the focus group video recorded. The age of the S&CC participants was 31.1 ± 4.82 years, with a wide experience in sports performance (8.1 ± 4.78 years of experience) and, in particular, in futsal performance (4.8 ± 3.31 years of experience). Table 1 presents the participants' characteristics.

Table 1. Participant characteristics.

Category	Classification	Number of Participants
Gender	Male	7
	Female	1
Age	<30	3
	30–35	4
	>35	1
Team category	First division	3
	Second division	5
Team gender	Male	4
	Female	4

Participation in the focus group was voluntary. If, at any time during the focus group, any participant considered that any of the topics being discussed were inappropriate or put them in an uncomfortable situation, they were free to leave the discussion or group without providing any justification.

For participants to be included in the study, they were required to meet the following inclusion criteria: (1) actively working during the data collection period; (2) employed by teams competing in the first or second division; (3) eligible regardless of team gender; and (4) possess at least a Bachelor's degree in sport sciences. The Clinical Research Ethics Committee of Aragon (CEICA) approved the research project. Ethics was initially obtained for this study in November 2023 (PI23-456), but because this intervention was integrated into a research project that included other experimental trials, an addendum was made to our initial ethics application in April 2024 (PI23-456). The research project was conducted in accordance with the ethical standards of the 1975 Declaration of Helsinki (revised at the

64th General Assembly, Fortaleza, Brazil, October 2013). Confidentiality was guaranteed following legal regulations on data confidentiality established by Organic Law 15/1999 of 13 December, Protection of Personal Data, and Organic Law 3/2018 of 5 December, Protection of Personal Data and Guarantee of Digital Rights.

2.3. Procedures

Once the participants who met the inclusion criteria were selected and their consent was obtained, each participant was randomly assigned to one of the two focus groups. Both groups were required to include S&CCs from both the men's and women's teams. The focus groups began by explaining the research's aim, the topics to be discussed, and the estimated duration. In addition, participants were informed of the anonymity and confidentiality of their information, opinions, comments, and use. Each S&CC participated in a 90-min virtual focus group composed of four S&CCs conducted through Microsoft Teams (v. 25044.2407.3474.4587, Microsoft Corporation, Redmond, WA, USA) and led by the investigator. The structure was similar in both focus groups, and S&CCs could provide additional information during the dynamics. The focus groups were videotaped and transcribed verbatim. Participants did not receive any financial or other compensation for their participation in the focus group. Figure 1 shows the data collection process.

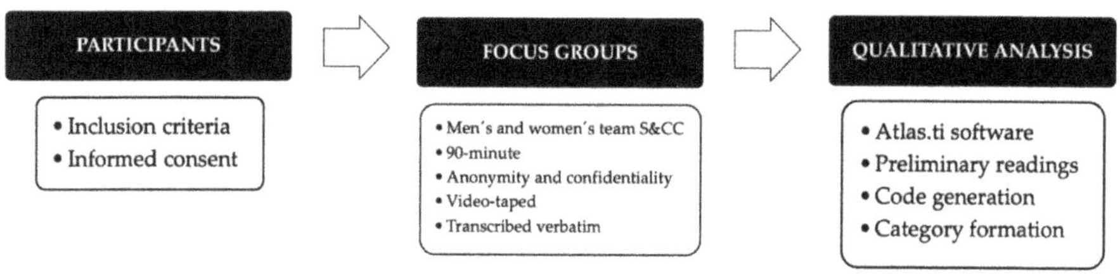

Figure 1. Data collection process.

2.4. Qualitative Analysis

A combined thematic and structural analysis of the focus group data was conducted to examine not only what was said but also how it was communicated by the participants [46]. The thematic analysis focused on capturing the meaning, description, and interpretation of the data's content, while the structural analysis explored the connotative aspects of language, including the use of specific expressions and linguistic forms [46]. Before starting the analysis, all data were prepared by verbatim transcription, anonymization, and aggregation of the information obtained using the aforementioned techniques.

For the qualitative analysis of the focus group's content, the texts were imported into the Atlas.ti qualitative analysis software (v.23.4.0, Berlin, Germany) to facilitate systematic coding and categorization. The analysis was performed by two independent researchers (RAA and OVG), who conducted three thorough preliminary transcript readings. During the subsequent coding phase, recurring quotes were identified, and keywords emerging from the text were used to create codes. These codes were then grouped into categories that encompassed similar thematic content, ensuring a systematic and comprehensive understanding of the focus group discussions [46]. Figure 2 illustrates the qualitative analysis process.

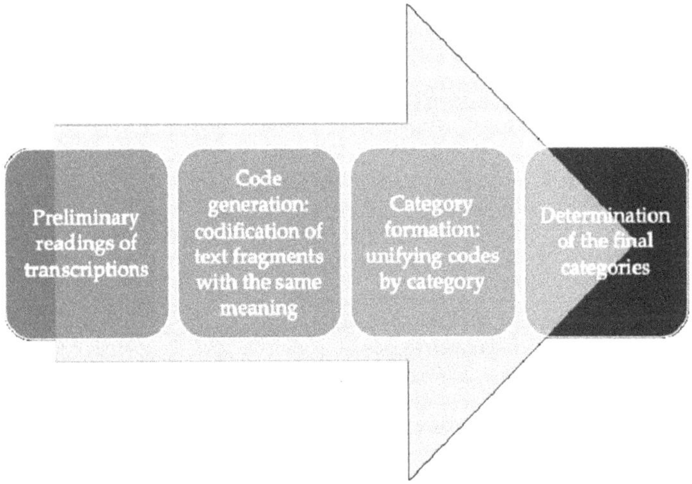

Figure 2. Qualitative analysis process.

2.5. Validity and Robustness

To ensure data quality, diverse triangulation techniques were used. In this study, triangulation involved a comprehensive search of the scientific literature and focus group interviews. The interview questions were developed based on the literature review, and data from the second focus group were triangulated with those from the first. Moreover, different members of the research team (RAA and OVG) independently conducted triangulation to compare and contrast the information and enhance credibility. This multifaceted approach enabled us to identify convergences and divergences in our data, thereby strengthening the validity of our findings. The reliability of the results was verified by including verbatim statements from the participants, and the entire work process was supervised by different team members who were not directly involved in the analysis of the results. In addition, the study's rigor was ensured by following the COREQ EQUATOR guidelines and applying the reliability criteria for qualitative research following Lincoln and Guba [47,48].

3. Results

The thoughtful analysis of the focus groups led to the following five general categories: (1) Analysis of the futsal performance model and competitive demands; (2) Load monitoring; (3) Injuries; (4) Contextual and relational factors; (5) Training methods and limitations. Table 2 presents a summary of the main results for each category identified through qualitative analysis.

Table 2. Overview of main results.

Categories	Subcategories	S&CC Current Practices and Key Considerations
Futsal performance model and competitive demands	Futsal performance	• Lower-body strength training • Intermittent training with incomplete and active recoveries to stress aerobic and anaerobic systems • Speed training, especially acceleration
	Competitive demands	• Playtime • Player position-specific actions • Distance covered

Table 2. *Cont.*

Categories	Subcategories	S&CC Current Practices and Key Considerations
Load Monitoring	Load control and monitoring	• Training load control • Periodization: short- and long-term • Questionnaire scores for wellness, RPE, TQR, and muscular quality • New technologies (GPS)
Injuries	Main injuries	• Ligament and muscle injuries • Ankle, knee, hip, quadriceps, and adductor • Women: higher prevalence of ACL and adductor injuries
	Strategies to minimize injury risk	• Individual and group preventive sessions • Strength training • Synergy among coaches, S&CCs, medical services, and players • Load control and periodization
	Measurements/Assessments	• Individual deficit test • Asymmetry, jumps, ankle dorsiflexion, movement quality assessment, progressive load, agonist–antagonist strength
Contextual and relational factors	Contextual factors	• Playing position • Season timing: schedule, trip, competitive density, and team ranking • Opponent level • Player context: age, body awareness, mood, previous sports education, and personal circumstances • Match results
	Interpersonal relationships	• Effective communication • Technical staff communication: multidisciplinary work • Player relationships: motivation and confidence
Training methods and limitations	Training methodologies	• Based on availability, resources, and contextual factors • Prioritize unilateral and dynamic training • Intermittent actions with slight recovery
	Individualization	• Essential for prescribing training programs • Account for individual player characteristics
	Limitations	• Lack of time • Suboptimal training facilities • Limited resources • Insufficient staff • Restricted player' availability • Individualization challenges

3.1. Analysis of Futsal Performance Model and Competitive Demands

3.1.1. Futsal Performance Model

Regarding the physical capacities that determine futsal performance, there was a consensus on the dominance of strength training, mainly of the lower body, and this was agreed to be used for both sports performance improvement and injury prevention. Aerobic training is also commonly performed through intermittent and repetitive high-intensity actions, prioritizing both aerobic and anaerobic energy systems. These actions occur continuously during competition and are characterized by brief, active, and incomplete recoveries. In addition, speed training, where acceleration plays a fundamental role, is crucial for player preparation. No sex differences (male and female) were found between the S&CC practices in this section.

> "Based on the current trends in futsal, training programs should consider strength training as a key element." I consider this one of the main pillars of training plans together with the aerobic-anaerobic training" (PT 1)

> "In addition to the previously mentioned strength and endurance training, (...) players should also be able to cover very short distances as quickly as possible, making acceleration a key component of their performance." (PT 5)

> "(...) and let's not forget it is essential to incorporate the ability to repeatedly perform high-intensity actions, such as accelerations, decelerations, fights, or offensive and defensive transitions, into training programs, as these are essential for player's physical conditioning" (PT 3)

In addition, one participant added that for the optimal development of all these capabilities and the prevention of injuries, we should not fail to include joint mobility and range of motion exercises in our training programs.

> "To complement the previously mentioned aspects, (...) I would emphasise that joint mobility and range of motion training should always be integrated into our training programs" (PT 4)

3.1.2. Competitive Demands

To identify whether S&CCs considered the competitive demands of program exercise training, we found that most of them prioritized playtime and player position, distance covered and specific actions. Additionally, these variables were mainly used to control the weekly individual and team workloads. It should be noted that only two of the participants had worked in their teams with advanced GPS technology, who highlighted that this technology enabled them to have a more real and precise quantification of numerous external load variables (accelerations, decelerations, distances covered, etc.). This method was claimed to help adjust training exercises and weekly loads more reliably based on the obtained data. There were no differences in S&CC practices according to sex. However, male teams generally have greater economic resources and a higher prevalence of GPS usage, which optimizes their training load monitoring.

> "Yes, I reckon the value of assessing competitive demands, but 'playing time' is the only variable I include, given my limited access to GPS technologies" (PT 1)

> "For instance, if one player participated 25 min and another 12 min in a match, an alternative strategy would be to individualize the first weekly training session to compensate the workload differences" (PT 5)

> "Each playing position has different physical demands in terms of strength, distance covered, and fighting actions. For instance, pivots engage in challenging actions to gain and maintain positions. Therefore, in addition to general training, these players require a greater emphasis on strength development" (PT 6)

> "I primarily focus on player profiles, which indirectly influence the training plan in terms of running distances. For instance, if I have a player whose role is pivot, I avoid programming excessive distances in a fixed pivot system. Therefore, I ensure that the prescribed distances closely align with the specific competitive demands. Additionally, in discussions with the coach, he specifically requests detailed insights into certain player's conditioning levels" (PT 2)

> "Using GPS technology provides us with a distinct advantage in understanding the actual competitive demands" (PT 3)

3.2. Load Monitoring

In the second block, participants shared their views on load control, its importance, and the tools they used to manage it. All participants, regardless of the sex of the team, agreed that having absolute control over training loads through proper periodization is crucial. Although training planning should always follow a holistic approach, it should be primarily focused on the short term to meet the immediate demands of competition.

> "It is essential to meticulously monitor loads and plan them at weekly or microcycle level, given the numerous demands of the season schedule" (PT 6)

Another aspect highlighted by the S&CCs, for both men's and women's teams, is the relevance of implementing different daily questionnaires (wellness, subjective perception of effort, muscular quality, quality of recovery, etc.) to check the players' physical condition and thus be able to adapt the training sessions. S&CCs working with women's teams reported that female athletes tend to be less accustomed to using these questionnaires compared to their male counterparts, thereby requiring additional time to familiarize themselves with the process.

> "The questionnaires provide me with a wealth of information about how the players are performing" (PT 5), and "based on the questionnaires, you can adjust the loads and modify the type of session" (PT 8)

New technologies, which are more prevalent in men's teams due to greater financial support, enable S&CCs to more precisely control training and match loads, allowing for adjustments not only in the load itself but also in recovery protocols and training exercises.

> "Now that I have GPS technology, I have access to plenty of information. Ultimately, this approach enables us to precisely identify competitive demands, resulting in significant improvements in load control and better structuring loads throughout the microcycle. For instance, you can verify whether you require more acceleration and deceleration on Tuesdays and whether you may need a more maximum-intensity distances on Wednesdays. Consequently, further adjustments can be made." (PT 4)

3.3. *Injuries*

This third category of results gathers the participants' perspectives on various topics of futsal injuries and the strategies employed by S&CCs to minimize injury risk.

3.3.1. Main Injury

Regarding the main injuries typically observed in male and female players, S&CCs predominantly highlight ligament and muscle injuries, most commonly located in the ankle, knee, hip, quadriceps, and adductors.

> "In my experience, I have encountered more ankle sprains than any other injury. Additionally, I have dealt with tendinopathies in various areas, most commonly in psoas and in the knee through patellar problems, and adductor overload" (PT 1)

> "Then in the knee, there have been lateral or medial sprains" (PT 6), and "regarding the quadriceps, I have mainly witnessed overload injuries, although occasionally there has been a tear" (PT 4)

> "Now I am concerned because I already have another case of pubalgia, an injury I experienced last year" (PT 7), "I have also encountered a case of pubalgia, a long and challenging injury to manage" (PT 6)

> "I would also note pain or discomfort in the lower back" (PT 6)

In this regard, some S&CC participants noted that some injuries could be linked to the type of court on which training sessions are conducted or to the athlete's gender.

> "The surface of the court is also a key factor in determining the type of injuries that can occur during the season. Last year we played on a very hard court, and three players suffered bone edema due to hard impacts against the court during different actions during the game. I had never seen this injury before, and it caused long-term absences of the players. In addition, some players suffered Achilles tendon discomfort due to the hardness of the court, especially when exposed to low temperatures during winter." (PT 4)

> "Girls are more exposed to a greater extent than men to suffer anterior cruciate ligament injuries due to their physical and anatomical characteristics." (PT 2)

> "In females, I have found a higher prevalence of discomfort and injuries in the adductor muscles." Anterior cruciate ligament injuries are also frequently observed, which is a very frequent injury in female players nowadays" (PT 3)

However, concerning the S&CCs' perception of injury incidence in futsal, they believe that the overall injury rate is low, regardless of sex. Most of the time, these injuries are minor and can be managed throughout the week, allowing the players to participate in the competition.

> "Given the current level of demand in futsal, I believe the injury rate is not excessive, especially considering the limited resources available, the long trips (generally in bus), the highly-demanding season schedule..." (PT 4)

3.3.2. Minimization of Injury Risk

The participants emphasized that the role of S&CCs is not to skip injuries fully, which is inherent in high-level sports, but to try to minimize injury risk through the various tools available and diverse strategies that can be implemented. They noted that these strategies extend beyond merely performing low-intensity exercises, which are commonly known as "preventive". Furthermore, some variables cannot be controlled and depend directly on the players and cannot be fully controlled by the S&CCs; thus, the responsibility for injuries is shared between the players, S&CCs, and the rest of the technical team.

"It is widely accepted in the futsal community that muscle injuries are physical trainers' fault, but this is not as simple; it is a responsibility shared equally between the physiotherapist, coach, player, and physical trainer. The physical trainer could potentially program a meticulous training plan with individualized loads, etc., but if the coach is not on the same page and works individually with his own training plan, it is impossible to build synergy and teamwork. I have worked with coaches who prepared down to the smallest detail: Which day do we train what? Which court size should we use, depending on the number of players? What time? However, I have worked with other coaches who say, "No, this is my way of training; we are going to do this, and that is it.". If, for example, an overtrained player could get the approval from the physiotherapist to keep training, then it turns out that he could not train and needed to rest. The same could also happen with me as a physical trainer: if I go beyond the limit, then the player may be training too much, and if the player does not take care of himself (adequate rest, nutrition, etc), then nothing works" (PT 4)

Furthermore, S&CCs emphasize that everything that is done during planning is preventive and that not only individual or group work performed at low intensity on certain structures or musculature can be considered preventive work. Instead, there are numerous factors to consider, and focusing solely on the "preventive" ones would provide a very simplistic and limited perspective.

> "Injury prevention is not something-specific; it includes everything we do. The pretense of finding specific exercises that focus on injury prevention is not correct.

> What prevents injuries and improves performance is a set of actions that we perform. We can implement many exercises, but if you do not sleep well, do not control the load, do not have minimum strength levels, etc., it does not matter what you do. And finally, training in court mimicking the specifics physical demands of competition is also highly preventive." (PT 6)

Considering the above, it is common for S&CCs to schedule these so-called "preventive" sessions, for both men's and women's teams and as a group (focusing on the main complementary structures that support sports performance and the general muscular and joint health of athletes), as well as individually (addressing each player's deficits and weaknesses to minimize them).

> "Even if we call it preventive, it is still good for me that we continue to train, for example, on ankle stability, ankle mobility, etc., even at low loads, regardless of the competitive demand" (PT 3), "maybe one day it's more mobility and stretching and another day it's more strength training with eccentrics exercise" (PT 4)

The prescription of this "preventive" session varies considerably. The number of individual or group sessions scheduled, as well as their location, depends on each team's weekly organization, player availability, or planned session type.

> "Some players do this preventive training before court training and others in the gym on their own, at their preferable convenience" (PT 1), "players have a preventive-compensatory routine before each training session that they have to do independently" (PT 7), "players perform this preventive training on the court" (PT 8), and "every day before training the players perform stretching and mobility, although some players prefer to stay after training to do so. In addition, some players prefer to perform eccentric exercises after training because they believe it is better for them" (PT 4)

3.3.3. Measurements

Another essential aspect of S&CCs when monitoring players is the performance of tests that identify any player deficits. The main assessments include asymmetries tests, jump tests, ankle dorsiflexion evaluation, movement quality assessment, progressive load tests using encoders, and agonist-antagonist strength tests using dynamometers. These are planned for both male and female teams.

> "First, we normally do different tests to assess how the player arrives" (PT 4), "We perform an initial assessment and then we follow up" (PT 1)

3.4. *Contextual and Relational Factors*

This section compiles the results regarding various contextual factors and the relevance of the different multidirectional relationships that occur within a team environment throughout the season, all of which should be considered when optimizing training and achieving peak athletic performance.

3.4.1. Contextual Factors

Unifying the participants' views, several contextual factors were identified that should be considered by coaches and S&CCs when conducting training sessions, designing workouts, or planning programming. Key factors include the playing position, the moment within the season (such as schedule, competitive density, trips, and team ranking), the level of the opponent, the player's context (age, body awareness, mood, previous sports education, and personal circumstances), or the results of the matches. It is important to note that these contextual factors are common to both male and female teams.

> "I also give a lot of relevance to age, the experience level, and the current state of the player" (PT 3), "I try to get to know the players as much as possible so I can help them and guide them to the best of my ability. Also, when they are young, I try to help and educate them for their professional future" (PT 4), "when we start working with a new player, the first thing we do is to examine her previous history and evaluate her fitness, and from there, we begin to prescribe training." (PT 4)

> "The season schedule is another key factor in establishing goals and allowing for an optimized periodization. However, initial planning may vary depending on the results during competition" (PT 7), "At certain times of the season, there is an increase in competitive density playing maybe five games in two weeks, which means playing every 3 or 4 days. In these cases, once this period of accumulation of games is over, I modify the type of training we do by changing, for example, the gym training or introducing more eccentric exercises that enable us to recover better. I also consider the most recent competitive weeks, the minutes played by athletes in competition, the moment of the season or of the amount of travelling" (PT 4), "the level of the opponent played on the weekend will also affect the weekly organization, as the players usually need more recovery time when playing against opponents in the upper part of the classification, which modifies the training sessions for that week." (PT 5)

> "Each position has specific demands. For example, a pivot has to do more wrestling actions to fight and win the position, so those players need a greater orientation towards increasing strength levels (. . .), and a wing should train more speed-oriented, without, of course, doing a well-loaded basic strength. Therefore, we have to adapt the training to the different playing positions." (PT 6)

3.4.2. Interpersonal Relationships

All participants, regardless of sex, agree that effective communication among team members is essential. These communications are multidirectional and include the relationships between the technical staff, which enable multidisciplinary work, and the relationships with the players, which are essential to achieving commitment, motivation, and confidence in their work.

> "I find the relationship with the coach very relevant and, above all, being aware of his coaching style, his actions. . . At the beginning, as we start to work together, this is especially important" (PT 4), "it is essential to know the coach and his method of training" (PT 3), and "effective communication with the coach is also crucial. In the end, no matter how much we (physical trainers) know or do, if we do not know how to communicate with the coach and if he does not understand us, or does not pay attention to us, our work is useless." (PT 6)

> "If you do a deadlift at 80% and then the coach wants to do transitions, then it is not well planned, no matter how good the transfer to real game may be" (PT 4)

> "The players are also very grateful for the feedback. If they realise that you make an effort, understand the training process, and see results, which in the end is the most important thing, they trust you greatly." (PT 4)

> "Beyond the conditional aspect, one of the most important things is to have the players' trust." Being able to talk to them, both about sporting and personal issues, and to set goals will be fundamental to our work. If we do not have the confidence of the players, the first ones who have to change are us because we are not helping to improve the team." (PT 8)

Regarding interpersonal relationships, S&C coaches of women's teams—each with prior experience in men's teams—highlighted that the dynamics between technical staff and female players are notably more complex and challenging. They argued that differences in communication styles, team dynamics, and expectations contribute to a more complex relational landscape in women's teams, which demands additional attention and tailored strategies to foster effective collaboration and performance.

> "My communication style with female players differs notably from the approach I previously used with male players" (PT 3), "I engage in more extensive communication with the women, as I believe it helps them manage the diverse demands they face throughout the season" (PT 5), "I believe that with female players it is essential to provide individual explanations for decisions they may find challenging, while also offering encouragement to sustain their efforts." (PT 7)

3.5. *Training Methods and Limitations*

Finally, this section presents the participants' perspectives on training methodologies and highlights the main limitations encountered in team management.

3.5.1. Training Methodologies

Each S&CC applies different training methodologies based on their availability, resources, and contextual factors (playing position, opponent level, or season time). However, they emphasize the importance of prioritizing unilateral and dynamic training, implementing it progressively, using varied stimuli, intermittent actions with slight recovery and including recreational tasks that "trick" the athlete into achieving particular goals. The training methodologies employed by S&CCs are influenced more by the abovementioned factors than by the team's gender.

> "During resistance training in the gym, I start with bilateral exercises and progress to unilateral, (...). In the court, I consider that almost everything is unilateral due to the characteristics of the sport itself" (PT 7)

> "During strength training, I often use intermittent training, which intense effort with short rest, to guide it to the court, and circuit training, which enables me to better control the players" (PT 8)

> "I mainly perform neuromuscular, plyometric, and speed training. In addition, I try to orient the task according to the game model of the weekend's opponent, if they play more with a fixed pivot or with four outsides" (PT 5)

3.5.2. Individualization

Individualization of training was undoubtedly the most frequently mentioned concept among all participants during the focus groups for both men's and women's teams, and they considered it essential for prescribing training programs. This individualization is transversal across all categories mentioned above, underscoring its fundamental importance and the need for both S&CCs and technical staff to integrate it into their planning.

> "Individualization is crucial because each player has his own needs and his particular stage in the season" (PT 8)

> "First of all, we have to assess the player to identify his deficits and be able to individualize the strength training (...), and during the competitive weeks, I try to individualize the load of each player based on the different variables that we monitor (minutes of play, RPE, wellness...)" (PT 3)

> "Ultimately, many aspects depend on the player, on the individual preventive training they have, on when they think they should do it, on exercises that give

> them the feeling of being well, etc. Some players perform eccentric training on the same day of the match because they feel better on the court, so in the end, we should individualize many aspects based on each player." (PT 4)

3.5.3. Limitations

S&CCs point out several key limitations: lack of time, particularly on the court, which often prevents them from providing adequate feedback, demonstrations, athletes' instruction or conducting more appropriate warm-ups, suboptimal training facilities, lack of knowledge of new players when team changes occur, interference from uncontrollable variables during training, small technical teams with limited availability, restricted players availability and challenges in individualizing training to address each athlete's specific needs. These limitations are widespread among S&CC teams in both men and women. However, participants noted that women's futsal is less developed than men's, and consequently, these limitations tend to be more pronounced.

> "Due to lack of time, some training content cannot be done during the session and you have to find other times to do it, with the difficulties that this entails." (PT 2), "I would like to have more time to warm up better and include compensatory and preventive content, but the reality is that I don't have it." (PT 6)

> "The players hardly ever do specific endurance work on the court with me. I have no time to train this with the players." (PT 1)

> "I use RIR to prescribe strength training, but it is difficult for players to understand it and use it correctly." (PT 2)

> "Many players do not know the correct exercise technique and I cannot always be present with them in the gym, which limits the exercise prescription and increases the injury risk of the players." (PT 1)

> "Educating the athlete is essential, but the day-to-day logistics and the hurry due to the lack of time available make it very complicated (...) I wish I had more time to talk to the players." (PT 6)

> "You must control many variables that are outside training" (PT 8)

> "Here, the training is over, and the physiotherapist is gone home in the first division. And then don't call him in the afternoon because he has his practice" (PT 4)

4. Discussion

To the authors' knowledge, this is the first study that analyzes the usual practices of futsal S&CCs through focus groups. This approach enables us to know in an open and unrestricted manner the opinions of these professionals in the development of their professional practice. Although a previous study analyzed the futsal S&CCs usual practice methodologies [15], this study was conducted through a survey with closed-ended answers, which inherently limited the participant responses. The present study aimed to investigate contemporary practices among futsal S&CCs and to understand how they integrate their theoretical formation and prior experience into diverse, evolving professional contexts. The findings of this study offer an overview of current futsal S&CC practices and highlight key elements that they consider essential for fulfilling their roles. The main findings of the study were as follows: (a) neuromuscular and strength training two days per week throughout the season as the cornerstone of the players' physical preparation and injury risk reduction; (b) meticulous monitoring of loads using different tools (e.g., GPS, LPS, RPE, Wellness assessments); (c) training individualization according to unique characteristics and contexts of each player and; (d) encouraging personal and professional relationships with the technical staff, which facilitated multidisciplinary collaboration in a productive and trust-based environment, as well as with the players, building mutual confidence and achieving greater implications and motivations.

Regarding the analysis of the performance model and competitive demands, S&CCs reported that strength, speed, and intermittent endurance are essential to futsal performance, a finding consistent with previous studies. Several studies have reported that lower limb strength plays a critical role in numerous game actions [49,50]. Enhanced lower limb strength increases motor unit recruitment, improves intra- and inter-muscular coordination, and boosts muscle mass, which is directly associated with better speed performance [30,51] and the execution of quick, explosive movements [52]. Meanwhile, other studies have indicated that movement speed is decisive in the game's critical moments for executing high-intensity, short-duration actions [2,53–55]. Likewise, other authors have confirmed the relevance of aerobic training due to the nature of the sport [2,56] and anaerobic metabolism due to the high physical demands of professional futsal and the requirement of this metabolism in decisive actions of the game, such as counter-attack situations, retrieving the ball, or attempts to avoid a goal [56–59]. In addition, S&CCs emphasized the importance of repeating these high-intensity actions throughout the match, which agrees with other studies that concluded that the ability to repeat multiple high-intensity efforts is essential because of the high repetition demands of high-intensity actions present in futsal matches [7,60]. In this sense, it is noteworthy that S&CCs rely on evidence from the scientific literature to determine the training content included in their sessions.

Concerning load monitoring, S&CCs underscored the relevance of precise load control, which enables a detailed record of the cumulative load and recovery dynamics experienced by the players throughout the season. This view aligns with other studies that have confirmed that optimal load control is essential for ensuring proper athlete adaptation and effectively managing the balance between training and recovery to optimize sports performance [61,62]. Although several studies have confirmed the importance of monitoring load through the complementation of various internal and external load variables [62], several limitations hinder the implementation of these tools in current high-level futsal environments [63]. This is in contrast with what happens in other sports, such as soccer, where heart rate monitoring and GPS are common [64,65]. These differences between sports could be explained by the fact that GPS technology is not applicable in indoor environments [63]. Additionally, local positioning systems (LPS) require fixed installation in the team's facilities, which poses practical challenges and renders them unsuitable for away matches. Moreover, LPS metrics are generally limited to accelerometry data, which restricts the analysis of distance and speed metrics [63]. The implementation of heart rate monitoring and GPS/accelerometry involves significant economic costs. Therefore, economic disparities between soccer and futsal may partly explain the limited use of these tools in futsal [15]. This, in turn, accounts for why S&CCs most commonly rely on RPE and wellness questionnaires for load monitoring, given their ease of use, implementation, and affordability. This approach is consistent with the findings of previous futsal studies [15] and other sports, such as rugby [66].

The injuries reported by the S&CCs were predominantly located in the lower body and were mainly muscular and ligamentous, which is consistent with findings from several previous studies [67–70]. Regarding the anatomical regions of these injuries, those affecting the ankle, knee, and thigh are predominant in both men and women, which is also in line with other studies [67–70]. Rui Pérez et al. [70] reported that the severity of injuries in futsal is usually slight (1–3 days) or mild (4–7 days), which enables most players to recover during the interval between games. This observation supports the perspective expressed by S&CCs in the focus groups. However, in contrast with other studies that reported most injuries in men's [67] and women's [68,71–73], futsal was moderate in severity (8–28 days). Among the multiple factors that could increase the risk of injury, S&CCs identified age as a particularly significant factor, which is in line with previous studies [72]. This underscores the need to consider age as a key factor in athlete preparation. Another important factor reported by S&CCs, which requires further research because of the lack of previous studies, is the type of court. According to the S&CCs, the playing surface appears to be associated with the occurrence of specific injuries, such as bone edemas or adductor muscle injuries. S&CCs have also reported a recent increase in anterior cruciate ligament (ACL) injuries, particularly in women's futsal, a trend that could alter the current understanding of futsal injury profiles in the scientific literature. S&CCs should implement their preventive strategies in consideration of the main futsal injuries as well as other relevant factors, such as player age or the type of court on which the sport is usually practiced.

For neuromuscular and strength training, prioritizing unilateral over bilateral exercises is emphasized, given the sport's predominantly one-leg demands (e.g., accelerations, changes of direction, shots). Although both training modalities enhance athletic performance [74,75], Stern et al. [76] highlighted the importance of unilateral specificity in soccer, and Gonzalo-Skok et al. [77] found that unilateral training yielded greater improvements in actions requiring unilateral force in basketball players. Ramirez-Campillo et al. [78] reported that unilateral training maximizes adaptations for game-specific, predominantly unilateral actions. Furthermore, studies by Gonzalo-Skok et al. [79,80] suggested that designing training based on the force vectors of specific movements is advantageous in team sports. The prescription of 2–3 days per week of these training sessions seems to be sufficient to achieve the sought adaptations. In addition, this training frequency was the most used by S&CCs, which is in line with that reported by other authors in several team sports [15,39].

S&CCs reported that their work is influenced by several contextual factors and relationships surrounding the context of the team in which they practice. Several studies have investigated the influence of playing position on player performance in futsal [35] and other sports, such as soccer [81], basketball [82], and rink hockey [83]. The incidence of schedule, ranking position, or match results has also been analyzed [35]. Several authors have also reported the importance of individual players' physical (age, injury history, or level of experience) [72] and psychological characteristics in sports performance and injury prevention [84–86]. Personal relationships within a sports team environment are critical for optimizing all team members, both the technical staff and the players [14,87]. Moreover, López-Gajardo et al. [36] reported that this factor is even more relevant in women's futsal than in men's. Scientific literature reinforces the opinion expressed by S&CCs regarding the relevance of various factors that influence their professional practice. However, further research is needed to analyze the interpersonal relationships within teams and their relationship with the professional practices of all team members. This is a key aspect that S&CCs emphasized during the focus groups.

S&CCs report that they must adapt their training methodologies to the context they face, which is limited by suboptimal facilities, lack of time, players' context, equipment, absence of advanced technology, or technical staff shortages. Spyrou et al. [15] reported that the primary concerns of futsal S&CCs were enhancing load monitoring capabilities (given the limitations of available technology), improving facilities, securing additional time, and expanding the technical staff. Weldon et al. [39] also found that limitations in technology, technical staff, facilities, equipment, and time were prevalent in other team sports, such as soccer or volleyball. The same results were found by Jones et al. [43] in rugby. In hockey, Ebben et al. [41] reported the need to improve training facilities and increase the influence over session design, underscoring the importance of strong personal and professional relationships within the technical staff. Therefore, S&CCs must adapt their practices to the particular conditions of each club.

Although analyzing the differences between male and female teams was not the primary objective of this study, the focus groups identified several key differences in the usual practices of S&CCs depending on the team's sex. While the training methodologies remain similar, female teams often face unique challenges due to their specific demands, as documented by previous studies [8]. Men's teams, although with their limitations as well, typically benefit from greater resources, which facilitate the adoption of advanced technologies (such as GPS), as evidenced in a recent systematic review [88]. In contrast, S&CCs working with women's teams noted that athletes are generally less familiar with monitoring tools like wellness questionnaires, necessitating additional time for proper familiarization. In addition, consistent with previous research, the injury profiles differed between genders, with women's teams exhibiting a higher prevalence of ACL injuries [30,51,53]. Moreover, in line with what was reported by Lopez-Gajardo et al. [36], interpersonal dynamics in women's teams were described as more complex, requiring tailored communication strategies. These differences highlight the importance of implementing gender-specific adaptations in training, protocols, and injury prevention to optimize performance across both contexts.

The main limitation of this study is the small number of participants in the focus groups. Moreover, all participants belonged to Spanish league teams, which may overlook certain cultural aspects of S&CC practices from other geographical areas. Future research should replicate these focus groups with participants from different leagues and geographic contexts and consider concentrating on a specific aspect of S&CC practices to provide more in-depth insights. Additionally, an independent study of each gender, male and female, could allow for a more thorough examination of potential differences between the two.

5. Conclusions

The study revealed that elite futsal strength and conditioning coaches structure their work around five central areas: analyzing competitive demands, monitoring training loads, mitigating injury risks, considering contextual and interpersonal factors and implementing performance-oriented training methodologies. Coaches prioritize neuromuscular and strength training—conducted typically two days per week—as essential for enhancing lower-limb power and minimizing injuries. They rely heavily on tools such as RPE and wellness questionnaires for load monitoring because of practical constraints in using more advanced technologies. Although the practices implemented are largely effective, the coaches face persistent limitations, including limited time, inadequate facilities, scarce resources and challenges in individualizing training protocols. These constraints highlight the need for further optimization in both the planning and implementation of training programs. The insights provided by the focus groups offer practical applications for both current and aspiring S&CCs, supporting the development of more individualized, multidisciplinary, and context-specific training strategies in elite futsal environments. These conclusions contribute to a better understanding of current practices and challenges in elite futsal training and underscore avenues for future research aimed at enhancing athletic performance while reducing injury risk.

Author Contributions: Conceptualization, R.A.-A., E.M.-P., B.M.-P. and G.V.-R.; methodology, R.A.-A., D.N.-V. and O.V.-G.; validation, R.A.-A. and O.V.-G.; formal analysis, R.A.-A. and O.V.-G.; investigation, R.A.-A., D.N.-V. and O.V.-G.; resources, R.A.-A., D.N.-V. and O.V.-G.; data curation, R.A.-A. and O.V.-G.; writing—original draft preparation, R.A.-A.; writing—review and editing, R.A.-A., E.M.-P., B.M.-P. and G.V.-R.; supervision, R.A.-A., E.M.-P., B.M.-P. and G.V.-R.; project administration, R.A.-A., E.M.-P., B.M.-P. and G.V.-R. All authors have read and agreed to the published version of the manuscript.

Funding: This research received no external funding.

Institutional Review Board Statement: The study was conducted in accordance with the Declaration of Helsinki and approved by The Clinical Research Ethics Committee of Aragon (CEICA) (PI23-456 on 8 November 2023).

Informed Consent Statement: Informed consent was obtained from all subjects involved in the study.

Data Availability Statement: The data that support the findings of this study are available from the corresponding author, upon reasonable request. The data are not publicly available due to privacy and ethical restrictions.

Acknowledgments: The authors thank all the S&CCs who participated in this study.

Conflicts of Interest: The authors declare no conflicts of interest.

References

1. Illa, J.; Fernandez, D.; Reche, X.; Carmona, G.; Tarragó, J.R. Quantification of an elite futsal team's microcycle external load by using the repetition of high and very high demanding scenarios. *Front. Psychol.* **2020**, *15*, 11. [CrossRef] [PubMed]
2. Spyrou, K.; Freitas, T.T.; Marín-Cascales, E.; Alcaraz, P.E. Physical and physiological match-play demands and player characteristics in futsal: A systematic review. *Front. Psychol.* **2020**, *11*, 569897. [CrossRef] [PubMed]
3. Barbero, J.C. Análisis cuantitativo de la dimensión temporal durante la competición en fútbol sala. *Eur. J. Hum. Mov.* **2003**, *10*, 143–163.
4. Martín Acero, R.; Seirul-lo Vargas, F.; Lago Peñas, C.; Lalin Novoa, C. Causas objetivas de planificación en deportes de equipo (I): Estado de forma y calendarios. *Rev. Entren. Deport.* **2013**, *27*, 1–19.
5. Barbero-Alvarez, J.C.; Soto, V.M.; Barbero-Alvarez, V.; Granda-Vera, J. Match analysis and heart rate of futsal players during competition. *J. Sports Sci.* **2008**, *26*, 63–73. [CrossRef]
6. Turner, A.N.; Stewart, P.F. Strength and conditioning for soccer players. *Strength Cond. J.* **2014**, *36*, 1–13. [CrossRef]
7. Ribeiro, J.N.; Gonçalves, B.; Coutinho, D.; Brito, J.; Sampaio, J.; Travassos, B. Activity profile and physical performance of match play in elite futsal players. *Front. Psychol.* **2020**, *24*, 11. [CrossRef] [PubMed]
8. Oliva-Lozano, J.M.; Muyor, J.M.; Puche Ortuño, D.; Rico-González, M.; Pino-Ortega, J. Analysis of key external and internal load variables in professional female futsal players: A longitudinal study. *Res. Sports Med.* **2023**, *31*, 309–318. [CrossRef]
9. Jones, T.W.; Howatson, G.; Russell, M.; French, D.N. Performance and neuromuscular adaptations following differing ratios of concurrent strength and endurance training. *J. Strength Cond. Res.* **2013**, *27*, 3342–3351. [CrossRef]
10. Gabbett, T.J.; Nassis, G.P.; Oetter, E.; Pretorius, J.; Johnston, N.; Medina, D.; Rodas, G.; Myslinski, T.; Howells, D.; Beard, A.; et al. The athlete monitoring cycle: A practical guide to interpreting and applying training monitoring data. *Br. J. Sports Med.* **2017**, *51*, 1451–1452. [CrossRef]
11. Gaudino, P.; Iaia, F.M.; Strudwick, A.J.; Hawkins, R.D.; Giampietro, A.; Atkinson, G.; Gregson, W. Factors influencing perception of effort (session-RPE) during elite soccer training. *Int. J. Sports Physiol. Perform.* **2015**, *10*, 860–864. [CrossRef] [PubMed]
12. Clemente, F.M.; Martinho, R.; Calvete, F.; Mendes, B. Training load and well-being status variations of elite futsal players across a full season: Comparisons between normal and congested weeks. *Physiol. Behav.* **2019**, *201*, 123–129. [CrossRef]
13. Jaspers, A.; Brink, M.S.; Probst, S.G.M.; Frencken, W.G.P.; Helsen, W.F. Relationships between training load indicators and training outcomes in professional soccer. *Sports Med.* **2017**, *47*, 533–544. [CrossRef] [PubMed]
14. Marques, J.; Chamari, K. Performance management in elite football: A teamwork modeling approach. *Int. J. Sports Physiol. Perform.* **2023**, *18*, 1371–1373. [CrossRef] [PubMed]
15. Spyrou, K.; Freitas, T.T.; Herrero Carrasco, R.; Marín-Cascales, E.; Alcaraz, P.E. Load monitoring, strength training, and recovery in futsal: Practitioners' perspectives. *Sci. Med. Footb.* **2024**, *8*, 76–83. [CrossRef]
16. Newton, M.; Owen, A.L.; Baker, J.S. Monitoring external and internal training loads: Relationships with injury risk in professional soccer: A Review. *EC Orthopaed.* **2019**, *10*, 686–697.
17. Foster, C.; Rodriguez-Marroyo, J.A.; De Koning, J.J. Monitoring training loads: The past, the present, and the future. *Int. J. Sports Physiol. Perform.* **2017**, *12*, S22–S28. [CrossRef]
18. Borresen, J.; Lambert, M.I. The quantification of training load, the training response and the effect on performance. *Sports Med.* **2009**, *39*, 779–795. [CrossRef]
19. Rodrigues, V.M.; Ramos, G.P.; Mendes, T.T.; Cabido, C.E.T.; Melo, E.S.; Condessa, L.A.; Coelho, D.B.; Garcia, E.S. Intensity of official futsal matches. *J. Strength Cond. Res.* **2011**, *25*, 2482–2487. [CrossRef]
20. Ali, A.; Farrally, M. Recording soccer players' heart rates during matches. *J. Sports Sci.* **1991**, *9*, 183–189. [CrossRef]

21. Bekris, E.; Gioldasis, A.; Gissis, I.; Katis, A.; Mitrousis, I.; Mylonis, E. Effects of a futsal game on metabolic, hormonal, and muscle damage indicators of male futsal players. *J. Strength Cond. Res.* **2022**, *36*, 545–550. [CrossRef] [PubMed]
22. Ribeiro, J.; Gantois, P.; Moreira, V.; Miranda, F.; Romano, N.; Nakamura, F.Y. Individual-based Creatine Kinase reference values in response to soccer match-play. *Int. J. Sports Med.* **2022**, *43*, 533–537. [CrossRef] [PubMed]
23. Stochi de Oliveira, R.; Borin, J.P. Monitoring and behavior of biomotor skills in futsal athletes during a season. *Front. Psychol.* **2021**, *28*, 661262. [CrossRef]
24. Chen, Y.S.; Clemente, F.M.; Pagaduan, J.C.; Crowley-McHattan, Z.J.; Lu, Y.X.; Chien, C.H.; Bezerra, P.; Chiu, Y.W.; Kuo, C.D. Relationships between perceived measures of internal load and wellness status during overseas futsal training camps. *PLoS ONE* **2022**, *17*, e0267227. [CrossRef] [PubMed]
25. Akubat, I.; Barrett, S.; Abt, G. Integrating the internal and external training loads in soccer. *Int. J. Sports Physiol. Perform.* **2014**, *9*, 457–462. [CrossRef]
26. Pino-Ortega, J.; Bastida-Castillo, A.; Gómez-Carmona, C.D.; Rico-González, M. Validity and reliability of an eight antennae ultra-wideband local positioning system to measure performance in an indoor environment. *Sports Biomech.* **2024**, *23*, 145–155. [CrossRef]
27. Nicolella, D.P.; Torres-Ronda, L.; Saylor, K.J.; Schelling, X. Validity and reliability of an accelerometer-based player tracking device. *PLoS ONE* **2018**, *13*, e0191823. [CrossRef]
28. Villanueva-Guerrero, O.; Lozano, D.; Roso-Moliner, A.; Nobari, H.; Lago-Fuentes, C.; Mainer-Pardos, E. Effects of different strength and velocity training programs on physical performance in youth futsal players. *Heliyon* **2024**, *10*, e30747. [CrossRef]
29. Yanci, J.; Castillo, D.; Iturricastillo, A.; Ayarra, R.; Nakamura, F.Y. Effects of two different volume-equated weekly distributed short-term plyometric training programs on futsal players' physical performance. *J. Strength Cond. Res.* **2017**, *31*, 1787–1794. [CrossRef]
30. Torres-Torrelo, J.; Rodríguez-Rosell, D.; González-Badillo, J.J. Light-load maximal lifting velocity full squat training program improves important physical and skill characteristics in futsal players. *J. Sports Sci.* **2017**, *35*, 967–975. [CrossRef]
31. Marques, D.L.; Travassos, B.; Sousa, A.C.; Gil, M.H.; Ribeiro, J.N.; Marques, M.C. Effects of low-moderate load high-velocity resistance training on physical performance of under-20 futsal players. *Sports* **2019**, *7*, 69. [CrossRef]
32. Halson, S.L. Monitoring training load to understand fatigue in athletes. *Sports Med.* **2014**, *44*, 139–147. [CrossRef]
33. Kasper, K. Sports training principles. *Curr. Sports Med. Rep.* **2019**, *18*, 95–96. [CrossRef] [PubMed]
34. Bahr, R.; Krosshaug, T. Understanding injury mechanisms: A key component of preventing injuries in sport. *Br. J. Sports Med.* **2005**, *39*, 324–329. [CrossRef] [PubMed]
35. Spyrou, K.; Freitas, T.T.; Marín-Cascales, E.; Herrero-Carrasco, R.; Alcaraz, P.E. External match load and the influence of contextual factors in elite futsal. *Biol. Sport* **2022**, *39*, 349–354. [CrossRef] [PubMed]
36. López Gajardo, M.Á.; Flores Cidoncha, A.; Rubio Morales, A.; Díaz García, J.; González Ponce, I. Factors that determine the achievement of performance in elite football: Qualitative orientation with professional players. *Retos* **2022**, *46*, 789–800. [CrossRef]
37. Serrano, C.; Felipe, J.L.; Garcia-Unanue, J.; Ibañez, E.; Hernando, E.; Gallardo, L.; Sanchez-Sanchez, J. Local positioning system analysis of physical demands during official matches in the Spanish futsal league. *Sensors* **2020**, *20*, 4860. [CrossRef] [PubMed]
38. Illa, J.; Fernandez, D.; Reche, X.; Serpiello, F.R. Positional differences in the most demanding scenarios of external load variables in elite futsal matches. *Front. Psychol.* **2021**, *12*, 625126. [CrossRef]
39. Weldon, A.; Duncan, M.J.; Turner, A.; Laplaca, D.; Sampaio, J.; Christie, C.J. Practices of strength and conditioning coaches: A snapshot from different sports, countries, and expertise levels. *J. Strength Cond. Res.* **2022**, *36*, 1335–1344. [CrossRef]
40. Ebben, W.P.; Blackard, D.O. Strength and conditioning practices of National Football League strength and conditioning coaches. *J. Strength Cond. Res.* **2001**, *15*, 48–58.
41. Ebben, W.P.; Carroll, R.M.; Simenz, C.J. Strength and conditioning practices of National Hockey League strength and conditioning coaches. *J. Strength Cond. Res.* **2004**, *18*, 889–897.
42. Ebben, W.P.; Hintz, M.J.; Simenz, C.J. Strength and conditioning practices of Major League Baseball strength and conditioning coaches. *J. Strength Cond. Res.* **2005**, *19*, 538–546.
43. Jones, T.W.; Smith, A.; Macnaughton, L.S.; French, D.N. Strength and conditioning and concurrent training practices in elite rugby union. *J. Strength Cond. Res.* **2016**, *30*, 3354–3366. [CrossRef]
44. Weldon, A.; Duncan, M.J.; Turner, A.; Sampaio, J.; Noon, M.; Wong, D.P.; Lai, V.W. Contemporary practices of strength and conditioning coaches in professional soccer. *Biol. Sport* **2021**, *38*, 377–390. [CrossRef]
45. Barrera-Díaz, J.; Figueiredo, A.J.; Field, A.; Ferreira, B.; Querido, S.M.; Silva, J.R.; Ribeiro, J.; Pinto, I.; Cornejo, P.; Torres, H.; et al. Contemporary practices of physical trainers in professional soccer: A qualitative study. *Front. Psychol.* **2023**, *19*, 1101958. [CrossRef]
46. Berenguera, A.; Fernández de Sanmamed, M.J.; Pons, M.; Pujol, E.; Rodríguez, D.; Saura, S. Escuchar, observar y comprender. Recuperando la narrativa en las Ciencias de la Salud. Aportaciones de la investigación cualitativa. *Inst. Univ. D'investigació En. Atenció Primària Jordi Gol.* **1994**, *1*, 224.

47. Lincoln, Y.S.; Guba, E.G.; Pilotta, J.J. Naturalistic inquiry: Beverly Hills. *Int. J. Intercult. Rel* **1985**, *9*, 438–439. [CrossRef]
48. Tong, A.; Sainsbury, P.; Craig, J. Consolidated criteria for reporting qualitative research (COREQ): A 32-item checklist for interviews and focus groups. *Int. J. Qual. Health Care* **2007**, *19*, 349–357. [CrossRef]
49. Baena-Raya, A.; García-Ortega, D.; Sánchez-López, S.; Soriano-Maldonado, A.; Reyes, P.J.; Rodríguez-Pérez, M.A. The influence of sprint mechanical properties on change of direction in female futsal players. *J. Hum. Kinet.* **2021**, *79*, 221–228. [CrossRef]
50. Jiménez-Reyes, P.; García-Ramos, A.; Cuadrado-Peñafiel, V.; Párraga-Montilla, J.A.; Morcillo-Losa, J.A.; Samozino, P.; Morin, J.B. Differences in sprint mechanical force-velocity profile between trained soccer and futsal players. *Int. J. Sports Physiol. Perform.* **2019**, *14*, 478–485. [CrossRef]
51. de Oliveira, R.S.; Borin, J.P.; Fernandes, P.T.; Uchida, M.C.; de Oliveira Borges, T. Descrição de 18 semanas de treinamento integrado sobre a velocidade de deslocamento em atletas brasileiros de futsal. *Rev. Bras. Ciênc. Esporte* **2019**, *41*, 308–313. [CrossRef]
52. Medina, J.Á.; Marqueta, P.M.; Salillas, L.G.; Corona Virón, P. Entrenamiento, rendimiento y control de la vía anaeróbico aláctica y de la fuerza en futbol sala. *Arch. Med. Deporte* **2004**, *21*, 307–315.
53. Augusto Barbieri, R.; Moura Zagatto, A.; Milioni, F.; Augusto Barbieri, F. Specific futsal training program can improve the physical performance of futsal players. *Sport Sci. Health* **2016**, *12*, 247–253. [CrossRef]
54. Makaje, N.; Ruangthai, R.; Arkarapanthu, A.; Yoopat, P. Physiological demands and activity profiles during futsal match play according to competitive level. *J. Sports Med. Phys. Fit.* **2012**, *52*, 366–374.
55. Nakamura, F.Y.; Pereira, L.A.; Rabelo, F.N.; Ramirez-Campillo, R.; Loturco, I. Faster futsal players perceive higher training loads and present greater decreases in sprinting speed during the preseason. *J. Strength Cond. Res.* **2016**, *30*, 1553–1562. [CrossRef]
56. Álvarez, J.C.B.; D'Ottavio, S.; Vera, J.G.; Castagna, C. Aerobic fitness in futsal players of different competitive level. *J. Strength Cond. Res.* **2009**, *23*, 2163–2166. [CrossRef] [PubMed]
57. Matzenbacher, F.; Pasquarelli, B.N.; Rabelo, F.N.; Stanganelli, L.C.R. Demanda fisiológica no futsal competitivo. Características físicas e fisiológicas de atletas profissionais. *Rev. Andal. Med. Deport.* **2014**, *7*, 122–131. [CrossRef]
58. Ferrari Bravo, D.; Impellizzeri, F.M.; Rampinini, E.; Castagna, C.; Bishop, D.; Wisloff, U. Sprint vs. interval training in football. *Int. J. Sports Med.* **2008**, *29*, 668–674. [CrossRef]
59. Castagna, C.; D'Ottavio, S.; Vera, J.G.; Álvarez, J.C.B. Match demands of professional Futsal: A case study. *J. Sci. Med. Sport* **2009**, *12*, 490–494. [CrossRef]
60. Ohmuro, T.; Iso, Y.; Tobita, A.; Hirose, S.; Ishizaki, S.; Sakaue, K.; Yasumatsu, M. Physical match performance of japanese top-level futsal players in different categories and playing positions. *Biol. Sport* **2020**, *37*, 359–365. [CrossRef]
61. Bourdon, P.C.; Cardinale, M.; Murray, A.; Gastin, P.; Kellmann, M.; Varley, M.C.; Gabbett, T.J.; Coutts, A.J.; Burgess, D.J.; Gregson, W.; et al. Monitoring athlete training loads: Consensus statement. *Int. J. Sports Physiol. Perform.* **2017**, *12*, 161–170. [CrossRef] [PubMed]
62. Vanrenterghem, J.; Nedergaard, N.J.; Robinson, M.A.; Drust, B. Training load monitoring in team sports: A novel framework separating physiological and biomechanical load-adaptation pathways. *Sports Med.* **2017**, *47*, 2135–2142. [CrossRef] [PubMed]
63. Torres-Ronda, L.; Beanland, E.; Whitehead, S.; Sweeting, A.; Clubb, J. Tracking systems in team sports: A narrative review of applications of the data and sport specific analysis. *Sports Med. Open* **2022**, *8*, 15. [CrossRef]
64. Akenhead, R.; Nassis, G.P. Training load and player monitoring in high-level football: Current practice and perceptions. *Int. J. Sports Physiol. Perform.* **2016**, *11*, 587–593. [CrossRef]
65. Loturco, I.; Freitas, T.T.; Alcaraz, P.E.; Kobal, R.; Hartmann Nunes, R.F.; Weldon, A.; Pereira, L.A. Practices of strength and conditioning coaches in Brazilian elite soccer. *Biol. Sport* **2022**, *39*, 779–791. [CrossRef] [PubMed]
66. Griffin, A.; Kenny, I.C.; Comyns, T.M.; Lyons, M. Training load monitoring in amateur rugby union: A survey of current practices. *J. Strength Cond. Res.* **2021**, *35*, 1568–1575. [CrossRef]
67. Lopes, M.; Martins, F.; Brito, J.; Figueiredo, P.; Tomás, R.; Ribeiro, F.; Travassos, B. Epidemiology of injuries in elite male futsal players. *Clin. J. Sport Med.* **2023**, *33*, 527–532. [CrossRef] [PubMed]
68. Lago-Fuentes, C.; Jiménez-Loaisa, A.; Padrón-Cabo, A.; Calvo, M.M.; García-Pinillos, F.; Rey, E. Epidemiology of injuries in elite female futsal players: A prospective cohort study. *Int. J. Sports Med.* **2020**, *41*, 885–890. [CrossRef]
69. Ruiz-Pérez, I.; López-Valenciano, A.; Jiménez-Loaisa, A.; Elvira, J.L.L.; Croix, M.D.S.; Ayala, F. Injury incidence, characteristics and burden among female sub-elite futsal players: A prospective study with three-year follow-up. *PeerJ* **2019**, *7*, e7989. [CrossRef]
70. Ruiz-Pérez, I.; López-Valenciano, A.; Elvira, J.L.; García-Gómez, A.; De Ste Croix, M.; Ayala, F. Epidemiology of injuries in elite male and female futsal: A systematic review and meta-analysis. *Sci. Med. Footb.* **2021**, *5*, 59–71. [CrossRef]
71. Gayardo, A.; Matana, S.B.; da Silva, M.R. Prevalence of injuries in female athletes of Brazilian futsal: A retrospective study. *Rev. Bras. Med. Esporte* **2012**, *18*, 186–189. [CrossRef]
72. Uluöz, E. Investigation of sport injury patterns in female futsal players. *Int. J. Sci. Cult. Sport* **2016**, *4*, 474–488. [CrossRef]
73. Angoorani, H.; Haratian, Z.; Mazaherinezhad, A.; Younespour, S. Injuries in Iran futsal national teams: A comparative study of incidence and characteristics. *Asian J. Sports Med.* **2014**, *5*, e23070. [CrossRef]

74. Ramírez-Campillo, R.; Burgos, C.H.; Henríquez-Olguín, C.; Andrade, D.C.; Martínez, C.; Álvarez, C.; Castro-Sepúlveda, M.; Marques, M.C.; Izquierdo, M. Effect of unilateral, bilateral, and combined plyometric training on explosive and endurance performance of young soccer players. *J. Strength Cond. Res.* **2015**, *29*, 1317–1328. [CrossRef]
75. Liao, K.F.; Nassis, G.P.; Bishop, C.; Yang, W.; Bian, C.; Li, Y.M. Effects of unilateral vs. bilateral resistance training interventions on measures of strength, jump, linear and change of direction speed: A systematic review and meta-analysis. *Biol. Sport* **2022**, *39*, 485–497. [CrossRef] [PubMed]
76. Stern, D.; Gonzalo-Skok, O.; Loturco, I.; Turner, A.; Bishop, C. A comparison of bilateral vs. unilateral-biased strength and power training interventions on measures of physical performance in elite youth soccer players. *J. Strength Cond. Res.* **2020**, *34*, 2105–2111. [CrossRef]
77. Gonzalo-Skok, O.; Tous-Fajardo, J.; Suarez-Arrones, L.; Arjol-Serrano, J.L.; Casajús, J.A.; Mendez-Villanueva, A. Single-leg power output and between-limbs imbalances in team-sport players: Unilateral versus bilateral combined resistance training. *Int. J. Sports Physiol. Perform.* **2017**, *12*, 106–114. [CrossRef]
78. Ramirez-Campillo, R.; Sanchez-Sanchez, J.; Gonzalo-Skok, O.; Rodríguez-Fernandez, A.; Carretero, M.; Nakamura, F.Y. Specific changes in young soccer player's fitness after traditional bilateral vs. unilateral combined strength and plyometric training. *Front. Physiol.* **2018**, *9*, 265. [CrossRef] [PubMed]
79. Gonzalo-Skok, O.; Sánchez-Sabaté, J.; Izquierdo-Lupón, L.; Sáez de Villarreal, E. Influence of force-vector and force application plyometric training in young elite basketball players. *Eur. J. Sport Sci.* **2019**, *19*, 305–314. [CrossRef]
80. Gonzalo-Skok, O.; Tous-Fajardo, J.; Valero-Campo, C.; Berzosa, C.; Bataller, A.V.; Arjol-Serrano, J.L.; Moras, G.; Mendez-Villanueva, A. Eccentric-overload training in team-sport functional performance: Constant bilateral vertical versus variable unilateral multidirectional movements. *Int. J. Sports Physiol. Perform.* **2017**, *12*, 951–958. [CrossRef]
81. Martín-García, A.; Casamichana, D.; Gómez Díaz, A.; Cos, F.; Gabbett, T.J. Positional differences in the most demanding passages of play in football competition. *J. Sports Sci. Med.* **2018**, *17*, 563. [PubMed]
82. Vázquez-Guerrero, J.; Ayala, F.; Garcia, F.; Sampaio, J. The most demanding scenarios of play in basketball competition from elite under-18 teams. *Front. Psychol.* **2020**, *11*, 552. [CrossRef] [PubMed]
83. Cuenca-Fernández, F.; Batalha, N.M.; Ruiz-Navarro, J.J.; Morales-Ortiz, E.; López-Contreras, G.; Arellano, R. Quantification of external load of elite rink hockey players in official matches. *J. Sports Med. Phys. Fit.* **2020**, *60*, 1526–1535.
84. Gimeno, F.; Buceta, J.M.; Pérez-Llantada, M.C. Influencia de las variables psicológicas en el deporte de competición: Evaluación mediante el cuestionario Características psicológicas relacionadas con el rendimiento deportivo. *Psicothema* **2007**, *19*, 667–672.
85. González Campos, G.; Valdivia-Moral, P.; Cachón Zagalaz, J.; Zurita Ortega, F.; Romero, O. Influencia del control del estrés en el rendimiento deportivo: La autoconfianza, la ansiedad y la concentración en deportistas. Retos: Nuevas tendencias en educación física, deporte y recreación. *Psicothema* **2017**, *32*, 3–6.
86. Thelwell, R.C.; Greenlees, I.A.; Weston, N.J.V. Using psychological skills training to develop soccer performance. *J. Appl. Sport Psychol.* **2006**, *18*, 254–270. [CrossRef]
87. Reid, C.; Stewart, E.; Thorne, G. Multidisciplinary sport science teams in elite sport: Comprehensive servicing or conflict and confusion? *Sport Psychol.* **2004**, *18*, 204–217. [CrossRef]
88. Albalad-Aiguabella, R.; Mainer-Pardos, E.; Casajús, J.A.; Vicente-Rodríguez, G.; Muniz-Pardos, B. Analysis of external load variables defining competitive demands in elite futsal through monitoring with tracking systems: A systematic review. *Strength Cond. J.* 2025, *in press*. [CrossRef]

sports

MDPI

Article

Sports Supplement Use in Road Cycling: A Comparative Analysis by Sex and Competitive Category †

Jesús García-Durán [1,2], David Romero-García [3], José Miguel Martínez-Sanz [4], José Antonio González-Jurado [1,2,*] and Antonio Jesús Sánchez-Oliver [2,5]

1 Faculty of Sports Science, Pablo de Olavide University, 41013 Seville, Spain; jgardur@alu.upo.es
2 Research Center on Physical and Sports Performance, Pablo de Olavide University, 41013 Seville, Spain; sanchezoliver@us.es
3 Optics, Pharmacology and Anatomy Department, Faculty of Sciences, University of Alicante, 03690 Alicante, Spain; david.romero@gcloud.ua.es
4 Nursing Department, Faculty of Health Sciences, University of Alicante, 03690 Alicante, Spain; josemiguel.ms@ua.es
5 Departamento de Motricidad Humana y Rendimiento Deportivo, Universidad de Sevilla, 41013 Seville, Spain
* Correspondence: jagonjur@upo.es
† This is a part of PhD thesis of Jesús García-Durán in Pablo de Olavide University, Seville, Spain.

Abstract: This study analyzes and compares sports supplement (SS) consumption among federated road cyclists, considering sex and competition category. The aim is to identify key factors influencing SS use and provide insights for developing nutritional strategies in cycling. A cross-sectional, descriptive study was conducted, involving 1503 cyclists (1231 men and 272 women). Data were collected through a validated questionnaire assessing anthropometric data, training habits, SS consumption patterns, and sources of information. Results indicate that 64.3% of cyclists currently use SS. Women reported a significantly higher consumption rate (88.2%) compared to men (59.1%), although men had a higher average SS intake than women (8.28 ± 9.36 vs. 6.76 ± 5.96). Additionally, SS use decreased with age and competition level, with elite cyclists showing the highest prevalence (76.3%) and master 50 the lowest (58.4%). Group A supplements (scientifically supported) were the most frequently used, while Group C supplements (limited evidence) and Group D substances (prohibited) were more commonly consumed by men. Findings highlight significant differences in SS consumption based on sex and competition level, with elite cyclists and women reporting higher prevalence. However, men reported a higher average number of SS consumed. The study underscores the need for targeted nutritional education, particularly among master cyclists, to promote evidence-based SS use and minimize the risks of ineffective or unsafe supplementation. Future research should explore the long-term effects of SS consumption in cycling and the effectiveness of educational interventions for safe and optimized supplementation practices.

Keywords: endurance performance; sport nutrition; road cycling; ergogenic aids; doping

1. Introduction

Road cycling has experienced significant growth [1,2], characterized by high physical and metabolic demands, particularly in aerobic capacity and lactate threshold [3,4]. These factors, alongside biomechanical and psychological aspects, are key to competitive success [5,6], making nutritional planning essential for optimizing performance and recovery [7,8].

 https://doi.org/10.3390/sports13040122

One of the most relevant elements in cyclists' nutritional planning is the consumption of sports supplements (SSs), which have been widely used to improve energy and macronutrient availability, optimize performance, and prevent nutritional deficiencies [8,9]. Excessive or misguided supplementation can lead to financial waste, ineffective performance enhancement, or even adverse health and sport performance effects [10,11].

The Australian Institute of Sport (AIS) categorizes SS into four groups based on scientific evidence: Group A (strong scientific support), Group B (emerging evidence), Group C (limited evidence), and Group D (prohibited or contaminant substances) [9]. While Group A supplements are widely recommended, the inappropriate use of substances from Groups C and D raises concerns regarding efficacy, safety, and the risk of unintentional doping [9]. Despite the availability of scientifically backed supplements, the misuse of banned substances has been observed, with a high prevalence among federated road cyclists [12].

SSs are often used inappropriately due to concerns about their safety, efficacy, and legality, as well as their consumption in unsuitable situations [13]. To ensure responsible use, supplementation should be justified based on specific needs and adapted to the athlete's age and life cycle [14]. Key reasons for SS use include correcting nutrient deficiencies, addressing inadequate energy intake, supporting restrictive diets, managing food allergies or intolerances, optimizing training adaptations, enhancing performance, and ensuring adequate nutrition during travel to areas with food availability or safety concerns [15].

The scarce existing literature suggests that SS consumption varies by sex and competition level among cyclists. Studies indicate that female cyclists report a higher prevalence of SS use than their male counterparts [12,16], though men often consume a greater number of supplements [8,12,16,17]. Additionally, competitive category influences SS intake, with elite athletes showing a higher reliance on evidence-based ergogenic aids, while lower-category cyclists may be more prone to using supplements with limited scientific backing [12,16]. Understanding these patterns is essential for developing targeted nutritional education and policies to promote safe and effective supplementation practices and to address the distinct needs of male and female cyclists at different levels of competition [18,19].

To date, no study has specifically examined a sample of federated road cyclists to compare SS consumption by sex and competition category. The present study aims to analyze and compare SS consumption among federated road cyclists, with a focus on sex and competition category. By addressing existing gaps in the literature, this study seeks to provide insights into the factors influencing SS use in cycling, contributing to evidence-based recommendations for optimizing nutritional strategies in cycling.

2. Materials and Methods

2.1. Study Design and Participants

This study follows a quantitative, cross-sectional, and descriptive design, focusing on the analysis of SS consumption among federated road cyclists. Participant selection was conducted through the Andalusian Cycling Federation, as well as cycling clubs and sports associations in the region. A non-probabilistic sampling method was employed, and the final sample included cyclists of both sexes, distributed across various competition categories: elite, master 30, master 40, and master 50. Table 1 presents descriptive data on the sample, including age, basic anthropometric characteristics, and sports-related aspects, segmented by sex and category.

The sample size was determined using the Australian Bureau of Statistics (https://www.abs.gov.au/websitedbs/D3310114.nsf/home/Sample+Size+Calculator, accessed on 15 January 2025) Sample Size Calculator, with a 95% confidence level. According to FAC data from 2023, the target population consisted of 8189 federated cyclists (371 women and

7818 men). Assuming an expected proportion of 0.5, the final sample included 1503 cyclists (men: $n = 1231$; women: $n = 272$), with a confidence interval of 0.02, a standard error of 0.01, and a relative standard error of 2.33.

Table 1. Descriptive data of the sample by sex and competition category.

	Sex (M ± SD)		Category (M ± SD)			
	Women (n = 272)	**Men (n = 1231)**	**Elite (n = 312)**	**Master 30 (n = 386)**	**Master 40 (n = 444)**	**Master 50 (n = 361)**
Age (years)	40.2 ± 9.6	41.6 ± 9.9	29.3 ± 4.0	34.7 ± 2.9	44.6 ± 2.9	54.7 ± 3.0
Height (cm)	162.7 ± 7.0	171.1 ± 7.3	170.8 ± 7.7	171.0 ± 7.9	170.5 ± 8.9	166.0 ± 5.6
Body Mass (kg)	60.0 ± 7.3	65.0 ± 7.2	61.9 ± 6.9	63.9 ± 8.0	65.5 ± 8.3	64.5 ± 5.5
Years Licensed	7.7 ± 3.0	7.0 ± 3.1	6.2 ± 2.9	5.4 ± 2.9	7.6 ± 3.2	9.3 ± 1.8
Weekly Training Days	4.2 ± 1.1	4.4 ± 0.9	4.7 ± 0.9	4.4 ± 1.0	4.3 ± 0.8	4.5 ± 0.8
Daily Training Hours	2.4 ± 0.6	4.2 ± 1.2	4.8 ± 1.4	4.0 ± 1.2	3.6 ± 1.1	3.2 ± 0.9
No. Competitions in the Season	9.1 ± 3.1	9.8 ± 2.5	10.8 ± 1.9	10.5 ± 1.9	10.0 ± 2.1	7.4 ± 3.0

M: mean; SD: standard deviation.

2.2. Data Collection Instrument

For data collection, a previously validated questionnaire was used and underwent a content, structure, and applicability review [20]. The questionnaire consisted of three main sections: (a) anthropometric and personal data (age, weight, height, years of federation, weekly training days and hours, number of competitions per year); (b) sports practice, including information on competition category and experience level; (c) SS consumption habits, which assessed types of supplements used, reasons for consumption, sources of information, purchasing locations, consumption frequency, and perceived results [21].

The questionnaire used in this study was reviewed and classified among the validated instruments included in the systematic review and meta-analysis conducted by Knapik et al. (2016), which assessed its adequacy for obtaining accurate data on SS use among athlete populations [17].

2.3. Procedure

Participants were contacted through the FAC and sports clubs via email, where they received detailed study information and a link to the questionnaire. Additionally, data collection was conducted in person at various competitions held between January and May 2024. For the in-person data collection, we used tablets to administer the questionnaire via Google Forms, with responses being automatically recorded in a Google Sheet.

Participation was voluntary and anonymous, ensuring compliance with the principles of the Declaration of Helsinki for research involving human subjects. Before participating, all subjects in the study were fully informed and consented. The study protocol was approved by the Ethics Committee of the Pablo de Olavide University (reference number: 27/7-3).

2.4. Statistical Analysis

To assess variable distribution and homoscedasticity, the Kolmogorov–Smirnov and Levene tests were applied. After confirming a normal distribution, a descriptive analysis was performed, presenting mean and standard deviation (Mean ± SD).

Differences in SS consumption by sex (women vs. men), based on the categories established by the AIS [9], were analyzed using Student's t-test, and the effect size was calculated using Cohen's d coefficient. To examine differences across competition categories (elite, master 30, master 40, and master 50), a one-way ANOVA was conducted, with effect size calculated using partial eta squared (ηp^2). Subsequently, Bonferroni-adjusted pairwise comparisons were performed for variables showing significant differences. The level of significance was set a priori at $p < 0.05$.

For qualitative variables, including current SS consumption and supplements used by more than 10% of the sample, a chi-square test (X^2) was applied to assess potential differences based on sex and competition category. Residuals and Cramér's V were also calculated to evaluate the association between different groups. The level of significance was set a priori at $p < 0.05$. All statistical analyses were conducted using the Statistical Package for Social Sciences (SPSS) v.25 (IBM, Armonk, NY, USA).

3. Results

Of the total sample, 64.3% reported currently consuming some type of SS. Regarding sex, significant differences were found between women and men ($p < 0.001$), with women showing a higher consumption rate (88.2% vs. 59.1%). Regarding the competition category, significant differences were also observed ($p < 0.001$), indicating that SS consumption decreased as the age category increased, with elite cyclists reporting the highest consumption (76.3%, 64.2%, 60.8%, 58.4%).

Table 2 shows that men consumed significantly more total SS, Group A ergogenic aids, and Group C and D supplements than women. When looking at competition categories, there were significant differences in consumption for all analyzed variables.

Table 2. Number of SSs used based on the level of evidence established by the AIS [9], segmented by sex and competition category.

		Sex (M ± SD)					Categories (M ± SD)						
		Women	Men	t	*p*	d Cohen	Elite	M 30	M 40	M 50	F	*p*	ηp2
Total SS		6.8 ± 6.0	8.3 ± 9.4	−3.39	<0.001	8.85	11.3 ± 10.8	10.0 ± 10.0	6.5 ± 7.4	4.9 ± 5.0	43.63	<0.001	0.08
Group A	Total	4.8 ± 3.1	4.8 ± 4.7	−0.23	0.815	4.46	7.0 ± 5.4	5.1 ± 4.3	4.1 ± 4.1	3.5 ± 3.4	43.19	<0.001	0.08
	Sport foods	3.0 ± 1.6	2.9 ± 2.7	0.74	0.458	2.50	4.3 ± 2.9	3.0 ± 2.2	2.5 ± 2.4	2.2 ± 2.1	47.67	<0.001	0.09
	Medical Sup.	1.0 ± 1.3	1.0 ± 1.2	0.36	0.720	1.21	1.4 ± 1.3	1.0 ± 1.2	0.8 ± 1.1	0.8 ± 1.2	19.15	<0.001	0.04
	Ergogenic aids	0.8 ± 1.0	1.0 ± 1.3	−2.47	0.014	1.22	1.4 ± 1.5	1.1 ± 1.3	0.9 ± 1.2	0.5 ± 0.7	36.05	<0.001	0.07
Group B		0.4 ± 0.9	0.5 ± 0.9	−1.88	0.060	0.93	0.8 ± 1.2	0.4 ± 1.0	0.5 ± 0.8	0.4 ± 0.7	17.81	<0.001	0.03
Group C		1.6 ± 2.9	2.0 ± 3.4	−2.28	0.023	3.29	3.0 ± 4.1	2.2 ± 3.7	1.8 ± 3.0	0.9 ± 1.5	23.93	<0.001	0.05
Group D		0.0 ± 0.1	0.9 ± 1.7	−18.28	<0.001	1.55	0.5 ± 1.0	2.3 ± 2.3	0.2 ± 0.5	0.0 ± 0.2	248.12	<0.001	0.33

Post hoc pairwise comparisons between different categories, adjusted using the Bonferroni correction and considering variables with significant differences by competition level, revealed significant differences between elite cyclists and all other categories ($p < 0.001$–0.008) for most variables analyzed, with elite cyclists consistently showing the highest SS consumption. The only exception was observed in Group D, where no significant differences were found when comparing elite cyclists with the master 30 category. Additionally, no significant differences were found when comparing elite and master 30 cyclists in terms of total SS consumption ($p = 0.215$).

When comparing master 30 with master 40 and master 50, significant differences were found in most analyzed variables ($p < 0.001$–0.037), with master 30 cyclists showing higher consumption levels. However, no significant differences were observed when comparing master 30 vs. master 50 in medical supplements ($p = 0.174$), master 30 vs. master 40 and 50 in Group B supplements ($p = 1.000$), or master 30 vs. master 40 in Group C supplements ($p = 0.499$). Finally, when comparing master 40 and master 50, significant differences were found in total SS consumption, ergogenic aids from Group A, and Group C supplements

($p < 0.001$–0.037), with higher consumption in master 40 cyclists. No significant differences were observed for the remaining variables ($p = 0.294$–1.000).

The post hoc analysis also showed that elite cyclists reported significantly higher SS consumption compared to master categories, especially when compared to master 40 and master 50 ($p < 0.001$). In Group A, elite cyclists consumed more sports foods, medical supplements, and ergogenic aids compared to master categories. In particular, ergogenic aids were more frequently used by elite cyclists than by those in master 40 and master 50 categories ($p < 0.001$), whereas differences between master 30 and master 40 were smaller.

In Group B, significant differences were found between elite cyclists and master categories in most cases, with lower consumption levels as age increased. A similar pattern was observed in Group C, where elite cyclists used more supplements with little scientific evidence compared to master cyclists. Finally, in Group D (prohibited or high-risk substances), higher consumption was identified in the master 30 category compared to other categories, highlighting the need for greater control and nutritional education in these groups.

Tables 3 and 4 present the SS consumed by at least 10% of the total sample, segmented by sex and competition level. Regarding sex, significant differences were observed for most SS analyzed, except for gels, iron, multivitamins, probiotics, beta-alanine, or glutamine. Regarding competition categories, significant differences were found for most analyzed SS, except for melatonin. SS consumption decreased as age categories increased, with elite cyclists reporting the highest intake levels. The consumption of sports drinks, sports bars, electrolytes, caffeine, beta-alanine, creatine, nitrates, BCAAs, mineral complexes, and spirulina showed a progressive decline across older categories, with elite cyclists consuming the most. Carbohydrate gainers, gels, iron, vitamin C, and citrulline malate were significantly more consumed in the elite category. Casein and multivitamins were more frequently consumed by elite and master 30 cyclists. Probiotics were consumed more frequently by the elite and master 50 categories. Finally, vitamin D, magnesium, and glutamine had a higher consumption rate in the master 40 category.

Table 3. Distribution (%) of the most consumed SS by sample, based on sex and according to the level of evidence established by the AIS [9].

Category			Total	Women	Residual	Men	Residual	X^2	p	V Cramer
Group A	Sport foods	Sports bars	61.9	80.5	7.0	57.8	7.0	48.591	<0.001	0.180
		Sport gels	60.8	64.7	1.5	60.0	−1.5	2.113	0.146	0.037
		Sports drinks	53.4	73.9	7.5	48.8	−7.5	56.283	<0.001	0.194
		CG	44.1	27.2	−6.2	47.8	6.2	38.501	<0.001	0.160
		Electrolytes	36.1	46.0	3.8	33.9	−3.8	14.102	<0.001	0.097
		Casein	15.0	4.0	−5.6	17.5	5.6	31.411	<0.001	0.145
	Medical Supplements	Multivitamin	39.3	36.8	−1.0	39.9	1	0.910	0.340	0.025
		Iron	23.8	21.7	−0.9	24.2	0.9	0.779	0.377	0.023
		Vitamin D	15.3	19.5	2.1	14.4	−2.1	4.482	0.034	0.055
		Probiotics	17.3	15.4	−0.9	17.7	0.9	0.801	0.371	0.023
	Ergogenic aids	Caffeine	40.4	49.6	3.4	38.3	−3.4	11.793	<0.001	0.089
		Nitrates	16.2	3.3	−6.4	19.0	6.4	40.515	<0.001	0.164
		CM	16.0	4.4	−5.8	18.6	5.4	33.322	<0.001	0.149
		Beta-alanine	14.5	11.0	−1.8	15.3	1.8	3.234	0.072	0.046
Group B		Vitamin C	24.2	11.0	−5.6	27.1	5.6	31.476	<0.001	0.145

potentially harmful products [9]. Ensuring equitable access to specialized guidance is particularly crucial for master cyclists, who reported lower consumption of scientifically supported supplements. Moreover, even though most supplements consumed by the sample belonged to Group A, supported by scientific evidence, they did not utilize other supplements with demonstrated potential to enhance performance in endurance sports, such as sodium bicarbonate and glycerol [32,33]. In addition, collagen and omega-3 (e.g., fish oil) may be beneficial in the nutritional management of musculoskeletal injuries in athletes, but further research is required [34].

Despite sports supplements are commonly used by athletes, their implementation is frequently suboptimal and inadequate [13,15]. Therefore, sports organizations, sports science and medicine practitioners, coaches, and athletes must adopt a practical and transparent approach that weighs the advantages and disadvantages of supplement use by evaluating their safety, effectiveness, and permissibility in sports [9]. This highlights the importance of conducting cost–benefit analyses to evaluate their responsible use, combined with personalized nutritional assessments tailored to athletes' specific contexts and requirements [14]. It is also critical to emphasize that supplements should not serve as a substitute for unbalanced diets or nutritional deficiencies [35]. Moreover, the excessive or unregulated consumption of these products poses serious risks, underscoring the need for educational initiatives starting at an early age to promote informed decision-making among athletes, coaches, and family members [15].

Although this study provides relevant information on SS consumption among federated cyclists according to competitive category and sex, several limitations must be considered when interpreting the results. First, although the study includes a large sample of federated cyclists across different competitive categories, data were collected at a single point in time. This limits the ability to extrapolate trends over the years, making it advisable to conduct longitudinal studies to analyze the evolution of SS consumption in this population. Second, the data are based on self-reported information obtained through a validated questionnaire, which may introduce biases in the reporting of supplement intake. Specifically, the low reported consumption of Group D substances could be influenced by participants being unwilling to disclose their use due to potential negative consequences or social stigma. Furthermore, individuals using such substances may have been less likely to participate in the survey altogether, leading to an underestimation of their prevalence. Finally, future research should explore the relationship between SS consumption and athletic performance in cyclists across different categories, which would allow for the identification of specific supplements and consumption patterns associated with various performance levels.

Future research should further investigate the underlying reasons for differences in SS consumption based on sex and competition level and explore the long-term impacts of supplementation on cycling performance and health. Evaluating the effectiveness of intervention strategies aimed at optimizing SS consumption in competitive cycling will be essential for promoting safe and effective nutritional practices. Additionally, future research should continue to monitor supplement consumption trends in road cycling, explore the motivations behind supplement choices, and evaluate the impact of educational interventions on athletes' nutritional practices.

5. Conclusions

This study reveals that sports supplement consumption is high among federated road cyclists, with notable variations influenced by both sex and competitive level. While women exhibit a higher overall prevalence of supplement use, men tend to consume a wider array and greater quantities of supplements. Supplementation patterns are also strongly linked to competition category, with elite cyclists demonstrating the highest engagement, which gradually declines across the master categories. Although supplements with strong scientific backing (Group A) are the most frequently used, the significant consumption of supplements with limited evidence (Group C) and potentially harmful or prohibited substances (Group D), particularly among men, raises concerns. These findings highlight the complex interplay between sex, competitive demands, and supplementation behaviors in road cycling.

Based on these conclusions, several recommendations can be made. Firstly, there is a clear need for targeted nutritional education programs tailored to the specific needs and consumption patterns of road cyclists, considering both sex and competition category. These programs should emphasize the importance of evidence-based supplementation and aim to discourage the use of ineffective or potentially risky products. Secondly, efforts should be made to ensure qualified sports nutrition professionals for cyclists at all levels, particularly for who may have less access to such resources. Sports organizations and coaches should play a proactive role in promoting informed decision-making regarding supplement use, emphasizing that supplements should complement, not replace, a balanced diet. Finally, given the concerning use of Group C and D supplements, stricter regulations and increased awareness campaigns regarding the risks associated with these substances may be warranted within the cycling community.

Author Contributions: Conceptualization, J.G.-D. and A.J.S.-O.; methodology, J.A.G.-J., J.M.M.-S. and A.J.S.-O.; validation, J.M.M.-S. and A.J.S.-O.; formal analysis, J.G.-D., D.R.-G. and A.J.S.-O.; investigation, J.G.-D.; data curation, J.G.-D., D.R.-G. and A.J.S.-O.; writing—original draft preparation, J.G.-D., J.M.M.-S. and A.J.S.-O.; writing—review and editing, J.A.G.-J., J.M.M.-S. and A.J.S.-O.; visualization, J.G.-D., J.A.G.-J., D.R.-G., J.M.M.-S. and A.J.S.-O.; supervision, J.G.-D., J.M.M.-S. and A.J.S.-O. All authors have read and agreed to the published version of the manuscript.

Funding: This research received no external funding.

Institutional Review Board Statement: This study was conducted following the Declaration of Helsinki, and it was approved by the Ethics Committee of Pablo de Olavide University (Seville, Spain) (protocol code: 23/7-3; date of approval: 17 November 2023).

Informed Consent Statement: Informed consent was obtained from all subjects involved in the study.

Data Availability Statement: In alignment with Research Data Policies promoting open science, the dataset from this study is accessible to interested researchers via the Figshare repository: doi:10.6084/m9.figshare.28400753, accessed on 13 February 2025.

Acknowledgments: The authors sincerely appreciate the support and collaboration of the Andalusian Cycling Federation (FAC) and the cycling clubs and associations involved in this study. This research represents a fundamental component of Jesús García Durán's doctoral thesis.

Conflicts of Interest: The authors declare no conflicts of interest.

Abbreviations

The following abbreviations are used in this manuscript:

AIS	Australian Institute of Sport
SS	Sports Supplement

References

1. Union Cycliste Internationale. Available online: https://www.uci.org/ (accessed on 11 June 2024).
2. Real Federación Española de Ciclismo. Available online: https://rfec.com/index.php/es/smartweb/seccion/seccion/rfec/home (accessed on 28 June 2024).

3. Mujika, I.; Padilla, S. Physiological and performance characteristics of male professional road cyclists. *Sports Med.* **2001**, *31*, 479–487. [CrossRef] [PubMed]
4. Atkinson, G.; Davison, R.; Jeukendrup, A.; Passfield, L. Science and cycling: Current knowledge and future directions for research. *J. Sports Sci.* **2003**, *21*, 767–787. [CrossRef] [PubMed]
5. Santalla, A.; Earnest, C.P.; Marroyo, J.A.; Lucia, A. The Tour de France: An updated physiological review. *Int. J. Sports Physiol. Perform.* **2012**, *7*, 200–209. [CrossRef]
6. Phillips, K.E.; Hopkins, W.G. Determinants of Cycling Performance: A Review of the Dimensions and Features Regulating Performance in Elite Cycling Competitions. *Sports Med. Open* **2020**, *6*, 23. [CrossRef]
7. Burke, L.M. Nutritional practices of male and female endurance cyclists. *Sports Med.* **2001**, *31*, 521–532. [CrossRef] [PubMed]
8. Maughan, R.J.; Burke, L.M.; Dvorak, J.; Larson-Meyer, D.E.; Peeling, P.; Phillips, S.M.; Rawson, E.S.; Walsh, N.P.; Garthe, I.; Geyer, H.; et al. IOC consensus statement: Dietary supplements and the high-performance athlete. *Br. J. Sports Med.* **2018**, *52*, 439–455. [CrossRef]
9. Australian Institute of Sport. Sports Supplement Framework. Available online: https://www.ais.gov.au/nutrition/supplements (accessed on 15 May 2024).
10. Martinez-Sanz, J.M.; Sospedra, I.; Ortiz, C.M.; Baladia, E.; Gil-Izquierdo, A.; Ortiz-Moncada, R. Intended or Unintended Doping? A Review of the Presence of Doping Substances in Dietary Supplements Used in Sports. *Nutrients* **2017**, *9*, 1093. [CrossRef]
11. Geyer, H.; Parr, M.K.; Koehler, K.; Mareck, U.; Schanzer, W.; Thevis, M. Nutritional supplements cross-contaminated and faked with doping substances. *J. Mass Spectrom.* **2008**, *43*, 892–902. [CrossRef]
12. García-Durán, J.; González-Jurado, J.A.; Sánchez-Oliver, A.J. Analysis of Sports Supplement Consumption in 1688 Federated Road Cyclists. *Nutrients* **2024**, *16*, 123. [CrossRef]
13. Maughan, R.J.; Shirreffs, S.M.; Vernec, A. Making Decisions About Supplement Use. *Int. J. Sport Nutr. Exerc. Metab.* **2018**, *28*, 212–219. [CrossRef] [PubMed]
14. Mata-Ordoñez, F.; Sánchez-Oliver, A.J.; Domínguez, R.; Villegas García, J.A. Suplementación en el deporte: Directrices desde la responsabilidad profesional. *Mot. Rev. Cienc. Act. Fís. Deport.* **2018**, *51*, 4–12.
15. Garthe, I.; Maughan, R.J. Athletes and Supplements: Prevalence and Perspectives. *Int. J. Sport Nutr. Exerc. Metab.* **2018**, *28*, 126–138. [CrossRef] [PubMed]
16. García-Durán, J.; González-Jurado, J.A.; Sánchez-Oliver, A.J. Sports Supplement Consumption in 316 Federated Female Road Cyclists. *Nutrients* **2024**, *16*, 2563. [CrossRef]
17. Knapik, J.J.; Steelman, R.A.; Hoedebecke, S.S.; Austin, K.G.; Farina, E.K.; Lieberman, H.R. Prevalence of Dietary Supplement Use by Athletes: Systematic Review and Meta-Analysis. *Sports Med.* **2016**, *46*, 103–123. [CrossRef]
18. Larrosa, M.; Gil-Izquierdo, A.; Gonzalez-Rodríguez, L.A.; Muñoz Alferez, M.J.; San Juan, A.; Sánchez-Gómez, A.; Calvo-Ayuso, N.; Ramos-Alvarez, J.J.; Fernández-Lázaro, D.; López-Grueso, R.; et al. Nutritional strategies for optimizing health, sports performance, and recovery for female athletes and other physically active women: A systematic review. *Nutr. Rev.* **2023**, *83*, nuae082. [CrossRef]
19. Sims, S.T.; Kerksick, C.M.; Smith-Ryan, A.E.; Janse de Jonge, X.A.K.; Hirsch, K.R.; Arent, S.M.; Hewlings, S.J.; Kleiner, S.M.; Bustillo, E.; Tartar, J.L.; et al. International society of sports nutrition position stand: Nutritional concerns of the female athlete. *J. Int. Soc. Sports Nutr.* **2023**, *20*, 2204066. [CrossRef]
20. Sanchez-Oliver, A.J. Suplementación Nutricional en la Actividad Físico-Deportiva. Análisis de la Calidad del Suplemento Proteico Consumido. Ph.D. Thesis, Universidad de Granada, Granada, Spain, 2013.
21. Sánchez-Oliver, A.J.; Domínguez, R.; Jiménez-Alfageme, R.; Romero-García, D.; Herrera-Puche, L.; Martínez Sanz, J.M.; Guerra-Hernández, E.J. Cuestionario Sobre Consumo de Suplementos Deportivos. Manual de Uso. 2024. Available online: http://hdl.handle.net/10045/144759 (accessed on 20 January 2025).
22. Huang, S.-H.S.; Johnson, K.; Pipe, A.L. The use of dietary supplements and medications by Canadian athletes at the Atlanta and Sydney Olympic Games. *Clin. J. Sport Med.* **2006**, *16*, 27–33. [CrossRef] [PubMed]
23. Loraschi, A.; Galli, N.; Cosentino, M. Dietary supplement and drug use and doping knowledge and attitudes in italian young elite cyclists. *Clin. J. Sport Med.* **2014**, *24*, 238–244. [CrossRef]
24. Baltazar-Martins, G.; Brito de Souza, D.; Aguilar-Navarro, M.; Muñoz-Guerra, J.; del Mar Plata, M.; Del Coso, J. Prevalence and patterns of dietary supplement use in elite Spanish atheltes. *J. Int. Soc. Sports Nutr.* **2019**, *16*, 30. [CrossRef]
25. Maughan, R.J.; Burke, L.M.; Dvorak, J.; Larson-Meyer, D.E.; Peeling, P.; Phillips, S.M.; Rawson, E.S.; Walsh, N.P.; Garthe, I.; Geyer, H.; et al. IOC consensus statement: Dietary supplements and the high-performance athlete. *Int. J. Sport Nutr. Exerc. Metab.* **2018**, *28*, 104–125. [CrossRef]
26. Jiménez-Alfageme, R.; Rubio-Quintanilla, N.; Romero-García, D.; Sanchez-Oliver, A.J.; Sospedra, I.; Martínez-Sanz, J.M. Are the Consumption Patterns of Sports Supplements Similar Among Spanish Mountain Runners? *Nutrients* **2023**, *15*, 262. [CrossRef] [PubMed]

27. Jiménez-Alfageme, R.; Domínguez, R.; Sanchez-Oliver, A.J.; Tapia-Castillo, P.; Martínez-Sanz, J.M.; Sospedra, I. Analysis of the Consumption of Sports Supplements in Open Water Swimmers According to the Competitive Level. *Nutrients* **2022**, *14*, 5211. [CrossRef]
28. Jiménez-Alfageme, R.; Martínez-Sanz, J.M.; Romero-García, D.; Giménez-Monzo, D.; Hernández Aparicio, S.; Sanchez-Oliver, A.J.; Sospedra, I. Do Spanish Triathletes Consume Sports Supplements According to Scientific Evidence? An Analysis of the Consumption Pattern According to Sex and Level of Competition. *Nutrients* **2023**, *15*, 1330. [CrossRef] [PubMed]
29. Hull, M.V.; Jagim, A.R.; Oliver, J.M.; Greenwood, M.; Busteed, D.R.; Jones, M.T. Gender Differences and Access to a Sports Dietitian Influence Dietary Habits of Collegiate Athletes. *J. Int. Soc. Sports Nutr.* **2016**, *13*, 38. [CrossRef] [PubMed]
30. Burke, L.; Deakin, V. *Clinical Sports Nutrition*, 6th ed.; McGraw-Hill Australia: Sydney, NSW, Australia, 2021.
31. Sánchez-Oliver, A.J.; Grimaldi-Puyana, M.; Domínguez, R. Evaluation and Behavior of Spanish Bodybuilders: Doping and Sports Supplements. *Biomolecules* **2019**, *9*, 122. [CrossRef] [PubMed]
32. Grgic, J.; Pedisic, Z.; Saunders, B.; Artioli, G.G.; Schoenfeld, B.J.; McKenna, M.J.; Bishop, D.J.; Kreider, R.B.; Stout, J.R.; Kalman, D.S.; et al. International Society of Sports Nutrition position stand: Sodium bicarbonate and exercise performance. *J. Int. Soc. Sports Nutr.* **2021**, *18*, 61. [CrossRef]
33. McCubbin, A.; Allanson, B.; Caldwell, J.; Cort, M.M.; Costa, R.J.S.; Cox, G.R.; Crawshay, S.T.; Desbrow, B.; Freney, E.G.; Gaskell, S.K.; et al. Sports Dietitians Australia position statement: Nutrition for exercise in hot environments. *Int. J. Sport Nutr. Exerc. Metab.* **2020**, *31*, 83–98. [CrossRef]
34. Giraldo-Vallejo, J.E.; Cardona-Guzman, M.A.; Rodriguez-Alcivar, E.J.; Koci, J.; Petro, J.L.; Kreider, R.B.; Cannataro, R.; Bonilla, D.A. Nutritional Strategies in the Rehabilitation of Musculoskeletal Injuries in Athletes: A Systematic Integrative Review. *Nutrients* **2023**, *15*, 819. [CrossRef]
35. Maughan, R.J.; Depiesse, F.; Geyer, H.; International Association of Athletics Federations. The use of dietary supplements by athletes. *J. Sports Sci.* **2007**, *25* (Suppl. S1), S103–S113. [CrossRef]

sports

MDPI

Article

Analysis of Magnitude and Direction of Body Composition Asymmetries in Male Brazilian Jiu-Jitsu Athletes: Pilot Study

Alex Ojeda-Aravena [1,*], Rafael L. Kons [2], Jairo Azócar-Gallardo [3,4], Xurxo Dopico-Calvo [5], Aida Fernández [6], Marcelo Tuesta-Roa [7], Mauricio Cresp-Barria [8], Jorge Olivares-Arancibia [9] and Eduardo Báez-San Martín [10,11]

1 Dirección de Docencia, Universidad de Los Lagos, Osorno 1305, Chile
2 Department of Physical Education, Faculty of Education, Federal University of Bahia, Salvador 40170-110, BA, Brazil; rafael.kons@ufba.br
3 Departamento de Ciencias de la Actividad Física, Universidad de Los Lagos, Osorno 1305, Chile; jairo.azocar@ulagos.cl
4 Programa de Investigación en Deporte, Sociedad y Buen Vivir (DSBv), Universidad de Los Lagos, Osorno 1305, Chile
5 Performance and Health Group, Department of Physical Education and Sport, Universidade da Coruña, 15001 A Coruña, Spain; xurxo.dopico@udc.es
6 Faculty of Education, Universidad Central de Chile, Santiago 8370292, Chile; aida.fernandez@ucentral.cl
7 Exercise and Rehabilitation Sciences Laboratory, School of Physiotherapy, Faculty of Rehabilitation Sciences, Universidad Andres Bello, Santiago 8370292, Chile; marcelo.tuesta@unab.cl
8 Department of Innovation and Education, Faculty of Education, Catholic University of Temuco Chile, Temuco 4810399, Chile; mcresp@uct.cl
9 AFySE Group, Research in Physical Activity and School Health, School of Physical Education, Faculty of Education, Universidad de las Américas, Santiago 8370292, Chile; jolivares@udla.cl
10 Carrera de Entrenador Deportivo, Escuela de Educación, Universidad Viña del Mar, Viña del Mar 2580022, Chile; eduardo.baez@upla.cl
11 Laboratorio de Evaluación y Prescripción de Ejercicio, Facultad de Ciencias de la Actividad Física y del Deporte, Universidad de Playa Ancha, Valparaíso 850, Chile
* Correspondence: aojeda.aravena@gmail.com

Abstract: In order to optimize body composition and its components, it is of interest to analyze inter-limb asymmetries in athletes of popular combat sports such as Brazilian Jiu-Jitsu (BJJ). This study aimed to assess the magnitude and direction of body composition asymmetry in competitive male BJJ athletes. Seventeen experienced and competitive male BJJ athletes (age 34.59 ± 8.00 years, 172.94 ± 5.46 cm, BJJ experience 7.88 ± 5.57 years, and 3.71 ± 1.05 days of weekly volume training), including Guard Fighters (n = 7) and Pass Fighters (n = 10), participated in this study. In a single session, whole-body and segmental upper limb and lower limb body composition (BC) was assessed utilizing dual-energy X-ray absorptiometry (DXA). The assessment included total mass (TM), fat mass (FM), fat mass percentage (%FM), fat-free mass (FFM), and bone mineral content (BMC). Absolute differences between limbs were analyzed using a paired t-test. A comparison of BC asymmetries according to combat styles was conducted using an independent t-test. The effect size (ES) was interpreted as Cohen's d. The main results revealed significant asymmetries in the upper limbs (ULs) of the total group; greater values were found on the left side for TM (p = 0.009, ES = 0.725), FM (p = 0.016, ES = 0.650), FFM (p = 0.026, ES = 0.594), and BMC (p < 0.001, ES = 0.993). In Pass Fighters, differences favored the right side in TM (p = 0.003, ES = 1.277), FM (p = 0.009, ES = 1.039), FFM (p = 0.011, ES = 1.000), and BMC (p < 0.001, ES = 1.916). In contrast, Guard Fighters showed no discrepancies in these parameters. No notable disparities were observed in the lower limbs. This pilot study reveals that BJJ athletes present significant asymmetries in BC, particularly in the ULs, with a marked predominance on the right side, especially in Pass Fighters.

Keywords: asymmetry; Brazilian Jiu-Jitsu; sports sciences; body composition

1. Introduction

Brazilian Jiu-Jitsu (BJJ) is a modern martial art and combat sport that focuses on subduing the opponent through submission and joint-lock techniques. BJJ athletes specialize in various fighting styles. Notably, there are Guard Fighters, who prefer to fight from the guard position on the ground, and Pass Fighters, who aim to overcome the guard to achieve a dominant position over their opponent [1]. It is important to note that Guard Fighters and Pass Fighters share several physical traits, such as flexibility, balance, isometric handgrip strength, endurance, and quadriceps and hamstring strength and the ability to perform well in specific BJJ physical tests [2]. However, Pass Fighters tend to excel in isometric trunk extension endurance, which can be attributed to the specific demands of their fighting style [2]. BJJ competitions are organized not only by weight categories but also by technical skill levels (grades or belts), which can lead to matchups between competitors of different weights and technical proficiency.

In this context, body composition (BC) is a critical factor in athletic performance and injury prevention in combat sports such as BJJ [3]. The optimal distribution of muscle mass, bone mass, and fat mass significantly influences an athlete's ability to execute effective techniques, maintain endurance during matches, and comply with weight categories [4]. Additionally, muscle and bone mass play fundamental roles in force production and transmission, whereas excess fat mass can negatively affect physical performance in combat sport athletes [3,4].

Specifically, bilateral asymmetries (i.e., differences in athletic performance and function between the two limbs) have emerged as a research topic, primarily derived from unilateral or bilateral strength tasks. The focus of this topic is on understanding how such discrepancies between limbs can influence performance and injury risk [5,6], as well as being a manifestation of fatigue [7]. Various equations are currently being discussed for determining asymmetries based on unilateral and bilateral tasks, although there is currently no consensus [8,9]. In sports such as judo, bilateral asymmetries have been observed to increase following the execution of sport-specific tests [10]. Meanwhile, in simulated combat in this sport, bilateral asymmetries do not appear to be significant to performance [10].

From this line of research, the analysis of body composition asymmetries (BC-ASs) has been extrapolated by comparing both limbs using advanced technologies including dual-energy X-ray absorptiometry (DXA) [11–14]. These asymmetries can affect an athlete's functionality and balance, thereby influencing their technical performance and increasing the risk of injuries [15–17]. However, most studies to date have only quantified the magnitude of BC-AS (quantification of the percentage difference between limbs), while the analysis of direction (i.e., which side of the body is less developed) is still in its early stages [18].

In BJJ, the preference for a certain laterality during combat movements can lead to predominant unilateral development, exacerbating BC-AS [19]. Therefore, it is reasonable to suggest that BJJ athletes may present BC-AS. Consequently, it is important to understand that asymmetries in body composition can have a negative impact on physical performance given their relationship to muscle strength and the biomechanics of movement in this sport. Despite the importance of this research topic, there is limited information regarding studies related to the prevalence, magnitude, and direction of BC-AS in BJJ athletes. An individualized approach is essential to accurately and meaningfully assess asymmetries as it allows training and injury prevention programs to be adapted to the specific needs of each athlete. These findings provide valuable information for optimizing training programs, preventing injuries, and improving performance. Coaches and sports professionals can use this information to design specific interventions that address asymmetries and enhance the physical capabilities of athletes by considering their fighting styles and skill levels.

Therefore, this study aimed to assess the magnitude and direction of body composition asymmetry in competitive male BJJ athletes.

2. Materials and Methods

2.1. Participants

Seventeen male BJJ athletes (age 34.59 ± 8.00 years, 172.94 ± 5.46 cm, BJJ experience 7.88 ± 5.57 years, and 3.71 ± 1.05 days of weekly volume training) participated in this pilot study. Seven athletes were self-declared Guard Fighters and ten Pass Fighters. Ten athletes had black belts, while seven had blue- or purple-level belts. The inclusion criteria were (i) training a minimum of three times per week; (ii) having at least two years of continuous BJJ training; (iii) possessing at least a blue belt; (iv) competing regularly during the last two years; (v) participation in at least one annual International Brazilian Jiu-Jitsu Federation (IBJJF) competition; and (vi) no injuries or health conditions that could affect their performance in this study. The research methodology adhered to the ethical principles of the Declaration of Helsinki and was approved by the local Ethics Committee (CODE: BIOPUCV-H 520-2022). The procedures, benefits of participation, and risks associated with X-ray exposure were communicated one week prior to the assessments.

2.2. Measures and Procedures

Anthropometric and Body Composition Measures

The athletes participated in two assessment sessions during a one-day period, conducted in an exercise and sports science laboratory maintained at a temperature of 21 °C. DXA-certified professionals measured the anthropometric and BC variables. Athlete height (±0.1 cm) was measured using a stadiometer (Seca 217; Hamburg, Germany) following standard protocols. Subsequently, BC was evaluated using DXA (General Electric Lunar iDXA, Boston, MA, USA). Briefly, the athletes removed any metal or jewelry and laid supine on a scanning table. A whole-body scan was performed in standard mode, following the manufacturer's recommended procedures. The standard thickness mode was determined by using an automatic scanning function. The results were analyzed using GE EnCORE 2015 v18 software (GE Healthcare) [14]. Each athlete's race/ethnicity was selected from available software options to accurately reflect their ancestry. Quality assurance was maintained through daily calibrations performed before all scans, using a calibration block provided by the manufacturer. All DXA measurements were performed by a laboratory technician certified in X-ray procedures by the Ministry of Health. Standardized athlete positioning procedures were employed [20]. The BC results included total mass (TM), fat mass (FM), percentage of fat mass (%FM), fat-free mass (FFM), and bone mineral content (BMC) for the total body, upper limbs (ULs), and lower limbs (LLs).

2.3. Statistical Analysis

Data were entered in Microsoft Excel and subsequently analyzed using the statistical software JASP version 0.17.3 (JASP Team, 2023, Amsterdam, The Netherlands). Continuous BC descriptors are presented as the mean ± standard deviation with a 95% confidence interval (CI95%). Categorical data were expressed as absolute and relative frequencies in percentage terms. Initially, the assumptions of normality were assessed using the Shapiro–Wilk test and homoscedasticity using the Levene test. The magnitude of asymmetry was described as the percentage difference between the upper and lower limbs, separately based on the higher or lower score obtained, using the equation (([Strongest − Weakest]/Strongest) × 100) [21] modified to higher and lower values according to Bishop et al. [22]. To represent the direction of asymmetries between individual limbs, an IF function was added to Microsoft Excel at the end of the formula *IF(left < right, 1, −1) without altering the magnitude [18]. The mean differences between body segments were determined using a paired sample *t*-test. Differences in the proportions of BC-AS were analyzed using a contingency table with Fisher's exact test and the Odds Ratio (OR) [23]. Asymmetries based on fighting style were evaluated using an independent sample *t*-test. The magnitude of differences or effect size (ES) was interpreted using Cohen's d, where values of 0.2, 0.5, and 0.8 indicate small, medium, and large effects, respectively. A p value of <0.05 was established as the significance threshold.

3. Results

In the normality analysis using the Shapiro–Wilk test, the evaluated variables did not show significant deviations from a normal distribution. In the homogeneity of variance analysis using the Levene test, none of the evaluated variables showed significant differences between the groups ($p > 0.05$).

3.1. Global Analysis of Differences and Asymmetries

Table 1 and Figure 1 provide a detailed description of the differences and asymmetries observed in the BC of the analyzed BJJ athletes. Regarding TM in the ULs, statistically significant differences were observed between the right and left limbs ($p = 0.009$, ES = 0.725). A total of 70.59% of participants showed greater TM in the right limb and 23.53% in the left limb, and 5.88% presented symmetry favoring the right side (OR = 9.0, $p = 0.012$). Conversely, in the LLs, no significant differences were found ($p = 0.239$), although 64.71% of athletes exhibited greater FFM in the right leg and 23.53% in the left leg, and 11.76% showed symmetry, slightly favoring the right side (OR = 7.56, $p = 0.027$).

Table 1. Inter-limb differences and body composition asymmetries in BJJ athletes analyzed ($n = 17$).

BC Variables	LIMBS	SIDE	Mean	SD	BC-AS ± SD	t	p	ES
TM (kg)	ULs	L	5.141	0.833	5.236 ± 2.969	2.991	0.009 **	0.725
		R	4.953	0.802				
	LLs	L	12.876	1.746	3.236 ± 2.766	1.222	0.239	0.296
		R	12.724	1.704				
%FM	ULs	L	17.259	4.889	5.484 ± 4.372	1.580	0.134	0.383
		R	16.782	5.082				
	LLs	L	18.494	4.303	3.345 ± 2.983	0.164	0.872	0.040
		R	18.324	4.333				
FM (kg)	ULs	L	0.841	0.283	9.198 ± 5.839	2.678	0.016 **	0.650
		R	0.785	0.262				
	LLs	L	2.269	0.689	5.860 ± 2.833	1.590	0.131	0.386
		R	2.215	0.657				
FFM (kg)	ULs	L	4.052	0.725	5.107 ± 2.804	2.449	0.026 *	0.594
		R	3.929	0.717				
	LLs	L	9.989	1.468	3.317 ± 2.848	1.081	0.296	0.262
		R	9.881	1.446				

Table 1. *Cont.*

BC Variables	LIMBS	SIDE	Mean	SD	BC-AS ± SD	*t*	*p*	ES
BMC (kg)	ULs	L	0.249	0.043	4.605 ± 3.194	4.094	<0.001 ***	0.993
		R	0.240	0.043				
	LLs	L	0.610	0.086	2.780 ± 3.352	0.164	0.872	0.040
		R	0.609	0.091				

SD: standard deviation. BC-ASs: body composition asymmetries. p: statistical significance value (* $p < 0.05$, ** $p < 0.01$, *** $p < 0.001$). BC: body composition. LIMBS: limbs (upper limbs—ULs—upper body; lower limbs—LLs—lower body). Side (L: left; R: right). ES: effect size expressed as Cohen's d. TM: Total mass. %FM: fat mass percentage. FM (kg): fat mass. FFM: fat-free mass. BMC: bone mineral content.

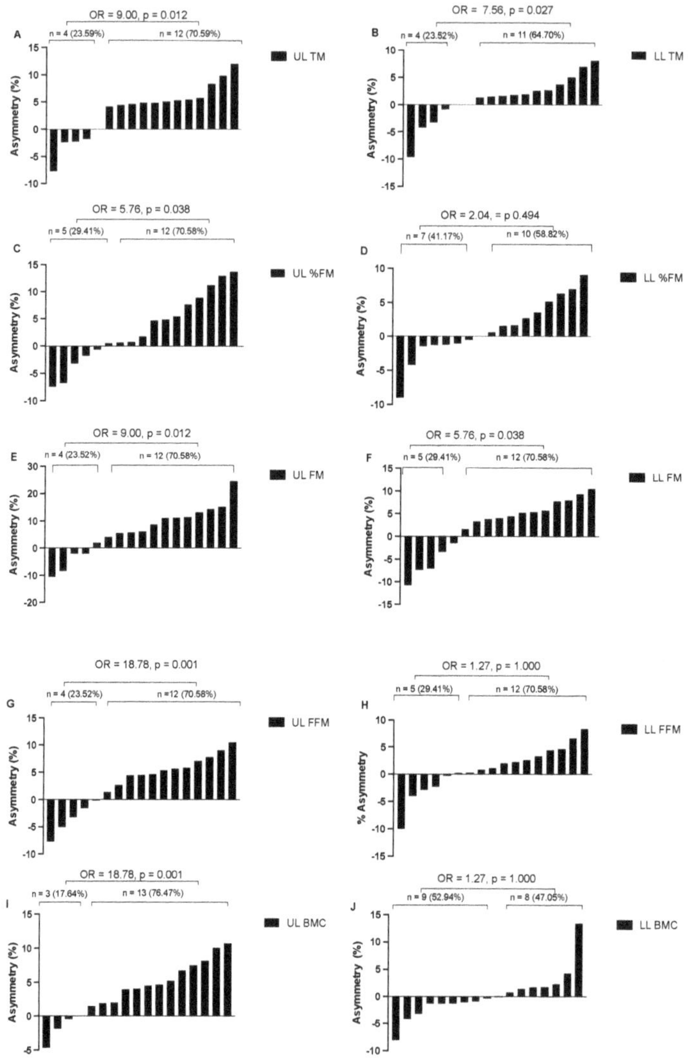

Figure 1. This figure shows the magnitude and direction of the asymmetry percentages in the body composition asymmetries of the athletes. (**A**): UL TM (kg); (**B**): LL TM (kg); (**C**): UL%FM; (**D**): LL FM%; (**E**): UL FM (kg); (**F**): LL FM; (**G**): UL FFM (kg); (**H**): LL FFM (kg); (**I**): UL BMC (kg); (**J**): LL BMC (kg).

Concerning %FM, no significant differences were found in the ULs, although 70.59% exhibited a higher %FM in the right limb (OR = 5.76, p = 0.038) compared to 29.41% in the left limb. Similarly, no significant differences were observed in the LLs (p = 0.872, ES = 0.040), with 58.82% favoring the right leg and 41.18% favoring the left leg (OR = 2.04, p = 0.494).

FM in the ULs showed a significant difference (p = 0.016, ES = 0.650), with 70.59% of participants presenting a greater FM in the right limb and 23.53% in the left limb and 5.88% showing symmetry (OR = 9.0, p = 0.012). In the LLs, no significant differences were found (p = 0.131, ES = 0.386), although 70.59% of athletes presented a greater FM in the right leg and 29.41% in the left leg (OR = 5.76, p = 0.038).

FFM in the ULs revealed a significant difference (p = 0.026, ES = 0.594), with 76.47% of participants presenting a greater FFM in the right limb (OR = 18.78, p = 0.001) and 17.65% in the left limb and 5.88% showing no asymmetry. In the LLs, no statistical differences were observed (p = 0.296, ES = 0.262), with a relatively balanced distribution of asymmetries between the right leg (52.94%) and the left leg (47.06%; OR = 1.27, p = 1.000).

Lastly, BMC in the ULs showed significant differences (p < 0.001, ES = 0.993), with 76.47% of athletes presenting a greater BMC in the right limb (OR = 18.78, p = 0.001) and 17.65% in the left limb and 5.88% showing symmetry. In the LLs, no significant differences were observed (p = 0.872, ES = 0.040), with asymmetry proportions evenly distributed between the right leg (52.94%) and the left leg (47.06%; OR = 1.27, p = 1.000).

3.2. *Comparative Analysis by Fighting Style*

Tables 2 and 3 present a detailed comparison of body composition asymmetries by fighting style (i.e., Guard Fighters vs. Pass Fighters). Regarding TM, the ULs showed similar mean values between Guard Fighters (5.339%) and Pass Fighters (5.164%), without significant differences (p = 0.909, ES = 0.057). For the LLs, Guard Fighters presented a higher mean value (4.262%) compared to Pass Fighters (2.518%), although this difference was not significant (p = 0.211, ES = 0.644), suggesting a possible trend warranting further analysis. In absolute terms, no significant differences were reported in Guard Fighters for either limb, whereas in Pass Fighters, significant differences were observed in the ULs (p = 0.003, ES = 1.277).

Regarding %FM, global asymmetries in the ULs were similar between Guard Fighters (5.965%) and Pass Fighters (5.149%), with no significant differences (p = 0.718, ES = 0.181). In the LLs, Guard Fighters also presented slightly higher values (3.961%) compared to Pass Fighters (2.915%), though without statistical significance (p = 0.495, ES = 0.345). In absolute terms, no significant differences were reported by fighting style for either limb.

In terms of FM, Guard Fighters recorded a higher mean percentage of asymmetry in the ULs (9.974%) compared to Pass Fighters (8.655%), though this difference was not significant (p = 0.661). In the LLs, Guard Fighters presented higher average values (7.434%) compared to Pass Fighters (4.759%), without significant results (p = 0.052) and a large effect size (ES = 1.041). In absolute terms, significant differences were reported only in Pass Fighters for the ULs (0.862 kg vs. 0.799 kg; p = 0.009, ES = 1.039) and the LLs (2.318 kg vs. 2.230 kg; p = 0.011, ES = 1.016).

For FFM, Guard Fighters presented a mean asymmetry percentage in the ULs (5.141%) similar to that of Pass Fighters (5.084%), with no significant differences (p = 0.909, ES = 0.057). In the LLs, Guard Fighters exhibited a higher average percentage (4.771%) compared to Pass Fighters (2.300%), though this difference was not statistically significant (p = 0.211, ES = 0.644). In absolute terms, Pass Fighters presented significant differences in the ULs (4.138 kg vs. 3.970 kg; p = 0.011, ES = 1.000).

Table 2. Absolute inter-limb differences according to fighting style.

BC Variables	Limbs	RIGHT	SD	LEFT	SD	*t*	*p*	95% CI Lower	95% CI Upper
GUARD FIGHTERS (n = 10)									
TM (kg)	ULs	4.957	0.665	4.857	0.648	0.810	0.449	−0.202	0.402
	LLs	12.586	1.551	12.500	1.493	0.318	0.761	−0.574	0.745
%FM	ULs	17.100	3.237	16.614	3.154	0.860	0.423	−0.896	1.867
	LLs	18.400	2.346	18.543	2.472	−0.406	0.699	−1.004	0.718
FM (kg)	ULs	0.811	0.191	0.766	0.158	1.009	0.352	−0.064	0.153
	LLs	2.200	0.338	2.195	0.348	0.066	0.950	−0.171	0.180
FFM (kg)	ULs	3.928	0.558	3.870	0.581	0.610	0.564	−0.175	0.291
	LLs	9.796	1.320	9.663	1.259	0.618	0.559	−0.393	0.658
BMC (kg)	ULs	0.233	0.023	0.229	0.026	1.020	0.347	−0.006	0.014
	LLs	0.579	0.060	0.589	0.074	−1.117	0.307	−0.033	0.012
PASS FIGHTERS									
TM (kg)	ULs	5.270	0.945	5.020	0.922	4.038	0.003 **	0.110	0.390
	LLs	13.080	1.924	12.880	1.900	1.762	0.112	−0.057	0.457
%FM	ULs	17.370	5.956	16.900	6.265	1.324	0.218	−0.333	1.273
	LLs	18.560	5.407	18.170	5.407	2.169	0.058	−0.017	0.797
FM (kg)	ULs	0.862	0.342	0.799	0.324	3.287	0.009 **	0.020	0.106
	LLs	2.318	0.872	2.230	0.828	3.212	0.011 *	0.026	0.151
FFM (kg)	ULs	4.138	0.841	3.970	0.827	3.163	0.011 **	0.048	0.289
	LLs	10.124	1.619	10.033	1.611	0.977	0.354	−0.120	0.302
BMC (kg)	ULs	0.260	0.051	0.247	0.052	6.059	<0.001 ***	0.008	0.018
	LLs	0.632	0.097	0.623	0.103	1.101	0.300	−0.010	0.028

Differences in body limbs in terms of body composition between BJJ fighting styles. Definitions: *: $p < 0.05$, **: $p < 0.005$; ***: $p < 0.001$; t = t value; p = p value. Definitions: ULs: upper limbs. LLs: lower limbs. TM: total mass. %FM: percentage of fat mass. FM: fat mass. FFM: fat-free mass. BMC: bone mineral content.

Table 3. Comparison of body composition asymmetries according to BJJ fighting style (n = 17).

BC Variables	Limbs	BJJ Style	AS% Mean	SD	*t*	*p*	Mean Difference	Lower	Upper	ES
TM	ULs	Guard Fighters	5.339	3.494	0.116	0.909	0.175	−3.045	3.396	0.057
		Pass Fighters	5.164	2.744						
	LLs	Guard Fighters	4.262	3.361	1.307	0.211	1.744	−1.099	4.587	0.644
		Pass Fighters	2.518	2.163						
%FM	ULs	Guard Fighters	5.965	4.563	0.368	0.718	0.816	−3.906	5.538	0.181
		Pass Fighters	5.149	4.450						
	LLs	Guard Fighters	3.961	3.171	0.700	0.495	1.046	−2.139	4.232	0.345
		Pass Fighters	2.915	2.937						
FM	ULs	Guard Fighters	9.974	7.673	0.447	0.661	1.319	−4.974	7.612	0.220
		Pass Fighters	8.655	4.536						
	LLs	Guard Fighters	7.434	2.851	2.113	0.052	2.675	−0.024	5.373	1.041
		Pass Fighters	4.759	2.363						

Table 3. *Cont.*

BC Variables	Limbs	BJJ Style	AS% Mean	SD	*t*	*p*	Mean Difference	Lower	Upper	ES
FFM	ULs	Guard Fighters	5.141	3.124	0.116	0.909	0.175	−3.045	3.396	0.057
		Pass Fighters	5.084	2.734						
	LLs	Guard Fighters	4.771	3.163	1.307	0.211	1.744	−1.099	4.587	0.644
		Pass Fighters	2.300	2.227						
BMC	ULs	Guard Fighters	3.674	3.178	−1.006	0.330	−1.583	−4.937	1.771	−0.496
		Pass Fighters	5.257	3.203						
	LLs	Guard Fighters	3.108	2.452	0.328	0.748	0.558	−3.067	4.182	0.162
		Pass Fighters	2.550	3.979						

t: Student's *t*-test value. *p*: statistical significance value. Difference: mean difference between groups. CI: confidence interval for mean difference. ES: effect size expressed as Cohen's d. Definitions: ULs: upper limbs. LLs: lower limbs. TM: total mass. %FM: percentage of fat mass. FM: fat mass. FFM: fat-free mass. BMC: bone mineral content.

Finally, BMC in the ULs showed a lower mean value in Guard Fighters (3.674%) compared to Pass Fighters (5.257%), though the difference was not significant ($p = 0.330$), with a moderate negative effect size (ES = −0.496). In the LLs, differences between both styles were minimal ($p = 0.748$, ES = 0.162). In absolute terms, significant differences were reported only in Pass Fighters for the ULs (0.260 kg vs. 0.247 kg; $p < 0.001$, ES = 1.916).

4. Discussion

This study is the first to explore the prevalence, magnitude, and direction of BC-AS in BJJ athletes. To date, most studies have focused on analyzing asymmetries from a functional perspective using bilateral or unilateral strength tasks. However, BC-AS has emerged as an area of study that focuses on understanding the morphological impact of BJJ athlete characteristics. Our main results showed significant differences between both limbs for the ULs in TM, FFM, and BMC, with ES ranging from moderate to large (ES = 0.594 to 1.19). BC-AS could originate from the specific demands and unilateral movement patterns inherent to BJJ, where athletes often use one side of the body more frequently to execute grip, submission, and opponent control techniques.

The predominance towards the right side suggests functional laterality, possibly related to hand dominance and specific BJJ techniques that favor one arm over the other. This finding contrasts with those of other studies in similar sports. For example, Mala et al. [24] observed less pronounced asymmetries in FFM in judokas than in sports that emphasize unilateral limb use, such as fencing and karate, in which athletes showed significant differences between dominant and non-dominant limbs in the arms ($t = -4.24$, $p < 0.01$) and legs ($t = -6.07$, $p < 0.01$). Greater muscle and bone mass on the dominant side could provide advantages in strength and endurance, but it is also proposed that they could generate musculoskeletal imbalances, increase susceptibility to overuse or compensatory injuries on the less developed side, and potentially influence sports performance, although the results to date are inconclusive [17,25].

In the LLs, differences were not statistically significant in most parameters, except in the TM, where the proportions of asymmetry favored the right side (OR = 7.56, $p = 0.027$). The lower magnitude of asymmetries in the LLs could be due to BJJ techniques requiring a more balanced involvement of both legs for movements, such as sweeps, leverages, and displacements. Interestingly, although this study did not directly evaluate functional asymmetries, research in similar sports, such as judo, has reported increases in asymmetries after simulated combats. Kons et al. [10] analyzed the effects of successive judo combats on inter-limb asymmetries and bilateral deficit, finding that the magnitude of asymmetry in unilateral countermovement jump height increased after the second combat ($p = 0.001$).

When considering fighting style, a tendency was observed in the FM of the LLs between Guard Fighters and Pass Fighters ($t = 2.113$, $p = 0.052$, ES = 1.041). Guard Fighters who prefer to fight from the guard position on the ground and extensively use their legs to control and manipulate the opponent might develop greater asymmetries in the fat mass and FFM of the LLs. These differences may be related to the technical and tactical characteristics of each style. Báez et al. [1] observed that Guard Fighters presented a higher percentage of fat mass compared to Pass Fighters, which aligns with our findings. However, Pass Fighters tend to excel in isometric trunk extension endurance, which can be attributed to the specific demands of their fighting style [2].

This highlights the potential differences in morphological terms between fighting styles, which deserves further study. The limitations of this study include the sample size, the absence of female participants, the varying levels of practice among the athletes in the sample, and the lack of consideration of athlete laterality (dominance). These limitations restrict the generalization of the results. Future studies should aim to increase the sample size, include female athletes, and incorporate the assessment of laterality to provide a more comprehensive understanding of asymmetries in sports performance.

Although our study focused on body composition asymmetries, we acknowledge that other factors such as neuromuscular coordination, specific sport techniques, and fatigue also play crucial roles in sports performance and the manifestation of asymmetries. Moreover, while laterality was not directly evaluated in this study, it is a recognized factor that can significantly influence the observed asymmetries. Dominance can affect strength, coordination, and movement efficiency, thereby impacting both performance and injury risk. Therefore, future research should include the evaluation of athlete laterality to better understand its impact on asymmetries and overall performance.

Regardless of the above, coaches, strength professionals, and conditioning professionals should consider BC-AS when designing training programs. This includes incorporating exercises that promote muscular and functional balance between both sides of the body. The inclusion of unilateral training and specific strength exercises could help correct these imbalances and improve performance [5,6]. Additionally, the regular monitoring of body composition and asymmetries can serve as a tool for adjusting training and rehabilitation programs. Ojeda-Aravena et al. [14] highlighted the importance of relating body composition asymmetries to specific performances such as taekwondo, suggesting that individualized assessments can contribute to the optimal development of athletes.

Several coaches emphasize the importance of specific training for increasing sports performance, highlighting its role in metabolic and neuromuscular improvement. Hence, specific training and the repetition of technical gestures and combat actions often create bilateral deficits by working more on the dominant side. While specificity is crucial for enhancing sports performance, it can also lead to more pronounced bilateral deficits, characteristic of high-performance athletes.

In a study by Turnes et al. [26], it was concluded that bilateral symmetry was not associated with better performance in a handgrip strength test carried out with a sample of judokas. On the other hand, when athletes were categorized based on the years of training experience specific to judo, those with the greatest lateral deficit were those who performed more hours of specific training, suggesting that practice and training time may contribute to the deficit. This finding was verified in both studies. However, this deficit should not increase to a level that compromises the athlete's sporting performance, injury risk, or health, highlighting the importance of studying asymmetry in the upper and lower limbs.

However, a systematic review on the relationship between asymmetry and injury risk by Helme et al. [27] concluded that the evidence supporting the functional asymmetry of the lower limbs as a risk factor for sports injuries was of moderate to low quality. Despite evidence showing that some measures were statistically associated with injury risk in different sporting populations, this field of research is still limited by a high degree of variation in methodological approaches and quality. Researchers should be mindful of these observations before implementing athletic interventions. From this review, it was identified that more research is needed that adopts key recommendations specifically addressing standardized injury definitions, the quantification of asymmetry, and the adoption of a multivariate approach, encapsulating exposure among other variables, within a sample of sufficient size. Without this investigation, no clear results are apparent for accepting or rejecting upper or lower limb functional asymmetry as a risk to sports participation.

Consequently, the topic of BC-AS and its impact on performance, injury risk, and fatigue holds significant potential for further study. This is based on their relevance to the structural morphology and force production of different body limbs. Future research should focus on analyzing the longitudinal effects of BC-AS through strength programs and/or specific BJJ training. Additionally, the efficacy of training programs designed to reduce asymmetries and their impact on performance and injury prevention should be investigated. Furthermore, structural asymmetries could be related to functional measures such as strength, power, and balance to better understand their influence on sports performance. Importantly, future studies should also consider the laterality of athletes, as dominance can significantly influence asymmetries. Including female athletes and athletes with different skill levels would broaden the generalizability of the findings.

5. Conclusions

BJJ athletes exhibited significant asymmetries in body composition, especially in the ULs, with a predominance towards the right side. Guard Fighters showed greater asymmetries in the LLs, possibly because of the increased use of the legs in their fighting style. These asymmetries appear to be influenced by the specific demands of the sport and the fighting style.

Author Contributions: Conceptualization, A.O.-A.; methodology, A.O.-A.; software, A.O.-A.; validation, A.O.-A., M.C.-B. and M.T.-R.; formal analysis, A.O.-A.; investigation, A.O.-A., R.L.K., J.A.-G., X.D.-C., A.F., M.T.-R. and M.C.-B.; resources, A.O.-A., R.L.K., J.A.-G. and X.D.-C.; data curation, A.O.-A., R.L.K., J.A.-G. and X.D.-C.; writing—original draft preparation, A.O.-A.; writing—review and editing A.O.-A., R.L.K., J.A.-G., X.D.-C., A.F., M.T.-R., J.O.-A., E.B.-S.M. and M.C.-B.; visualization A.O.-A.; supervision, A.O.-A. All authors have read and agreed to the published version of the manuscript.

Funding: This research received no external funding.

Institutional Review Board Statement: CODE: BIOPUCV-H 520-2022).

Informed Consent Statement: Informed consent was obtained from all subjects involved in the study.

Data Availability Statement: Data may be requested from the corresponding author.

Conflicts of Interest: The authors declare no conflict of interest.

References

1. Báez, E.; Franchini, E.; Ramírez-Campillo, R.; Cañas-Jamett, R.; Herrera, T.; Burgos-Jara, C.; Henríquez-Olguín, C. Anthropometric Characteristics of Top-Class Brazilian Jiu Jitsu Athletes: Role of Fighting Style. *Int. J. Morphol.* **2014**, *32*, 1043–1050. [CrossRef]
2. Lima Kons, R.; da Silva Athayde, M.S.; da Silva Junior, J.N.; da Silva Tavares, W.; Detanico, D. Vertical Jump Performance in Judo and Brazilian Jiu-Jitsu Athletes: An Approach with Different Training Levels. *Ido Mov. Cult. J. Martial Arts Anthropol.* **2017**, *17*, 25–31.

3. Reale, R.; Burke, L.M.; Cox, G.R.; Slater, G. Body Composition of Elite Olympic Combat Sport Athletes. *Eur. J. Sport Sci.* **2020**, *20*, 147–156. [CrossRef] [PubMed]
4. Ojeda-Aravena, A.; Azocar-Gallardo, J.; Galle, F.; García-García, J.M. Relación Entre Las Características de La Composición Corporal y El Rendimiento Físico General y Específico En Competidores de Taekwondo Chilenos de Nivel Nacional de Ambos Sexos: Un Estudio Observacional. *Rev. Esp. Nutr. Humana Dietética* **2020**, *24*, 154–164. [CrossRef]
5. Afonso, J.; Peña, J.; Sá, M.; Virgile, A.; García-de-Alcaraz, A.; Bishop, C. Why Sports Should Embrace Bilateral Asymmetry: A Narrative Review. *Symmetry* **2022**, *14*, 1993. [CrossRef]
6. Bishop, C.; Turner, A.; Read, P. Effects of Inter-Limb Asymmetries on Physical and Sports Performance: A Systematic Review. *J. Sports Sci.* **2018**, *36*, 1135–1144. [CrossRef]
7. Kons, R.L.; Orssatto, L.B.D.R.; Sakugawa, R.L.; da Silva Junior, J.N.; Diefenthaeler, F.; Detanico, D. Effects of Stretch-Shortening Cycle Fatigue Protocol on Lower Limb Asymmetry and Muscle Soreness in Judo Athletes. *Sports Biomech.* **2023**, *22*, 1079–1094. [CrossRef] [PubMed]
8. Bishop, C.; Read, P.; Chavda, S.; Turner, A. Asymmetries of the Lower Limb: The Calculation Conundrum in Strength Training and Conditioning. *Strength Cond. J.* **2016**, *38*, 27. [CrossRef]
9. Bishop, C.; Read, P.; Lake, J.; Chavda, S.; Turner, A. Interlimb Asymmetries: Understanding How to Calculate Differences from Bilateral and Unilateral Tests. *Strength Cond. J.* **2018**, *40*, 1–6. [CrossRef]
10. Kons, R.L.; Pupo, J.D.; Gheller, R.G.; Costa, F.E.; Rodrigues, M.M.; Bishop, C.; Detanico, D. Effects of Successive Judo Matches on Interlimb Asymmetry and Bilateral Deficit. *Phys. Ther. Sport Off. J. Assoc. Chart. Physiother. Sports Med.* **2021**, *47*, 15–22. [CrossRef]
11. Bell, D.R.; Sanfilippo, J.L.; Binkley, N.; Heiderscheit, B.C. Lean Mass Asymmetry Influences Force and Power Asymmetry during Jumping in Collegiate Athletes. *J. Strength Cond. Res.* **2014**, *28*, 884–891. [CrossRef] [PubMed]
12. Chapelle, L.; Bishop, C.; Clarys, P.; D'Hondt, E. International vs. National Female Tennis Players: A Comparison of Upper and Lower Extremity Functional Asymmetries. *J. Sports Med. Phys. Fitness* **2021**, *62*, 944–952. [CrossRef]
13. Chapelle, L.; Rommers, N.; Clarys, P.; D'Hondt, E. Whole-Body Morphological Asymmetries in High-Level Female Tennis Players: A Cross-sectional Study. *J. Sports Sci.* **2021**, *39*, 777–782. [CrossRef]
14. Ojeda-Aravena, A.; Warnier-Medina, A.; Brand, C.; Morales-Zúñiga, J.; Orellana-Lepe, G.; Zapata-Bastias, J.; Tuesta, M. Relationship between Body Composition Asymmetry and Specific Performance in Taekwondo Athletes: A Cross-Sectional Study. *Symmetry* **2023**, *15*, 2087. [CrossRef]
15. Polletta, J.; Leung, K.; Diaz, D.; Branum, N.; Mokha, M. Influence of Interlimb Lean Muscle Mass Asymmetry on Countermovement Jump Neuromuscular Performance Qualities Among American Football Players. *J. Strength Cond. Res.* **2024**. [CrossRef]
16. Sanchis-Moysi, J.; Dorado, C.; Vicente-Rodríguez, G.; Milutinovic, L.; Garces, G.L.; Calbet, J.A.L. Inter-Arm Asymmetry in Bone Mineral Content and Bone Area in Postmenopausal Recreational Tennis Players. *Maturitas* **2004**, *48*, 289–298. [CrossRef] [PubMed]
17. Vaillancourt, N.; Montpetit, C.; Carile, V.; Fortin, M. DEXA Body Composition Asymmetry Analysis and Association to Injury Risk and Low Back Pain in University Soccer Players. *Int. J. Environ. Res. Public Health* **2024**, *21*, 559. [CrossRef] [PubMed]
18. Bishop, C.; Lake, J.; Loturco, I.; Papadopoulos, K.; Turner, A.; Read, P. Interlimb Asymmetries: The Need for an Individual Approach to Data Analysis. *J. Strength Cond. Res.* **2021**, *35*, 695–701. [CrossRef]
19. Loffing, F.; Deeken, O.; Schorer, J. Lateral Preference in Complex Combat Situations: Prevalence and Relationship with General Measures of Hand and Foot Preference. *Laterality* **2024**, *29*, 37–62. [CrossRef] [PubMed]
20. Ackland, T.R.; Lohman, T.G.; Sundgot-Borgen, J.; Maughan, R.J.; Meyer, N.L.; Stewart, A.D.; Müller, W. Current Status of Body Composition Assessment in Sport: Review and Position Statement on Behalf of the Ad Hoc Research Working Group on Body Composition Health and Performance, Under the Auspices of the I.O.C. Medical Commission. *Sports Med.* **2012**, *42*, 227–249. [CrossRef]
21. Mertz, K.H.; Reitelseder, S.; Jensen, M.; Lindberg, J.; Hjulmand, M.; Schucany, A.; Binder Andersen, S.; Bechshoeft, R.L.; Jakobsen, M.D.; Bieler, T.; et al. Influence of Between-Limb Asymmetry in Muscle Mass, Strength, and Power on Functional Capacity in Healthy Older Adults. *Scand. J. Med. Sci. Sports* **2019**, *29*, 1901–1908. [CrossRef] [PubMed]
22. Bishop, C.; Turner, A.N.; Gonzalo-Skok, O.; Read, P. Inter-Limb Asymmetry during Rehabilitation Understanding Formulas and Monitoring the "Magnitude" and "Direction". *Aspetar Sports Med. J.* **2020**, *9*, 18–22.
23. Azócar-Gallardo, J.; Ojeda-Aravena, A.; Báez-San Martín, E.; Herrera-Valenzuela, T.; Tuesta, M.; González-Rojas, L.; Calvo-Rico, B.; García-García, J.M. Effect of a Concurrent Training Program with and Without Metformin Treatment on Metabolic Markers and Cardiorespiratory Fitness in Individuals with Insulin Resistance: A Retrospective Analysis. *Biomolecules* **2024**, *14*, 1470. [CrossRef] [PubMed]
24. Mala, L.; Maly, T.; Cabell, L.; Cech, P.; Hank, M.; Coufalova, K.; Zahalka, F. Composición Corporal y Asimetría Morfológica de Miembros En Competidores En Seis Artes Marciales. *Int. J. Morphol.* **2019**, *37*, 568–575. [CrossRef]

25. Cohen, T.R.; Rosenstein, B.; Rizk, A.; Frenette, S.; Fortin, M. Body Composition Asymmetry in University Rugby Players: Influence of Sex, Position, and Injury. *J. Sport Rehabil.* **2023**, *32*, 385–394. [CrossRef]
26. Turnes, T.; Silva, B.A.; Kons, R.L.; Detanico, D. Is Bilateral Deficit in Handgrip Strength Associated With Performance in Specific Judo Tasks? *J. Strength Cond. Res.* **2022**, *36*, 455–460. [CrossRef]
27. Helme, M.; Tee, J.; Emmonds, S.; Low, C. Does Lower-Limb Asymmetry Increase Injury Risk in Sport? A Systematic Review. *Phys. Ther. Sport* **2021**, *49*, 204–213. [CrossRef]

sports

MDPI

Commentary

The Women's Tennis Association (WTA) Multidisciplinary Education and Treatment Protocol for the Female Athlete Triad (1996–2022)

Emily A. Ricker [1,2,3], Kristen J. Koltun [3,4], Carol L. Otis [5], Anna S. Peavler [6] and Mary Jane De Souza [3,*]

1 Consortium for Health and Military Performance, Department of Military and Emergency Medicine, F. Edward Hébert School of Medicine, Uniformed Services University, 4301 Jones Bridge Rd., Bethesda, MD 20814, USA; emily.ricker.ctr@usuhs.edu
2 Henry M. Jackson Foundation for the Advancement of Military Medicine, Inc., 6720A Rockledge Dr., Bethesda, MD 20817, USA
3 Women's Health and Exercise Lab, Department of Kinesiology, Penn State University, 104 Noll Laboratory, University Park, PA 16802, USA; kjk116@pitt.edu
4 Neuromuscular Research Laboratory/Warrior Human Performance Research Center, Department of Sports Medicine and Nutrition, University of Pittsburgh, 3860 S. Water St., Pittsburgh, PA 15203, USA
5 Development Advisory Panel, The Women's Tennis Association, St. Petersburg, Fl 33701, USA; carolotis921@gmail.com
6 Performance Health Department, The Women's Tennis Association, St. Petersburg, FL 37701, USA; apeavler@wtatennis.com
* Correspondence: mjd34@psu.edu; Tel.: +1-814-863-0045

Abstract

Elite female tennis players are among those at high risk for developing the Female Athlete Triad (Triad), characterized by three interrelated conditions: energy deficiency/low energy availability, menstrual dysfunction, and low bone mineral density. From 1996 to 2022, the Women's Tennis Association (WTA) developed and implemented prevention, education, and management plans for female athletes at risk for, or exhibiting symptoms of, the Triad. This article reviews the WTA Triad protocol, developed in 2018 and utilized through 2022, in collaboration with subject matter experts in the Women's Health and Exercise Laboratory at The Pennsylvania State University. The WTA Triad protocol (1996–2022) includes prevention and management programs implemented by a multidisciplinary Performance Health Team to include screening for "red flags" during annual physicals or upon clinical presentation of a menstrual problem, bone disorder, or nutritional concern; targeted education for players, coaches, and other support team members with handouts and lectures on nutrition and body image to prevent energy deficiency; and a multidisciplinary protocol to guide treatment and return-to-play decisions. Other sport governing bodies can adopt similar multi-layered programs and practices for their athletes, coaches, and support teams to educate, screen, manage, and help to prevent the development of the Triad.

Keywords: energy deficiency; low energy availability; nutrition; body image; amenorrhea; bone health; injury prevention; coaching; player monitoring

1. Introduction

Since 1996, the Women's Tennis Association (WTA), the governing body of the international professional women's tennis circuit (i.e., WTA Tour), has been among the first international women's sports organizations to develop and implement comprehensive prevention, education, and treatment plans for female athletes with components of the Female

https://doi.org/10.3390/sports13070205

Athlete Triad (Triad), the syndrome encompassed by the following three interrelated conditions: (1) energy deficiency/low energy availability (ED/LEA) with or without an eating disorder, (2) menstrual dysfunction (e.g., functional hypothalamic amenorrhea), and (3) low bone mineral density (BMD) [1,2]. This article briefly summarizes the basic physiology underlying the Triad and subsequently reviews the WTA Performance Health programs and practices created to educate, prevent, screen, and manage professional female tennis athletes at risk of or exhibiting symptoms of the Triad. These specific practices have been expanded upon since 2022, with emerging research, but for the purpose of this article, the focus will be on the Triad and the WTA practices from 1996 to 2022.

1.1. History of the Female Athlete Triad

The Triad was first defined by an expert panel in 1992 [3], with the first official position stand published in 1997 [4] and updated in 2007 [2]. Causal evidence obtained through human [5–7] and animal studies [8,9] has demonstrated that ED/LEA is the underlying cause of menstrual disturbances and poor bone health in women with the Triad [1,2]. The Triad affects 16–60% of exercising women [10]; certain subpopulations of athletes, such as those who participate in sports that emphasize leanness for competitive or aesthetic purposes, can be at an elevated risk [11–14]. In 2014, the International Olympic Committee introduced a new model, Relative Energy Deficiency in Sports (REDs), which proposed an expanded model portraying additional physiological and performance effects of ED/LEA (e.g., immunological, cardiovascular, etc.) [15,16]. The elements of the Triad model (energy status, reproductive function, and bone health) continue to be the REDs outcomes with the highest prevalence and the most evidence supporting a causal relationship between energy and clinical outcomes [17–19]. As such, the WTA focused on preventing, screening for, diagnosing, and treating the Triad in its athletes from 1996 to 2022 due to the clinical importance and urgency of early intervention to prevent deleterious outcomes.

1.2. The Basic Physiology Underlying the Triad

As mentioned, ED/LEA is the underlying cause of the Triad. ED/LEA occurs when energy intake (i.e., calories from food eaten) is insufficient to meet the demands of energy expenditure, including that of exercise. In response to the energy "mismatch," metabolic adaptations occur to conserve energy and preserve functions vital for survival (e.g., thermoregulation, locomotion, cellular maintenance) at the expense of less vital functions (e.g., reproduction, growth) [20]. ED/LEA can result from any behaviors that result in inadequate caloric intake: disordered eating, clinical eating disorders, unintentional undereating, or intentional dietary restriction without disordered eating/eating disorders [1]. With respect to reproduction, menstrual dysfunction in younger women can present as primary amenorrhea, or failure to achieve menarche by age 15 [21]. In women who have achieved menarche, menstrual disturbances can range from subclinical, in the case of luteal phase defects or anovulatory cycles [22–24], to clinical, in the case of functional hypothalamic amenorrhea (absence of menses for $\geq$90 days) or oligomenorrhea (long, irregular cycles, 36–89 days). These menstrual disturbances are accompanied by underlying suppression in ovarian steroid hormones, namely estrogen and progesterone, with the severity of menstrual disturbance proportional to both the degree of hormone suppression and degree of energy deficiency [25]. ED/LEA impacts bone health through direct and indirect mechanisms. Directly, insufficient energy results in uncoupling of bone turnover such that bone resorption outpaces bone formation, which may ultimately lead to bone loss [26–29]. Indirectly, hypoestrogenism in response to ED/LEA impacts bone, as estrogen plays a role in preventing excess bone resorption and promoting bone formation [30]. Therefore, the combination of both ED/LEA and menstrual disturbances can be especially harmful to bone [31,32]. Importantly, the Triad is considered a spectrum disorder, as each component (energy status, reproductive function, and bone health) can range from optimal to subclinical to pathological clinical endpoints, and the presence of any one clinical (e.g., osteoporosis) or subclinical (e.g., luteal phase defect) condition may warrant further investigation and an eventual diagnosis [1,2].

1.3. The Triad in Tennis Athletes

Elite female tennis players are exposed to media pressures (portraying a thin, idealized body image) and pressure from coaches or other stakeholders to lose weight (in a mistaken belief that "thinner is faster"). These athletes are among those at high risk for the development of disordered eating, ED/LEA, and the Triad [33–35]. Although there are only a few studies assessing Triad components in elite tennis players, one study described a high prevalence of Triad-related conditions in 24 adolescent Brazilian tennis players: 91.7% of the athletes met criteria for disordered eating and/or ED/LEA, 33.3% for menstrual irregularities, and 25% for low bone mass [36]. Further, a greater percentage of tennis players than sedentary controls presented with Triad components, and one athlete presented with all three components of the Triad [36]. Similarly, in a study of 26 elite French professional tennis players, 46% had disordered eating attitudes based on standardized questionnaire assessments [37]. Additionally, those with disordered eating attitudes had lower energy intake and body mass index (BMI) and higher state anxiety than in the group without disordered eating attitudes [37]. In addition to health concerns relating to menstrual dysfunction (hypoestrogenism) and suboptimal BMD, ED/LEA and the Triad are also associated with increased risk of injury, such as stress fracture [38], and hindered sport performance [39].

1.4. Development of a WTA Triad Protocol

Identifying athletes at risk for, or exhibiting symptoms of, the Triad was crucial in order to intervene early and properly treat, manage, and prevent the progression of the condition, ultimately preserving optimal health and performance in the athlete. From 1996 to 2022, the WTA took a proactive approach to Triad prevention and management. In 1996, an independent scientific commission found that young female players needed support from minimum age rules for professional sport participation and education programs to help ease athletes into the international arena of professional women's tennis [40]. The approach has evolved to include protocols and programs managed by the WTA Performance Health Team (PHT). Education specific to the Triad is implemented by a PHT consisting of primary health care providers (PHCPs, including athletic trainers and physical therapists), massage therapists, mental health care providers, medical advisors, and sport dietitians. Stakeholders (players, coaches, parents, and agents) in the WTA tennis community digitally receive various performance health education topics. Additionally, players and their coaches who are entering the WTA are required to complete education modules on nutrition, hydration, injury prevention, and other health-related topics. Individual education and intervention for the Triad, specifically, began with the WTA player being screened for Triad "red flags" [1,2] (Table 1) at her annual physical and also upon clinical presentation of a menstrual problem, bone disorder, or nutritional concern. These red flags include a combination of research-documented symptoms of the Triad and indicators deemed relevant by those with clinical experience treating athletes with the Triad. This article summarizes the Triad programs and policies in place in the WTA from 1996 to 2022 and provides a successful example for other sporting organizations developing protocols to prevent and manage the Triad and other related syndromes.

Table 1. Indicators or "red flags" for each component of the Triad used by the WTA.

Low Energy Availability	Menstrual Disturbances	Low Bone Mineral Density
Fatigue	Long and irregular menstrual cycles of 36–90 days, defined as oligomenorrhea	Family history of osteoporosis
Irritability and mood changes	Complete absence of menstrual cycles, defined as amenorrhea	Stress fracture and/or other secondary clinical risk factors for fracture, previous fractures [41]
Difficulty handling travel or time zone changes	Difficulty conceiving or maintaining pregnancy	Nutrition: low calcium intake and/or low vitamin D status, restrictive calories or recent weight loss, restrictive diets (veganism, vegetarianism, etc.), history of eating disorders
Poor recovery after training	Initiation of hormonal contraceptive use in response to irregular/absent menstrual cycles	Medication: corticosteroid medications for 3+ months [42]
Difficulty healing from minor injuries	Primary amenorrhea (no menses by age 15 years) [21,43,44]	Hormonal deficiencies: amenorrhea (primary and secondary), low testosterone, hypoestrogenism (estrogen is important in building and maintaining bone mass)
History of recent dieting or comments about needing to lose weight		Medical conditions that can reduce bone mass: lupus, cirrhosis, alcoholism, atherosclerosis, thyroid disease, hyperparathyroidism, celiac disease
Restrictive eating patterns, food faddism		
Preoccupation with weight		
Unable to get into "high gear" during training or a match		
Lack of energy or fading in long matches		
Failing to improve performance despite ongoing training		
Changes in menstrual cycle		
Frequent illness		

WTA: Women's Tennis Association; Triad: Female Athlete Triad.

2. Triad Prevention and Education

The WTA approach to Triad prevention involves first educating and empowering the PHT with specific protocols and policies written in consultation with experts in the field and approved by WTA legal. In 2018, a Triad protocol was developed for the WTA in collaboration with subject matter experts in the Women's Health and Exercise Laboratory at The Pennsylvania State University. The protocol is summarized in a clinical decision-making tree (Figure 1) that outlines procedures for assessment and diagnosis of the three interrelated conditions of the Triad, i.e., menstrual function, energy status, and bone health. All WTA PHCPs are expected to know, understand, and implement the protocol. The protocol may also be shared with a player's individual physician and WTA tournament physicians around the world to further educate physicians on the WTA Triad treatment process.

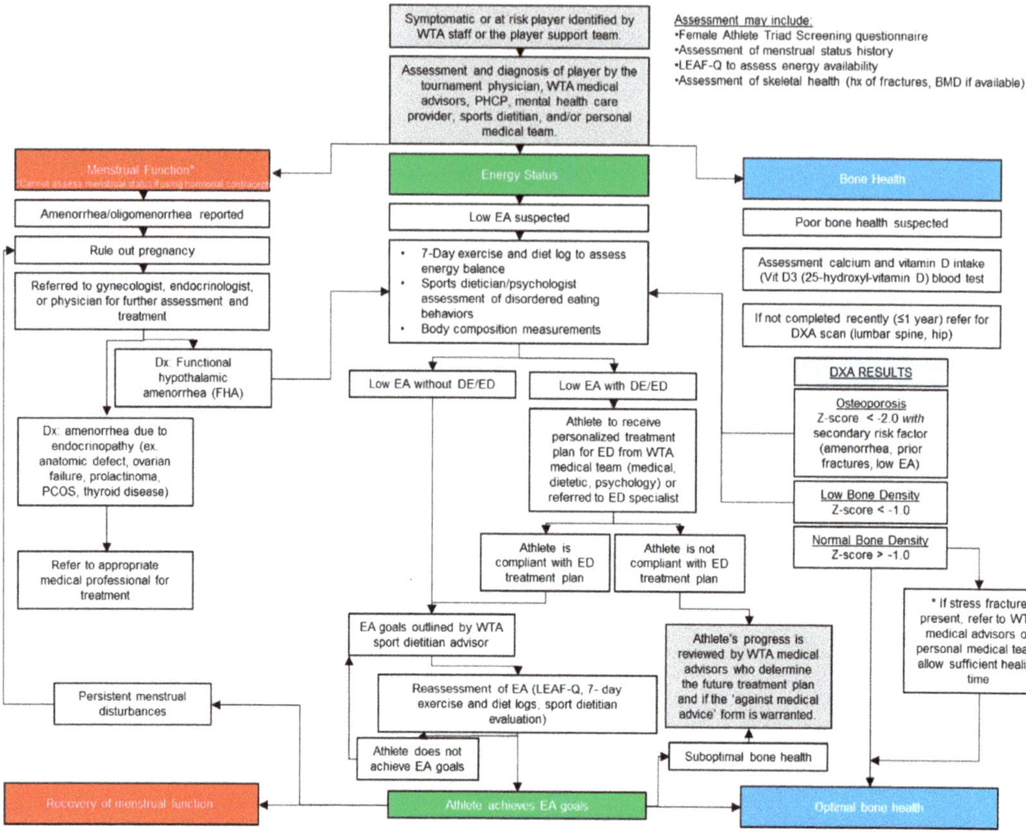

Figure 1. WTA clinical decision-making tree. This diagram is part of the WTA protocol and is used by the WTA multidisciplinary team when there is suspicion of red flags or risk factors for the Female Athlete Triad. Energy availability (EA); eating disorder (ED); disordered eating (DE) Reprinted with permission from the Women's Tennis Association.

Additionally, members of the PHT are trained in part by the WTA University, an online private learning platform, covering topics such as nutrition, female health, and bone stress injuries to ensure they are equipped with the necessary knowledge and tools to assess athletes presenting with aspects of the Triad. Players and support team members receive targeted education with handouts and lectures on health, nutrition, and body image. In addition, an online series, titled "*Physically Speaking*", was also developed by the PHT and leading medical providers to provide more in-depth information on health topics and can be given to athletes on an as-needed basis. Another WTA educational strategy includes informational signs posted at every tournament on topics such as hydration techniques, proper recovery routines, and fueling for matches. Posting educational and referral information in highly viewed areas, such as on the back of bathroom doors in tournament locker rooms, is another method used and mentioned by players as a useful avenue for education.

Since ED/LEA is the causative factor underlying the Triad, it is essential that education and prevention strategies focus on ensuring the athlete and her support team are aware of the importance of performance fueling. Signs specific to nutrition and fueling are purposefully posted in the dining areas and often spark the interest of players, coaches, and fitness trainers. Athletes and player support team members can also receive specific dietary advice from the on-site WTA sports dietitians and have individualized meal plans created to help meet energy requirements. Notably, sports dietitians play an integral role in Triad prevention by enabling players to adequately fuel to meet their energy expenditure needs. For tournaments, 7-day meal plans are developed that include low-fat and high-carbohydrate choices, lean proteins, vegetarian and gluten-free options, healthy snacks, chocolate milk or recovery drinks, and international seasonings and condiments to ensure that athletes are fueling adequately and to their taste. There may be added fueling challenges for elite athletes who travel internationally, for which strategies have been developed by WTA sports dietitians. For example, if an athlete is traveling to a foreign country that may not have local cuisine tailored to an athlete's diet or if an athlete is worried about travel and food selections, WTA sports dietitians can provide one-on-one consultations to give tips on travel snacks and finding healthy food choices in different countries and provide a balanced meal plan for the athlete.

Body image concerns may also lead to suboptimal nutrition in elite athletes, especially due to perceived media pressure [45]. To combat this problem, the WTA provides media training to inform players about how social and mass media messages are constructed. For example, media may portray a thin ideal body image that can lead athletes to develop a high drive for thinness and intentionally restrict energy intake. Media training can empower the athlete with the knowledge needed and provide the skills to respond to inappropriate or unhealthy messages around body image [46].

3. Screening and Diagnosis of the Triad in Tennis Athletes

3.1. Screening

Screening and early detection among athletes at risk for the development of any component of the Triad is critical and requires a multidisciplinary health care team approach [47,48], which can include tournament physicians, medical advisors, PHCPs, mental health and performance team members, sports dietitians, and/or an athlete's personal medical team. In 1996, the WTA instituted annual mandatory physicals completed on-site by PHCPs, medical advisors, and sports dietitians that include Triad screening questions to detect "red flags" (Table 1). Specific questions currently used to screen for the Triad include questions related to menstrual regularity, hormonal medication use, weight concerns, eating disorder history, and stress fracture history. As of 2022, annual physicals also include dual energy X-ray absorptiometry (DXA) scanning to assess BMD and body composition [49]. Triad screening can also occur when an athlete presents with any of the Triad symptoms, such as a stress fracture or irregular menstrual cycle, or is identified by WTA staff or the player support team as being at risk for the Triad. For example, when an athlete presents in the training room with a possible bone stress injury, the PHT uses the WTA Triad protocol, specifically the decision tree (Figure 1), to confirm that all necessary steps are followed, including appropriate initial questioning, determining possible need for referral to a specialist, and athlete education. Through three intersecting diagrams, decision-making and treatment strategies should be made in a comprehensive manner to address all components of the Triad.

3.2. Diagnosis

Diagnosing each component of the Triad can be achieved by following recommendations published by the Female Athlete Triad Coalition [1]. Below, the recommendations are summarized, followed by a detailed description of the specific procedures implemented by the WTA for their athletes.

3.2.1. Energy Deficiency/Low Energy Availability

There are several methods for assessing ED/LEA. Initial indications of LEA include recent weight loss and a BMI < 17.5 kg/m^2 or <85% of expected body weight in adolescents (approximately age 10–19 years). However, weight stability or estimates of energy balance alone should not be used to diagnose ED/LEA, specifically, since physiological functions can be suppressed in the face of LEA and weight may remain stable, as has been observed in amenorrheic athletes [50]. Other measures can include those used specifically to assess physiological signs of a chronic energy deficiency and include low total triiodothyronine (TT_3) hormone levels [51,52], reduced resting metabolic rate (RMR) [53], and/or a ratio of measured to predicted resting metabolic rate (mRMR/pRMR) of less than a given threshold, which varies by RMR prediction method (i.e., Harris–Benedict ratio and Cunningham_{1980} ratio < 0.90, Cunningham_{1991} ratio < 0.92, DXA ratio < 0.94) [51].

EA, specifically, can be calculated based on food intake and energy expenditure records according to the following equation:

$$EA = [energy\ intake\ (kcal) - exercise\ energy\ expenditure\ (kcal)]/Fat\ Free\ Mass\ (FFM)\ (kg).$$

Physically active women should aim for at least 45 kcal/kg FFM/day to ensure adequate EA for all physiological functions [1]. A 3- to 7-day diet and exercise log can be used to assess energy intake and exercise energy expenditure; however, accurate dietary intake assessments can be difficult to acquire due to issues such as under- or over-reporting of intake, modified intake during reporting periods, and imprecise reporting of portion sizes [54,55]. To determine exercise energy expenditure, athletes may use heart rate monitoring or estimate exercise energy expenditure based on the Compendium of Physical Activities, where [56,57]

$$Exercise\ Energy\ Expenditure\ (kcal) = METs\left(kcal * kg^{-1} * hr^{-1}\right)\ x\ weight(kg)\ x\ duration(hrs).$$

To assess FFM, a total body DXA scan is optimal; however, other field measures can be substituted where necessary with varying degrees of error (air plethysmography, hydrostatic weighing, bioelectrical impedance, skinfold measurements) [58]. Importantly, in cases where an athlete may be at risk for nutrient deficiencies, a registered sports nutritionist should complete a comprehensive nutrition assessment.

The aforementioned methods of assessing EA may be difficult to obtain from a traveling tennis player; therefore, when ED/LEA or the Triad is suspected, WTA athletes meet in person or virtually with a licensed sports dietitian to evaluate their food intake, training routine, and recovery techniques. The athlete is asked to fill out an initial dietary consult and have the sports dietitian review the form. Upon completion of the initial dietary consult, the athlete may be asked to fill out a food diary and exercise log to monitor food intake and exercise energy expenditure during 7 days of practice and competition. An initial dietary consult combined with a 7-day food diary provides greater insight into eating behaviors and practices compared to either component alone, as estimating energy expenditure needs is essential to understanding and calculating EA and dietary intake needs. This consult is also a time when recovery snacks/drinks can be suggested. Additional components of Triad diagnosis may include body composition measurements and/or assessment of disordered eating behaviors by a sports dietitian or mental health practitioner. If appropriate, the athlete is also educated on the consequences of ED/LEA, such as fatigue, poor recovery, poor healing, bone loss, and impaired performance.

3.2.2. Menstrual Disturbances

Athletes who present with amenorrhea or oligomenorrhea are assessed by the PHCPs and then referred for further evaluations. The athlete is first evaluated to rule out pregnancy and other endocrinopathies, such as thyroid dysfunction, hyperprolactinemia or prolactinoma, primary ovarian insufficiency, hypothalamic and pituitary disorders, and hyperandrogenic disorders, such as polycystic ovary syndrome (PCOS) [43]. Amenorrhea secondary to ED/LEA is a diagnosis of exclusion, and the most common alternative causes can often be identified after a thorough medical history, physical examination, pregnancy test, and evaluation of labs such as thyroid-stimulating hormone, follicle-stimulating hormone, and prolactin [43]. In cases where there is evidence of androgen excess (i.e., hirsutism, acne, or androgenic alopecia), laboratory tests of total and free testosterone and dehydroepiandrosterone and its sulfate (DHEA-S) may be warranted, as well as a pelvic ultrasound to confirm polycystic ovaries or rule out virilizing ovarian tumors [59]. A position stand detailing functional hypothalamic amenorrhea diagnosis was published by the Endocrine Society in 2017 [43].

If an athlete is using hormonal contraception, it is not possible to assess menstrual status, as combined hormonal contraceptives suppress menstrual function. Many hormonal contraceptive options, including oral contraceptives ("the pill"), the transdermal patch, and the vaginal ring, are cyclically administered such that every month, the athlete will experience withdrawal bleeding during a hormone-free (placebo) week. Other types of hormonal contraception, such as progesterone intrauterine devices (IUDs) and/or progesterone subdermal (Nexplanon), can suppress menses altogether. As such, bleeding patterns that present in women using hormonal contraception are not reflective of endogenous reproductive hormone profiles and, therefore, are not indicative of an athlete's menstrual status or energy status [1,60]. In fact, withdrawal bleeding during hormone-free (placebo) phases of contraception or menstrual suppression due to continuous use of combined hormonal contraception pills may actually mask menstrual disturbances that are an important sign of ED/LEA and menstrual status. If an athlete who is using hormonal contraception is suspected to have ED/LEA, clinicians should take the appropriate steps to screen the athlete's nutritional status. Likewise, because hormonal contraception can mask ED/LEA-induced menstrual disturbances, hormonal contraception is not advised as a first-line strategy to treat menstrual disturbances in athletes. Hormonal contraceptives deliver suboptimal concentrations of estrogen, and the estrogen delivered (ethinyl estradiol) is not identical to the estrogen produced naturally (17-β estradiol). Further, oral administration of hormonal contraceptives can suppress the production of hormones important for bone, including insulin-like growth factor-1 (IGF-1), in a process called hepatic first-pass effects [61]. Together, the low-dose non-physiologic form of estrogen and first-pass effect of oral contraceptives may explain the lack of efficacy to improve BMD in athletes with pre-existing menstrual disturbances [62,63]. If athletes are in need of contraception, the risks and benefits of all available options should be weighed so that informed choices can be made for the athlete's health. The Female Athlete Triad Coalition has provided recommendations about very specific circumstances when to use estrogen therapy, which include worsening BMD or ongoing stress fractures, and involves transdermal administration of 17-beta estradiol with oral cyclic progesterone [1].

3.2.3. Low Bone Mineral Density

DXA scans are primarily used to evaluate BMD and can also be used to measure total body composition (fat mass, lean body mass, FFM). For adult athletes ≥ 20 years old, BMD should be assessed at weight-bearing sites (lumbar spine, total hip, and femoral neck). For adolescent athletes and women < 20 years old, bone mineral content (BMC) and BMD should be assessed at the lumbar spine and, if possible, the whole body less the head (otherwise, the whole body) [1]. DXA scans provide results in two scores: Z-score and T-score. The Z-score is the number of standard deviations a patient's BMD differs from the average BMD of their age, sex, and ethnicity. The T-score is a comparison of a patient's BMD to that of a healthy thirty-year-old of the same sex and ethnicity and is used in postmenopausal women because it better predicts risk of future fracture. Premenopausal women should have the Z-score assessed for the appropriate age, sex, and ethnicity [64]. The Female Athlete Triad Coalition recommends that athletes should receive DXA scans if they present with any of the following: (1) at least one "high-risk" Triad risk factor, (2) at least two "moderate-risk" Triad risk factors, (3) a history of at least one nonperipheral or at least two peripheral long bone traumatic (non-stress) fractures in the face of one or more moderate- or high-risk Triad risk factors, and/or (4) at least 6 months of use of medication that may impact bone [1]. "High-risk" Triad risk factors include a history of DSM-5-diagnosed eating disorder; BMI $\leq$ 17.5 kg/m^2, <85% estimated weight, or recent weight loss of $\geq$10% in 1 month; menarche $\geq$ 16 years old; current or history of <six menses in 12 months; two prior stress fractures, one high-risk stress fracture, or a low-energy nontraumatic fracture; and prior Z-score < -2.0 after at least 1 year from baseline DXA. "Moderate-risk" Triad risk factors include a current or history of disordered eating for $\geq$6 months; BMI between 17.5 and 18.5 kg/m^2, <90% estimated weight, or recent weight loss of 5–10% in 1 month; menarche between 15 and 16 years old; current or history of 6–8 menses in 12 months; one prior stress reaction/fracture; and prior Z-score between -1.0 and -2.0 (after at least a 1-year interval from baseline DXA) [1]. The recommendations for diagnosing low BMD and osteoporosis follow the guidelines from the International Society for Clinical Densitometry (ISCD), such that a combination of low BMD and a clinically significant fracture history are required for an osteoporosis diagnosis in children and adolescents, and premenopausal women require both low BMD and a secondary cause of osteoporosis, with the caveat that low BMD in adolescent and young adult female athletes in weight-bearing sports (such as tennis) can be defined as a Z-score < -1.0, rather than the typical threshold of Z-score < -2.0 [1,42,65].

When a WTA athlete is identified as having low BMD or at risk of having low BMD, her case is discussed with the WTA medical advisors to determine the appropriate next steps, including further diagnostic testing. Assessments of calcium and vitamin D are conducted via a food diary and blood test, respectively, and, if not completed within the past year, the athlete is referred for DXA screening. Additionally, if a bone stress injury is present, the athlete is referred to WTA medical advisors or her personal medical team for evaluation of underlying causes and treatment. She is also referred for a dietary consult, which includes food diary and exercise log completion. These data are reviewed by the sports dietitian and shared with the athlete's medical team in order to comprehensively assess if the athlete is receiving the adequate energy and nutrients to support bone health.

Beginning at the 2022 BNP Paribas Open in Indian Wells, CA, WTA athletes are offered BMD screening of the lumbar spine, total hip, and forearms (Hologic Horizon®, Hologic Inc., Bedford, MA, USA) during their annual physical examination [49]. DXA screening was used to establish baseline BMD and body composition values for WTA athletes, which, together with clinical history, may be useful in the evaluation and treatment of the Triad. Long term, the WTA intends to use the data collected from the baseline DXA scans to establish normal reference ranges for WTA professional tennis athletes and potentially provide predictive models for injury risk. More research will be needed to see if these normative values can be generalized to other weight-bearing sports.

The WTA Triad protocol (1996–2022) of assessing BMD Z-scores from DXA follows recommendations from the Female Athlete Triad Coalition and the ISCD and aligns with research demonstrating low BMD as a risk factor for bone stress injuries in female athletes (e.g., [38]). An additional measure of bone health that can now be derived from DXA imaging is Trabecular Bone Score (TBS), which evaluates grayscale variation in lumbar spine DXA images as a surrogate for bone microarchitecture [66]. This capability was developed in an effort to improve fracture risk prediction from DXA and has been used effectively in older postmenopausal women, in whom lower TBS scores are associated with increased risk of osteoporotic fracture [66]. However, in younger, premenopausal women, TBS has not demonstrated consistent associations with fracture risk, including osteoporotic fracture, all fractures, and stress fracture/bone stress injury [66–68]. For instance, in a study of male and female adults ages 20–39 years, TBS score was not associated with incident fracture risk [67]. However, in a sample of collegiate female athletes, a lower TBS score was associated with increased odds of bone stress injury, especially for trabecular-rich bone injury sites, but including TBS in the model did not improve the prediction of injury risk compared with the model that included spinal BMD alone [68]. Until more evidence demonstrates a consistent and reliable utility of TBS to improve bone health evaluation and risk assessment in younger athletic populations, the WTA supports and recommends other sporting organizations continue to abide by ISCD recommendations to only consider TBS in adults ages 40 years and older [66].

4. Treatment and Management

Recovery from each component of the Triad may occur at differing rates when an appropriate treatment strategy of increasing energy intake is initiated (Figure 2) [1]. Recovery of energy status is typically observed after days or weeks of increased energy intake and/or decreased energy expenditure, but the rate of recovery is dependent upon the degree of ED/LEA and the presence of disordered eating or eating disorder behaviors that require intervention. Recovery of menstrual status may be observed after months of increased energy intake and/or decreased energy expenditure, which improves energy status [69,70]. Recovery of BMD may not be observed until one or more years after recovery of energy status and until menstrual recovery has been achieved for several years [1,71]. It is also possible that bone may not fully recover if energy deficiency and menstrual dysfunction are prolonged, especially during the time of peak bone mineral accrual (adolescence to young adulthood) [72,73]. In a recently published randomized controlled trial called REFUEL, increasing energy intake by approximately 350 kcal/day for 12 months successfully resumed menstrual frequency in amenorrheic and oligomenorrheic athletes but was not adequate to significantly improve estrogen exposure or BMD, despite an increase in body weight, fat mass, and TT_3 [69,72]. More data are required at higher energy intakes (>350 kcal/d) to determine the adequacy of increased refueling in athletes with severe menstrual disturbances on recovery of BMD.

The best practice for management of the Triad is demonstrated by the incorporation of a multidisciplinary team. Player support team members who may become involved, at the discretion of the overseeing physician and athlete, may include the athlete's coach, family members, and other professionals involved in the athlete's career [1]. To approach a traveling professional tennis athlete about suspected Triad conditions, especially one linked to an eating disorder, body image, or menstrual cycle disturbance, it is necessary to have her confidence and trust and ensure confidentiality. To be a trusted team member, the WTA multidisciplinary team must not only be knowledgeable in their field, but they must also understand and be part of the world of the professional tennis player. The WTA therefore schedules members of the PHT to be present in the same environment as the player. The PHCPs, massage therapists, and mental health care providers travel with the players, living the same life of travel and unpredictable schedules. These professionals have a constant presence in each tournament training room, gaining trust from players while providing treatment and player education on an as-needed basis and as part of the athlete's daily experience. An athlete is assigned to one PHCP for continuity when the player is not traveling.

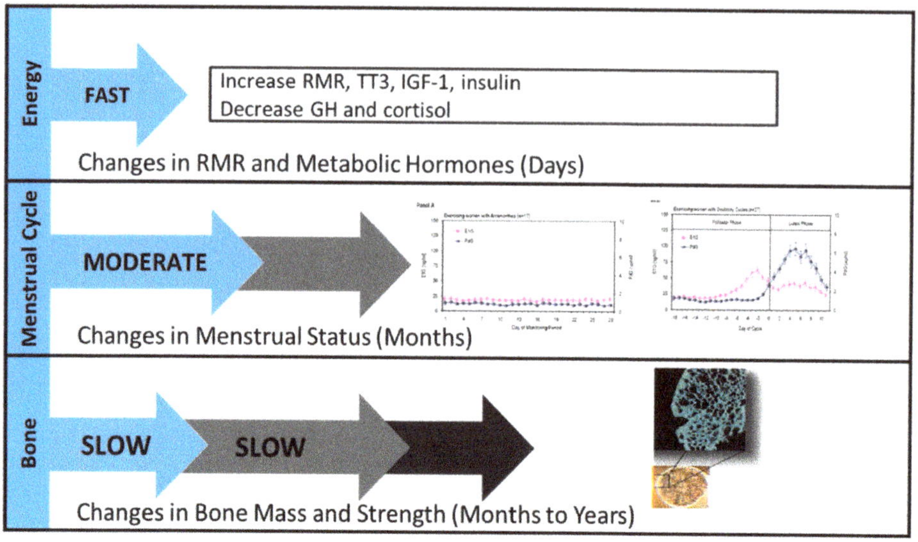

Figure 2. Recovery from the Female Athlete Triad. The three components of the Triad recover at different rates with the appropriate treatment.

If a WTA athlete has ED/LEA or any component of the Triad, early recognition and action are taken. The first approach is for the PHCP to meet with the athlete to reinforce the following:

- Regular periods can be an indicator ("barometer") of good health and adequate nutrition.
- Estrogen and progesterone are important hormones that regulate the female reproductive system. These hormones also help build and maintain strong bones.
- Menstrual disorders may contribute to difficulty conceiving or maintaining a pregnancy, but you could still get pregnant even if you are not getting a period. If that athlete is sexually active, contraception is advised.
- Not having a period could mean the athlete has an underlying health condition that needs to be investigated.
- Consequences of long-term amenorrhea, like low BMD, may not be completely reversible; thus, early diagnosis and intervention are critical.

To facilitate athlete participation in the treatment plan, the multidisciplinary team must develop a therapeutic alliance with the athlete [1]. The development of any Triad treatment plan should include and consider the goals of the athlete, her unique diet and training regimen, any coexisting conditions, mental health issues, and a systemic approach for monitoring changes. The overseeing physician must also take into account all aspects of the athlete's health when making the decision regarding safe return to play following diagnosis of any aspect of the Triad. Returning to competition too soon can be detrimental to an athlete's season and career longevity. Thus, return-to-play criteria include functional testing, approval from the overseeing dietitian and sports psychologist as necessary, and acknowledgement from the athlete and her team that maintaining communication with the WTA PHT throughout her career is critical to her overall well-being and success.

Professionals are encouraged to reference the 2014 Female Athlete Triad Coalition Statement on Treatment and Return to Play for detailed guidelines to this effect [1].

5. Future Directions and Protocol Modifications

Since the development and use of the WTA Triad protocol from 1996 to 2022, Triad science and associated clinical practice have continued to evolve. The following recommendations are provided as suggested modifications to the Triad protocol for other sporting organizations that wish to follow the example set forth by the WTA in creating a Triad protocol for their athletes.

Since weight/BMI can remain stable even in the presence of energy deficiency, we emphasize the use of serial measures of other markers of metabolic compensation, such as changes in metabolic hormones like TT3 or decreasing weight/BMI or body fat percentage. These objective metabolic biomarkers may be more reliable than calculating EA based on food and exercise logs, especially considering how food logs are prone to reporting inaccuracies [74] and accurate calculation of exercise energy expenditure requires sensitive, often expensive technology [75]. Regarding assessment of menstrual function and management of menstrual disturbances, more recent research has demonstrated that although previously amenorrheic women may resume menses with dietary intervention, menstrual quality may still be hampered, with many "recovered" women demonstrating anovulatory cycles and suppressed ovarian hormone profiles [69,76]. Thus, it is suggested that women continue to be monitored to ensure multiple consecutive cycles of normal length are achieved, as this more robust level of recovery is associated with improved cycle quality [76]. The WTA's continued efforts to assess BMD in their athletes is significant, as low Z-scores are a risk stratifier, and increased risk of bone stress injury is an important clinical outcome associated with the Triad [38,77–79]. This is particularly true for higher-grade bone stress injury and injury to trabecular bone sites, as return to play is often longer for these injuries [80]. As bone imaging technologies evolve to allow for more high-resolution, sensitive assessments of bone structure and microarchitecture, we recommend sporting organizations adopt such advances as they become clinically available and recommended [81,82]. Further, the WTA's use of multidisciplinary teams to prevent and manage the Triad in tennis athletes, especially the use of mental health professionals as needed, is a critical layer of this successful WTA program.

6. Conclusions

The WTA has been among the first international women's sports to develop and implement comprehensive education, recognition, and treatment plans for female athletes with components of the Triad in the 1996–2022 protocols. The programs are athlete-centered and coordinated by the PHCPs, who travel with the players. Comprehensive annual physicals screen for "red flags" for components of the Triad, and if one is recognized, the athlete is referred for appropriate care from the WTA PHT, which includes physical therapists, athletic trainers, mental health care providers, massage therapists, and sports dietitians and is coordinated with WTA medical advisors and tournament physicians. The PHT providers follow a Triad protocol developed specifically for the WTA athletes, their coaches, and their other support team members, who also receive targeted education on the topics related to the Triad, such as nutrition, menstrual health, body image, and the media.

This comprehensive overview of the 1996–2022 WTA Triad protocol exemplifies successful implementation of the Female Athlete Triad Coalition consensus guidelines [1,2], offering a model for other sporting organizations to optimize care for athletes with the Triad. The 1996–2022 WTA Triad protocol provides specific guidance for caring for elite tennis athletes, tailoring the broad recommendations from numerous professional sporting and medical organizations. For instance, a consensus statement from a collaboration of six major professional associations has published "*Female Athlete Issues for the Team Physician*," which overviews what team physicians ought to know with respect to female-specific musculoskeletal and medical conditions, including those included in the Triad (low energy availability, disordered eating, eating disorders, menstrual dysfunction, bone health, and bone stress injury) [83]. A similar collaborative consensus statement charges team physicians with the duty of establishing return-to-play processes that do not put the individual at undue risk for injury or illness [84]. The 1996–2022 WTA Triad protocol provides detailed guidance for the care and return-to-play decision-making process for tennis athletes in alignment with these consensus statements. The availability of nutritional professionals and guidance in the 1996–2022 WTA Triad protocol is supported by the National Athletic Trainers' Association's published "*Appropriate Medical Care Standards for Organizations Sponsoring Athletic Activity for the Secondary School Age Athlete*," which includes a standard that "education and counseling (be) provided for athletes on nutrition, hydration, and dietary supplementation" [85]. Similarly, nutrition assistance for the traveling tennis athlete follows the Health Care Guidelines for International Federation Events set forth by the Association of Summer Olympic International Federations (e.g., "...medical teams should ensure adequate and appropriate nutrition at international sporting events. Nutritional requirements should include...provision of a variety of food options to aid athlete recovery...food/menu options that meet the health and specific sports nutrition considerations of the athlete population...sufficient accessibility to support the overall nutrition needs of the athletic group and the logistics around training and competition schedules..." [86].

The WTA is committed to incorporating new and emerging research and science into their practices in order to ensure their players are provided with the highest quality and relevant care. In order to best support their athletes, the WTA PHT has updated its protocol as science and clinical recommendations have evolved. In the future, the WTA plans on providing outcomes based upon the implementation of their new WTA female athlete protocol in hopes of further setting the standard for female athlete care.

Author Contributions: Conceptualization, E.A.R., K.J.K., C.L.O., A.S.P. and M.J.D.S.; Methodology, E.A.R., K.J.K., C.L.O., A.S.P. and M.J.D.S.; Formal Analysis, E.A.R., K.J.K., C.L.O., A.S.P. and M.J.D.S.; Investigation, E.A.R., K.J.K., C.L.O., A.S.P. and M.J.D.S.; Writing—Original Draft Preparation, E.A.R., K.J.K., C.L.O., A.S.P. and M.J.D.S.; Writing—Review and Editing, E.A.R., K.J.K. and M.J.D.S.; Visualization, E.A.R., K.J.K., C.L.O., A.S.P. and M.J.D.S.; Supervision, C.L.O. and M.J.D.S.; Project Administration, C.L.O. and M.J.D.S. All authors have read and agreed to the published version of the manuscript.

Funding: This research received no external funding.

Acknowledgments: The authors would like to acknowledge Carlos L. Benitez, Ashley Keber, and Kathleen Stroia for their expert input on the contents of this article.

Conflicts of Interest: E.A.R., K.J.K., and M.J.D.S. are members of the Female and Male Athlete Triad Coalition.

References

1. De Souza, M.J.; Nattiv, A.; Joy, E.; Misra, M.; Williams, N.I.; Mallinson, R.J.; Gibbs, J.C.; Olmsted, M.; Goolsby, M.; Matheson, G.; et al. 2014 female athlete triad coalition consensus statement on treatment and return to play of the female athlete triad: 1st international conference held in San Francisco, California, May 2012 and 2nd international conference held in Indianapolis, Indiana, May 2013. *Br. J. Sports Med.* **2014**, *48*, 289. [CrossRef]
2. Nattiv, A.; Loucks, A.B.; Manore, M.M.; Sanborn, C.F.; Sundgot-Borgen, J.; Warren, M.P. American college of sports medicine position stand. The female athlete triad. *Med. Sci. Sports Exerc.* **2007**, *39*, 1867–1882. [CrossRef] [PubMed]
3. Yeager, K.K.; Agostini, R.; Nattiv, A.; Drinkwater, B. The female athlete triad: Disordered eating, amenorrhea, osteoporosis. *Med. Sci. Sports Exerc.* **1993**, *25*, 775–777. [CrossRef]
4. Otis, C.L.; Drinkwater, B.; Johnson, M.; Loucks, A.; Wilmore, J. American college of sports medicine position stand. The female athlete triad. *Med. Sci. Sports Exerc.* **1997**, *29*, i–ix. [CrossRef] [PubMed]
5. Loucks, A.B.; Verdun, M.; Heath, E.M. Low energy availability, not stress of exercise, alters lh pulsatility in exercising women. *J. Appl. Physiol.* **1998**, *84*, 37–46. [CrossRef] [PubMed]
6. Williams, N.I.; Helmreich, D.L.; Parfitt, D.B.; Caston-Balderrama, A.; Cameron, J.L. Evidence for a causal role of low energy availability in the induction of menstrual cycle disturbances during strenuous exercise training. *J. Clin. Endocrinol. Metab.* **2001**, *86*, 5184–5193. [CrossRef]
7. Bullen, B.A.; Skrinar, G.S.; Beitins, I.Z.; von Mering, G.; Turnbull, B.A.; McArthur, J.W. Induction of menstrual disorders by strenuous exercise in untrained women. *N. Engl. J. Med.* **1985**, *312*, 1349–1353. [CrossRef]
8. Williams, N.I.; Caston-Balderrama, A.L.; Helmreich, D.L.; Parfitt, D.B.; Nosbisch, C.; Cameron, J.L. Longitudinal changes in reproductive hormones and menstrual cyclicity in cynomolgus monkeys during strenuous exercise training: Abrupt transition to exercise-induced amenorrhea. *Endocrinology* **2001**, *142*, 2381–2389. [CrossRef]
9. Williams, N.I.; Berga, S.L.; Cameron, J.L. Synergism between psychosocial and metabolic stressors: Impact on reproductive function in cynomolgus monkeys. *Am. J. Physiol. Endocrinol. Metab.* **2007**, *293*, E270–E276. [CrossRef]
10. Gibbs, J.C.; Williams, N.I.; De Souza, M.J. Prevalence of individual and combined components of the female athlete triad. *Med. Sci. Sports Exerc.* **2013**, *45*, 985–996. [CrossRef]
11. Sundgot-Borgen, J.; Torstveit, M.K. Prevalence of eating disorders in elite athletes is higher than in the general population. *Clin. J. Sport Med.* **2004**, *14*, 25–32. [CrossRef]
12. Torstveit, M.K.; Sundgot-Borgen, J. Participation in leanness sports but not training volume is associated with menstrual dysfunction: A national survey of 1276 elite athletes and controls. *Br. J. Sports Med.* **2005**, *39*, 141–147. [CrossRef]
13. Sophia, B.; Kelly, P.; Ogan, D.; Larson, A. Self reported history of eating disorders, training, weight control methods, and body satisfaction in elite female runners competing at the 2020 U.S. Olympic marathon trials. *Int. J. Exerc. Sci.* **2022**, *15*, 721–732. [PubMed]
14. Martinsen, M.; Sundgot-Borgen, J. Higher prevalence of eating disorders among adolescent elite athletes than controls. *Med. Sci. Sports Exerc.* **2013**, *45*, 1188–1197. [CrossRef]
15. Mountjoy, M.; Sundgot-Borgen, J.; Burke, L.; Carter, S.; Constantini, N.; Lebrun, C.; Meyer, N.; Sherman, R.; Steffen, K.; Budgett, R.; et al. The IOC consensus statement: Beyond the female athlete triad—Relative energy deficiency in sport (RED-S). *Br. J. Sports Med.* **2014**, *48*, 491–497. [CrossRef] [PubMed]
16. Mountjoy, M.; Sundgot-Borgen, J.; Burke, L.; Ackerman, K.E.; Blauwet, C.; Constantini, N.; Lebrun, C.; Lundy, B.; Melin, A.; Meyer, N.; et al. International olympic committee (IOC) consensus statement on relative energy deficiency in sport (RED-S): 2018 update. *Int. J. Sport Nutr. Exerc. Metab.* **2018**, *28*, 316–331. [CrossRef]
17. De Souza, M.J.; Williams, N.I.; Nattiv, A.; Joy, E.; Misra, M.; Loucks, A.B.; Matheson, G.; Olmsted, M.P.; Barrack, M.; Mallinson, R.J.; et al. Misunderstanding the female athlete triad: Refuting the ioc consensus statement on relative energy deficiency in sport (RED-S). *Br. J. Sports Med.* **2014**, *48*, 1461–1465. [CrossRef] [PubMed]
18. Williams, N.I.; Koltun, K.J.; Strock, N.C.A.; De Souza, M.J. Perspectives for progress—Female athlete triad and relative energy deficiency in sport: A focus on scientific rigor. *Exerc. Sport Sci. Rev.* **2019**, *47*, 197–205. [CrossRef]
19. Jeukendrup, A.E.; Areta, J.L.; Van Genechten, L.; Langan-Evans, C.; Pedlar, C.R.; Rodas, G.; Sale, C.; Walsh, N.P. Does relative energy deficiency in sport (REDs) syndrome exist? *Sports Med.* **2024**, *54*, 2793–2816. [CrossRef]
20. Wade, G.N.; Schneider, J.E. Metabolic fuels and reproduction in female mammals. *Neurosci. Biobehav. Rev.* **1992**, *16*, 235–272. [CrossRef]
21. Committee on Adolescent Health Care. Committee opinion No. 651 summary: Menstruation in girls and adolescents: Using the menstrual cycle as a vital sign. *Obstet. Gynecol.* **2015**, *126*, 1328. [CrossRef] [PubMed]
22. De Souza, M.J.; Miller, B.E.; Loucks, A.B.; Luciano, A.A.; Pescatello, L.S.; Campbell, C.G.; Lasley, B.L. High frequency of luteal phase deficiency and anovulation in recreational women runners: Blunted elevation in follicle-stimulating hormone observed during luteal-follicular transition. *J. Clin. Endocrinol. Metab.* **1998**, *83*, 4220–4232. [CrossRef] [PubMed]

23. Koltun, K.J.; De Souza, M.J.; Scheid, J.L.; Williams, N.I. Energy availability is associated with luteinizing hormone pulse frequency and induction of luteal phase defects. *J. Clin. Endocrinol. Metab.* **2020**, *105*, 185–193. [CrossRef] [PubMed]
24. Beitins, I.Z.; McArthur, J.W.; Turnbull, B.A.; Skrinar, G.S.; Bullen, B.A. Exercise induces two types of human luteal dysfunction: Confirmation by urinary free progesterone. *J. Clin. Endocrinol. Metab.* **1991**, *72*, 1350–1358. [CrossRef]
25. De Souza, M.J.; Lee, D.K.; VanHeest, J.L.; Scheid, J.L.; West, S.L.; Williams, N.I. Severity of energy-related menstrual disturbances increases in proportion to indices of energy conservation in exercising women. *Fertil. Steril.* **2007**, *88*, 971–975. [CrossRef]
26. Ihle, R.; Loucks, A.B. Dose-response relationships between energy availability and bone turnover in young exercising women. *J. Bone Miner. Res.* **2004**, *19*, 1231–1240. [CrossRef]
27. Southmayd, E.A.; Williams, N.I.; Mallinson, R.J.; De Souza, M.J. Energy deficiency suppresses bone turnover in exercising women with menstrual disturbances. *J. Clin. Endocrinol. Metab.* **2019**, *104*, 3131–3145. [CrossRef]
28. Papageorgiou, M.; Elliott-Sale, K.J.; Parsons, A.; Tang, J.C.Y.; Greeves, J.P.; Fraser, W.D.; Sale, C. Effects of reduced energy availability on bone metabolism in women and men. *Bone* **2017**, *105*, 191–199. [CrossRef]
29. Papageorgiou, M.; Martin, D.; Colgan, H.; Cooper, S.; Greeves, J.P.; Tang, J.C.Y.; Fraser, W.D.; Elliott-Sale, K.J.; Sale, C. Bone metabolic responses to low energy availability achieved by diet or exercise in active eumenorrheic women. *Bone* **2018**, *114*, 181–188. [CrossRef]
30. Weitzmann, M.N.; Pacifici, R. Estrogen deficiency and bone loss: An inflammatory tale. *J. Clin. Investig.* **2006**, *116*, 1186–1194. [CrossRef]
31. De Souza, M.J.; West, S.L.; Jamal, S.A.; Hawker, G.A.; Gundberg, C.M.; Williams, N.I. The presence of both an energy deficiency and estrogen deficiency exacerbate alterations of bone metabolism in exercising women. *Bone* **2008**, *43*, 140–148. [CrossRef]
32. Southmayd, E.A.; Mallinson, R.J.; Williams, N.I.; Mallinson, D.J.; De Souza, M.J. Unique effects of energy versus estrogen deficiency on multiple components of bone strength in exercising women. *Osteoporos. Int.* **2017**, *28*, 1365–1376. [CrossRef] [PubMed]
33. Harris, M.B. Weight concern, body image, and abnormal eating in college women tennis players and their coaches. *Int. J. Sport. Nutr. Exerc. Metab.* **2000**, *10*, 1–15. [CrossRef] [PubMed]
34. Harris, M.; Foltz, S. Attitudes toward weight and eating in young women tennis players, their parents, and their coaches. *Eat. Disord.* **1999**, *7*, 191–205. [CrossRef]
35. Cignarelli, J. The skinny on athletic stardom: Disordered eating and body dissatisfaction in elite female tennis players. *J. Med. Sci. Tennis* **2019**, *24*, 6–10.
36. Coelho, G.M.; de Farias, M.L.; de Mendonca, L.M.; de Mello, D.B.; Lanzillotti, H.S.; Ribeiro, B.G.; Soares Ede, A. The prevalence of disordered eating and possible health consequences in adolescent female tennis players from Rio de Janeiro, Brazil. *Appetite* **2013**, *64*, 39–47. [CrossRef]
37. Filaire, E.; Massart, A.; Hua, J.; Le Scanff, C. Dietary intake, eating behaviors, and diurnal patterns of salivary cortisol and alpha-amylase secretion among professional young adult female tennis players. *Int. J. Sport Nutr. Exerc. Metab.* **2015**, *25*, 233–242. [CrossRef]
38. Barrack, M.T.; Gibbs, J.C.; De Souza, M.J.; Williams, N.I.; Nichols, J.F.; Rauh, M.J.; Nattiv, A. Higher incidence of bone stress injuries with increasing female athlete triad-related risk factors: A prospective multisite study of exercising girls and women. *Am. J. Sports Med.* **2014**, *42*, 949–958. [CrossRef]
39. Vanheest, J.L.; Rodgers, C.D.; Mahoney, C.E.; De Souza, M.J. Ovarian suppression impairs sport performance in junior elite female swimmers. *Med. Sci. Sports Exerc.* **2014**, *46*, 156–166. [CrossRef]
40. Otis, C.L. *A Review of the Age Eligibility Commission Report*; Fall Edition; USTA Sport Science Newsletter: Orlando, FL, USA, 1994; pp. 1–3.
41. Marx, R.G.; Saint-Phard, D.; Callahan, L.R.; Chu, J.; Hannafin, J.A. Stress fracture sites related to underlying bone health in athletic females. *Clin. J. Sport Med.* **2001**, *11*, 73–76. [CrossRef]
42. International Society for Clinical Densitometry (ISCD). 2023 ISCD Official Positions—Adults. Available online: https://iscd.org/wp-content/uploads/2024/03/2023-ISCD-Adult-Positions.pdf (accessed on 29 January 2025).
43. Gordon, C.M.; Ackerman, K.E.; Berga, S.L.; Kaplan, J.R.; Mastorakos, G.; Misra, M.; Murad, M.H.; Santoro, N.F.; Warren, M.P. Functional hypothalamic amenorrhea: An endocrine society clinical practice guideline. *J. Clin. Endocrinol. Metab.* **2017**, *102*, 1413–1439. [CrossRef]
44. Klein, D.A.; Paradise, S.L.; Reeder, R.M. Amenorrhea: A systematic approach to diagnosis and management. *Am. Fam. Physician* **2019**, *100*, 39–48. [PubMed]
45. Stoyel, H.; Delderfield, R.; Shanmuganathan-Felton, V.; Stoyel, A.; Serpell, L. A qualitative exploration of sport and social pressures on elite athletes in relation to disordered eating. *Front. Psychol.* **2021**, *12*, 633490. [CrossRef] [PubMed]
46. Martin, K.; Page, L. Managing athletes with eating issues: The WTA tour approach. *J. Med. Sci. Tennis* **2010**, *15*, 6–11.
47. Taylor, W.C. The preparticipation physical: The WTA experience and findings. In *Tennis Medicine*; Di Giacomo, G., Ellenbecker, T., Kibler, W., Eds.; Springer: Berlin/Heidelberg, Germany, 2018.

48. Wells, K.R.; Jeacocke, N.A.; Appaneal, R.; Smith, H.D.; Vlahovich, N.; Burke, L.M.; Hughes, D. The Australian institute of sport (AIS) and national eating disorders collaboration (NEDC) position statement on disordered eating in high performance sport. *Br. J. Sports Med.* **2020**, *54*, 1247–1258. [CrossRef]
49. A Healthy Innagural Season for the Hologic-WTA Partnership. Available online: https://www.wtatennis.com/news/2983829/a-healthy-inaugural-season-for-the-hologic-wta-partnership (accessed on 14 June 2025).
50. Myerson, M.; Gutin, B.; Warren, M.P.; May, M.T.; Contento, I.; Lee, M.; Pi-Sunyer, F.X.; Pierson, R.N., Jr.; Brooks-Gunn, J. Resting metabolic rate and energy balance in amenorrheic and eumenorrheic runners. *Med. Sci. Sports Exerc.* **1991**, *23*, 15–22. [CrossRef]
51. Strock, N.C.A.; Koltun, K.J.; Southmayd, E.A.; Williams, N.I.; De Souza, M.J. Indices of resting metabolic rate accurately reflect energy deficiency in exercising women. *Int. J. Sport Nutr. Exerc. Metab.* **2020**, *30*, 14–24. [CrossRef]
52. Loucks, A.B.; Heath, E.M. Induction of low-T3 syndrome in exercising women occurs at a threshold of energy availability. *Am. J. Physiol.* **1994**, *266*, R817–R823. [CrossRef]
53. Koehler, K.; De Souza, M.J.; Williams, N.I. Less-than-expected weight loss in normal-weight women undergoing caloric restriction and exercise is accompanied by preservation of fat-free mass and metabolic adaptations. *Eur. J. Clin. Nutr.* **2017**, *71*, 365–371. [CrossRef]
54. Burke, L.M.; Lundy, B.; Fahrenholtz, I.L.; Melin, A.K. Pitfalls of conducting and interpreting estimates of energy availability in free-living athletes. *Int. J. Sport Nutr. Exerc. Metab.* **2018**, *28*, 350–363. [CrossRef]
55. De Souza, M.J.; Koltun, K.J.; Strock, N.C.A.; Williams, N.I. Rethinking the concept of an energy availability threshold and its role in the female athlete triad. *Curr. Opin. Physiol.* **2019**, *10*, 35–42. [CrossRef]
56. Ainsworth, B.E.; Haskell, W.L.; Herrmann, S.D.; Meckes, N.; Bassett, D.R., Jr.; Tudor-Locke, C.; Greer, J.L.; Vezina, J.; Whitt-Glover, M.C.; Leon, A.S. 2011 compendium of physical activities: A second update of codes and met values. *Med. Sci. Sports Exerc.* **2011**, *43*, 1575–1581. [CrossRef]
57. Ainsworth, B.E.; Haskell, W.L.; Whitt, M.C.; Irwin, M.L.; Swartz, A.M.; Strath, S.J.; O'Brien, W.L.; Bassett, D.R., Jr.; Schmitz, K.H.; Emplaincourt, P.O.; et al. Compendium of physical activities: An update of activity codes and met intensities. *Med. Sci. Sports Exerc.* **2000**, *32*, S498–S504. [CrossRef] [PubMed]
58. Rose, G.L.; Farley, M.J.; Ward, L.C.; Slater, G.J.; Skinner, T.L.; Keating, S.E.; Schaumberg, M.A. Accuracy of body composition measurement techniques across the age span. *Appl. Physiol. Nutr. Metab.* **2022**, *47*, 482–494. [CrossRef] [PubMed]
59. The Rotterdam ESHRE/ASRM-Sponsored PCOS Consensus Workshop Group. Revised 2003 consensus on diagnostic criteria and long-term health risks related to polycystic ovary syndrome (PCOS). *Hum. Reprod.* **2004**, *19*, 41–47. [CrossRef]
60. Bergstrom, I.; Crisby, M.; Engstrom, A.M.; Holcke, M.; Fored, M.; Jakobsson Kruse, P.; Of Sandberg, A.M. Women with anorexia nervosa should not be treated with estrogen or birth control pills in a bone-sparing effect. *Acta Obstet. Gynecol. Scand.* **2013**, *92*, 877–880. [CrossRef]
61. Yakar, S.; Rosen, C.J.; Beamer, W.G.; Ackert-Bicknell, C.L.; Wu, Y.; Liu, J.L.; Ooi, G.T.; Setser, J.; Frystyk, J.; Boisclair, Y.R.; et al. Circulating levels of IGF-1 directly regulate bone growth and density. *J. Clin. Investig.* **2002**, *110*, 771–781. [CrossRef]
62. Ackerman, K.E.; Singhal, V.; Baskaran, C.; Slattery, M.; Campoverde Reyes, K.J.; Toth, A.; Eddy, K.T.; Bouxsein, M.L.; Lee, H.; Klibanski, A.; et al. Oestrogen replacement improves bone mineral density in oligo-amenorrhoeic athletes: A randomised clinical trial. *Br. J. Sports Med.* **2019**, *53*, 229–236. [CrossRef]
63. Ackerman, K.E.; Singhal, V.; Slattery, M.; Eddy, K.T.; Bouxsein, M.L.; Lee, H.; Klibanski, A.; Misra, M. Effects of estrogen replacement on bone geometry and microarchitecture in adolescent and young adult oligoamenorrheic athletes: A randomized trial. *J. Bone Miner. Res.* **2020**, *35*, 248–260. [CrossRef]
64. International Society for Clinical Densitometry (ISCD). *2019 ISCD Official Positions—Adult*; International Society for Clinical Densitometry (ISCD): Middletown, CT, USA, 2019.
65. International Society for Clinical Densitomtry (ISCD). 2019 ISCD Official Positions-Pediatrics. Available online: https://iscd.org/wp-content/uploads/2024/03/2019-ISCD-Pediatric-Postions.pdf (accessed on 29 January 2025).
66. Goel, H.; Binkley, N.; Boggild, M.; Chan, W.P.; Leslie, W.D.; McCloskey, E.; Morgan, S.L.; Silva, B.C.; Cheung, A.M. Clinical use of trabecular bone score: The 2023 ISCD official positions. *J. Clin. Densitom.* **2024**, *27*, 101452. [CrossRef]
67. Goel, H.; Binkley, N.; Hans, D.; Leslie, W.D. Bone density and trabecular bone score to predict fractures in adults aged 20–39 years: A registry-based study. *Osteoporos. Int.* **2023**, *34*, 1085–1091. [CrossRef]
68. Tenforde, A.S.; Carlson, J.L.; Sainani, K.L.; Chang, A.O.; Kim, J.H.; Diaz, R.; Golden, N.H.; Fredericson, M. Lower trabecular bone score and spine bone mineral density are associated with bone stress injuries and triad risk factors in collegiate athletes. *PM&R* **2021**, *13*, 945–953. [CrossRef]
69. De Souza, M.J.; Mallinson, R.J.; Strock, N.C.A.; Koltun, K.J.; Olmstead, M.; Ricker, E.A.; Scheid, J.L.; Allaway, H.C.; Mallinson, D.J.; Kuruppumullage Don, P.; et al. Randomized controlled trial of the effects of increased energy intake on menstrual recovery in exercising women with menstrual disturbances: The "refuel" study. *Hum. Reprod.* **2021**, *36*, 2285–2297. [CrossRef] [PubMed]
70. Arends, J.C.; Cheung, M.Y.; Barrack, M.T.; Nattiv, A. Restoration of menses with nonpharmacologic therapy in college athletes with menstrual disturbances: A 5-year retrospective study. *Int. J. Sport Nutr. Exerc. Metab.* **2012**, *22*, 98–108. [CrossRef] [PubMed]

71. Drinkwater, B.L.; Nilson, K.; Ott, S.; Chesnut, C.H., 3rd. Bone mineral density after resumption of menses in amenorrheic athletes. *JAMA* **1986**, *256*, 380–382. [CrossRef]
72. De Souza, M.J.; Ricker, E.A.; Mallinson, R.J.; Allaway, H.C.M.; Koltun, K.J.; Strock, N.C.A.; Gibbs, J.C.; Kuruppumullage Don, P.; Williams, N.I. Bone mineral density in response to increased energy intake in exercising women with oligomenorrhea/amenorrhea: The refuel randomized controlled trial. *Am. J. Clin. Nutr.* **2022**, *115*, 1457–1472. [CrossRef]
73. Cialdella-Kam, L.; Guebels, C.P.; Maddalozzo, G.F.; Manore, M.M. Dietary intervention restored menses in female athletes with exercise-associated menstrual dysfunction with limited impact on bone and muscle health. *Nutrients* **2014**, *6*, 3018–3039. [CrossRef]
74. Ravelli, M.N.; Schoeller, D.A. Traditional self-reported dietary instruments are prone to inaccuracies and new approaches are needed. *Front. Nutr.* **2020**, *7*, 90. [CrossRef]
75. Hills, A.P.; Mokhtar, N.; Byrne, N.M. Assessment of physical activity and energy expenditure: An overview of objective measures. *Front. Nutr.* **2014**, *1*, 5. [CrossRef]
76. Mallinson, R.J.; Williams, N.I.; Ricker, E.A.; Allaway, H.C.M.; De Souza, M.J. Multiple eumenorrheic cycles are necessary to observe a significant increase in estrogen exposure and ovulation in exercising females with functional hypothalamic oligo/amenorrhea: Insights from the REFUEL Study. *PM&R* **2024**. *submitted*.
77. Tenforde, A.S.; Carlson, J.L.; Chang, A.; Sainani, K.L.; Shultz, R.; Kim, J.H.; Cutti, P.; Golden, N.H.; Fredericson, M. Association of the female athlete triad risk assessment stratification to the development of bone stress injuries in collegiate athletes. *Am. J. Sports Med.* **2017**, *45*, 302–310. [CrossRef] [PubMed]
78. Tenforde, A.S.; Katz, N.B.; Sainani, K.L.; Carlson, J.L.; Golden, N.H.; Fredericson, M. Female athlete triad risk factors are more strongly associated with trabecular-rich versus cortical-rich bone stress injuries in collegiate athletes. *Orthop. J. Sports Med.* **2022**, *10*, 23259671221123588. [CrossRef] [PubMed]
79. Tenforde, A.S.; Parziale, A.L.; Popp, K.L.; Ackerman, K.E. Low bone mineral density in male athletes is associated with bone stress injuries at anatomic sites with greater trabecular composition. *Am. J. Sports Med.* **2018**, *46*, 30–36. [CrossRef]
80. Nattiv, A.; Kennedy, G.; Barrack, M.T.; Abdelkerim, A.; Goolsby, M.A.; Arends, J.C.; Seeger, L.L. Correlation of mri grading of bone stress injuries with clinical risk factors and return to play: A 5-year prospective study in collegiate track and field athletes. *Am. J. Sports Med.* **2013**, *41*, 1930–1941. [CrossRef]
81. Ackerman, K.E.; Putman, M.; Guereca, G.; Taylor, A.P.; Pierce, L.; Herzog, D.B.; Klibanski, A.; Bouxsein, M.; Misra, M. Cortical microstructure and estimated bone strength in young amenorrheic athletes, eumenorrheic athletes and non-athletes. *Bone* **2012**, *51*, 680–687. [CrossRef] [PubMed]
82. Ackerman, K.E.; Nazem, T.; Chapko, D.; Russell, M.; Mendes, N.; Taylor, A.P.; Bouxsein, M.L.; Misra, M. Bone microarchitecture is impaired in adolescent amenorrheic athletes compared with eumenorrheic athletes and nonathletic controls. *J. Clin. Endocrinol. Metab.* **2011**, *96*, 3123–3133. [CrossRef]
83. Female athlete issues for the team physician: A consensus statement-2017 update. *Med. Sci. Sports Exerc.* **2018**, *50*, 1113–1122. [CrossRef]
84. Herring, S.A.; Kibler, W.B.; Putukian, M. The team physician and the return-to-play decision: A consensus statement-2012 update. *Med. Sci. Sports Exerc.* **2012**, *44*, 2446–2448. [CrossRef]
85. National Athletic Trainers' Association. Appropriate Medical Care Standards for Secondary School-Aged Athletes. 2019. Available online: https://www.nata.org/sites/default/files/nata_appropriate_medical_care_standards.pdf (accessed on 29 January 2025).
86. Association of Summer Olympic International Federations. Health Care Guidelines for International Federation Events. 2020. Available online: https://www.asoif.com/sites/default/files/documents/main/health_care_guidelines_for_international_federation_events.pdf (accessed on 29 January 2025).

MDPI AG
Grosspeteranlage 5
4052 Basel
Switzerland
Tel.: +41 61 683 77 34

Sports Editorial Office
E-mail: sports@mdpi.com
www.mdpi.com/journal/sports

www.ingramcontent.com/pod-product-compliance
Lightning Source LLC
Chambersburg PA
CBHW061613210926
51850CB00009B/2313
9783725874569